NURSING SERVICE STAFF DEVELOPMENT

NURSING STAFF DEVELOPMENT

Current Competence, Future Focus

Nursing Staff Development
Current Competence, Future Focus

Karen J. Kelly, MS, RN, CNAA

President, Kelly Thomas Associates
Alexandria, VA

Formerly
Associate Director of Nursing,
Education, Research, and Development
Greater Southeast Community Hospital
Washington, D.C.

J. B. Lippincott Company   Philadelphia

Sponsoring Editor: Diana Intenzo
Production Manager: Lori J. Bainbridge
Editorial/Production: NB Enterprises
Cover Design: Lou Fuiano
Interior Design: Jill Feltham
Printer/Binder: R.R. Donnelley & Sons, Harrisonburg
Cover Printer: R.R. Donnelley & Sons, Harrisonburg

6 5 4 3 2 1

ISBN 0-397-54810-9

Library of Congress Cataloging-in-Publication Data

Nursing staff development : current competence, future focus / [edited by] Karen J. Kelly.
     p. cm.
    Includes bibliographical references and index.
    ISBN 0-397-54810-9
    1. Nurses—In-service training. 2. Nursing—Study and teaching (Continuing education) I. Kelly, Karen J.
    [DNLM: 1. Education, Nursing, Continuing—organization & administration.
2. Nursing Staff—education. 3. Staff Development—methods.   WY 18.5 N9735]
RT76.N85   1992
610.73'071'55—dc20
DNLM/DLC
for Library of Congress   92-6265
                                         CIP

For my parents—

Mary Hasson Stuhler
Richard C. Stuhler

Contributors

Susan E. Costello, DNSc, RN, is the Nursing Education and Research Director at Georgetown University Hospital in Washington, DC, as well as an Adjunct Assistant Professor at Georgetown University School of Nursing. At GUH, Susan has designed and implemented a clinical education program that promotes effective and efficient use of resources within a highly decentralized environment. Susan Costello holds a BSN from St. Anselm's College, an MSEd in Instructional Systems Design from Southern Illinois University–Edwardsville, and a DNSc from The Catholic University of America.

Karen J. Kelly MS, RN, CNAA, has 15 years of experience in nursing staff development in a variety of settings. In her recent role as Associate Director of Nursing for Education, Research and Development, she had a variety of responsibilities including leadership of the staff development program and its competency assessment program, administration of the clinical ladder program and research program, and direction of a dermal ulcer management initiative. As a member of the Executive Council, she participated in all policy and practice decisions regarding nursing and patient care at Greater Southeast Community Hospital in Washington, DC. Karen began a private consulting practice in November, 1991.

Karen has a diploma in nursing from Holy Name Hospital School of Nursing in Teaneck, New Jersey, a BSN from Regents College in Albany, New York, and an MS in Adult and Continuing Education from Virginia Polytechnic Institute and State University. She is currently enrolled in the doctoral program in nursing administration at George Mason University in Fairfax, Virginia.

Karen speaks to national groups on a regular basis about quality assurance, nursing staff development, strategic planning, instructional technology, creativity and innovation, and productivity. She has also published more than a dozen articles and chapters in books.

Karen serves on the editorial advisory board for the *Journal of Nursing Staff Development* and writes the Administrators Forum for that journal. She is a founding member and was elected the first President of a new organization for nursing staff development specialists called the National Nursing Staff Development Organization (NNSDO), which has recruited more than 1500 members since January 1990. Karen has also volunteered extensively with the American Heart Association, primarily in program development for BLS.

Phyllis J. Miller, RN, MS, FHCE, has more than ten years of staff development experience and received her baccalaureate degree at Eastern Mennonite College in Harrisonburg, Virginia. She pursued a master's degree at the University of Maryland in Baltimore, and was awarded an MS degree in Nursing Education with an emphasis in Staff Development in 1985.

As the Director of the Center for Nursing Education at Greater Southeast Community Hospital in Washington, DC, Phyllis is responsible for managing the nursing staff development program, which provides orientation, continuing education, management and leadership development and organizational development services. In 1987, Phyllis implemented the organizational development services in response to requests from nursing work groups for assistance in performing more effectively.

A member of the Board of Directors for the American Society for Healthcare Education and Training, she was awarded the distinction of Fellow, Healthcare Education in 1988, the highest award for professional excellence in healthcare education and training. Achievement of this designation reflects excellence through sustained contributions to healthcare organizations an to the field of healthcare education and training. A speaker for numerous organizations throughout the country, Phyllis focuses her presentations on the real and practical, and assists learners to engage in activities that move them from identification of problems to applying the information learned in the classroom directly to their work setting .

Belinda E. Puetz, PhD, RN, is president of the consulting firm Belinda E. Puetz & Associates, Inc., in Pensacola, Florida. A graduate of Henry Ford Hospital School of Nursing in Detroit, she obtained her BSN from Indiana University School of Nursing in Indianapolis. Her graduate degrees (MSEd and PhD) in adult education are from Indiana University in Bloomington.

Belinda has worked in nursing staff development and continuing education for nearly 20 years. She has extensive experience in consultation and teaching continuing education activities for nurses.

Belinda is founder and Editor-in-Chief of the *Journal of Nursing Staff Development*. She is a prolific writer, having published four books, one of which received the *American Journal of Nursing* Book of the Year Award. Her numerous articles have appeared in the nursing and education literature.

Belinda is the founder and administrator of the National Nursing Staff Development Organization. She has been recognized at the state, regional, and national levels for her contributions to continuing education in nursing.

Mary Cramer Simpson, MSN, RN, is a 1972 graduate of the College of Saint Teresa in Winona, Minnesota, and began her nursing practice in Milwaukee, Wisconsin. As a staff nurse in labor and delivery, community health and medical surgical settings, it became increasingly clear that education, be it staff or patient education, was the key to achievement of patient and practice outcomes. It was in Milwaukee that Mary began in staff development practice as coordinator of a nurse internship program in a 250-bed community hospital.

In 1977, Mary returned to her native state of Kentucky and continued her specialization in staff development as the Assistant Director of Nursing for Staff Development at the University of Kentucky Medical Center in Lexington. She received her MS in adult nursing from the University of Kentucky in 1981.

Since 1982, Mary has been the Director of Nursing Staff Development at The Ohio State University Hospitals in Columbus, Ohio. She is administratively responsible for a staff development program that supports the orientation, inservice, and continuing education needs of over 1200 nursing personnel. She has previously assumed responsibility for quality assurance, continuity of care, primary nursing, and clinical ladder programming.

Mary Cramer Simpson believes that the role of staff development within an organization is multifaceted and that the changing nature of health care is creating tremendous opportunities for staff development specialists to refine and extend their scope of practice.

Judith F. Warmuth, PhD, RN, is Director of Nursing Resources at Meriter Hospital in Madison, Wisconsin. Meriter is a new acute care institution created from the merger of two established Madison hospitals. Judith is responsible for all of the nonclinical areas in nursing including quality assurance, information systems, administrative coordinators (off-shift supervisors), resource nurses, nursing education, and clinical nurse specialists.

Judith's educational preparation includes a Master's in Medical-Surgical Nursing and a PhD in Adult Education from the University of Wisconsin-Madison. She is especially interested in the development of competence and the creation of nurse experts.

Judith is chair of the Commission on Accreditation of the American Nurses Credentialling Center, a member of the ANA Council on Continuing Education and Staff Development, and has been active in creating the National Nursing Staff Development Organization. She also serves as the nurse member of the Dane County Board of Health.

Francie J. Wolgin, MSN, RN, CNA, received her BSN and MSN from the University of Cincinnati College of Nursing and Health. She graduated with a major in clinical psychiatry and a minor in business administration.

Francie is the Director of Nursing Practice Development at Duke University Medical Center. She manages the professional resource programs and areas including quality assurance, intravenous and chemotherapy team, and patient satisfaction surveys, and serves as a liaison to the School of Nursing and the clinical specialists.

She was previously Director for Clinical Resources at the University of Cincinnati Hospital where she provided overall direction for nursing consultation and research, patient educational TV, quality assurance, staff development and education, and nursing recruitment and retention. She functioned as liaison between nursing and the College of Nursing and Health and facilitated all student placement contracts. Francie also provided leadership for the development and implementation of a four-tack, hospital-wide management development training program.

She holds a volunteer faculty appointment at Duke University and the UC College of Nursing and is on the Raymond Walters College Nursing Advisory Board. Current professional activities include serving as *JNSD* department editor for "Perspectives in Research," NNSDO, and Sigma Theta Tau research reviewer. She is past chairperson of the Ohio State Board of Nursing's Task Force to implement mandatory CNE. As past vice chairperson of ANA's Council on Continuing Education and Staff Development, she coauthored the ANA Standards for Nursing Staff Development. Francie has conducted and presented research, provides consultation, and has published several articles.

Foreword

As Karen Kelly indicates in her preface, much has happened in staff development during the past 20 years. An event that has enormous implication for future staff development educators was the 1991 JCAHO emphasis on competence assessment and maintenance. Even novices in the field of staff development will need to be prepared to address the practical implications of these expectations. No longer will it be sufficient to give the random programs, which I used to call, many years ago, "Wednesday matinees." Similarly, orientation must be more than a technical skills list and passive information provided by a "parade of stars," or random assortment of organizational representatives. Employee development activities will now need to be based on validated performance deficits and assessed needs, not "want-to-knows."

Additionally, as Kelly and others emphasize throughout this book, political savvy, organizational awareness, and recognition that staff development is a part of, not apart from, the business of health care is essential for staff developers' success. This success will not be based merely on how many programs are given or how many people attend classes, but rather on what contribution is made by agency employees to patients' care and well-being. Unfortunately, a difficult dilemma exists for the novice in staff development, that is, whom to please or satisfy—learners, managers, administrators, or other educators? Each of these groups has a different and sometimes conflicting perspective of needs and priorities. All can make considerable demands on staff developers' time, energy, and talent. And although there can never be complete resolution of any dilemma, thoughtful application of the content in this book's many chapters on planning, assessment, and organization will help address these thorny issues.

In Chapter 3, Wolgin writes about the importance of the existence of a staff development philosophy or statement of beliefs. Equally important is congruence between the organization's philosophy and the staff developer's personal philosophy. Although there may be organizational tolerance for a diversity of opinion, it is generally expected that employers will promote the stated mission and values. Also, knowing and understanding the relative importance or priority of these stated beliefs is essential if the staff development function is to be viewed as an important organizational contributor. Only then will the function consistently be supported with the resources needed to do the job.

As with most complex phenomena, there are no simple answers or solutions to the multiple issues, demands, priorities, and needs germane to organizational success. All employees, including those in staff development, need to engage in continuous learning activities that will assist in the acquisition of new skills and maintenance of current competence. This book makes an important contribution to such learning. As a veteran of staff development, I wish you success and enjoyment in an endeavor that may be both frustrating and gratifying—but never boring!

Dorothy J. del Bueno

Preface

By thinking about our current practice we can create our future. This text is a reflection of current nursing staff development practice. It is specifically written to help the nurse who is new to this specialty. Nurses who choose this field of practice rarely have formal preparation for the myriad tasks required, nor can they access one or two references to help as they develop programs needed by nursing departments in organizations. This book is intended to serve as a basic reference and help the new specialist learn about the practice of nursing staff development.

Nurses who begin staff development practice usually bring refined clinical skills to the new role. Sometimes they bring teaching experience from a previous role in academic settings. Other times the nurse will bring a strong interest and desire to teach but limited experience with planning and organizing a variety of programs for diverse groups of nurses. Occasionally, a nurse begins staff development practice with formal academic preparation for the role. Though graduate education is advocated for staff development practice, nursing graduate programs rarely prepare the nurse for this role. It is unusual to find course work related to program planning and evaluation in the nursing curriculum. Graduate programs in adult education may seem more relevant, yet course work specific to nursing and staff development is difficult to combine in most universities and still meet degree requirements. Some work in this area is beginning. The National Nursing Staff Development Organization (NNSDO) is engaged in a project to collect information about this topic. In the meantime, this text is designed to help the new staff development nurse make the transition to a specialist in this field.

Specific help is provided in a way that is familiar to all nurses. The nursing process is used as a familiar and primary organizing framework. Recalling strategies used to assess, plan, implement, and evaluate nursing care needs of patients, new staff development specialists are encouraged to use the same approach to diagnose performance problems of nursing staff and plan, implement, and evaluate programs to resolve these problems. Key to the application of the nursing process framework to staff development is the differentiation of performance problems and administrative or systems problems. Throughout the text, reference is made to validate performance problems with management and gain the support of the organization for the intervention planned. If organizational support and endorsement is not achieved, new behaviors will not be expected or reinforced.

The text begins with an overview of the field of practice to give the new specialist a flavor of the dynamic, diverse, and developing nature of this work. The second chapter lays the foundation for a theoretical framework for the focus of nursing staff development. In Chapter 3, Francie Wolgin discusses specific strategies that are helpful as the new specialist begins this role in the organization. Chapter 4, contributed by Susan Costello, provides basic curriculum design principles and standard program suggestions.

Chapters 5 through 8 discuss needs assessment, program planning, implementation and evaluation. The contributors, Belinda Puetz, Phyllis Miller and Judy Warmuth, have wide experience with these topics and demonstrate their expertise in their contributions. In Chapter 9, Mary Simpson describes a variety of programs often managed by staff development specialists and program administrators. Rationales for the inclusion of these programs in a nursing staff development department are discussed and help the new specialist gain an appreciation for the breadth of programming often generated to develop the competence of nurses.

Chapter 10 describes basic administration principles and considerations for the new program manager. This chapter is also written to help the new specialist in a large department gain a basic understanding of staff development administration. The nurse in a single-person department may also discover new information in this section. Chapter 11 is the result of several years experience with the management of quality within the staff development program. Written specifically to assist the new specialist understand the application of quality monitoring strategies, this chapter was added by popular demand for such a resource. The final chapter attempts to help staff development specialists with experience begin to look to the future. Experience seems to indicate that the specialist needs about two years to gain insight and comprehensive understanding regarding this field of practice. At this point, the specialist is ready to plan for long-range change. This chapter provides a strategic planning model to assist this process and help staff development specialists design a staff development program that will meet the future needs of nursing personnel and organizations.

Woven throughout the text are the organizational implications of staff development interventions. Stressed throughout is the need for strong liaisons to the organizations, usually as represented by the nurse manager. This theme is important for efficiency, productivity, and role effectiveness. A key understanding necessary early in the development of the new specialist is the interrelatedness of this role with so many other organizational roles. The staff development specialist crosses all boundaries. The specialist will be welcome if the role is perceived as helpful and not if it is thought to be obstructive. The perceptive staff development specialist will recognize the nurse manager or learner who needs help understanding the role of the staff development specialist and purpose of the program. Establishing a working relationship when roles and purposes are clearly understood will contribute to the success of the specialist in the organization. Many nurse managers do not understand or have experience with principles of nursing staff development and base their expectations on past experience.

Health care organizations have a right to expect a return on the investments made through nursing staff development programs. The astute specialist and program manager will recognize this need to link to organizational goals and imperatives. Staff development programs that contribute to the need to assess, maintain, and develop the competence of nursing personnel will enjoy success in the organization. This text will help specialists and program managers achieve that success.

Karen J. Kelly

Acknowledgments

The idea for this book began about seven years ago. At that time, the classic reference text that defined and described the evolving field of nursing staff development was out of print. This text, by Tobin, Yoder-Wise, and Hull titled *The Process of Staff Development: Components for Change* served as the classic reference. This book was last published in 1979. The first edition, published in 1974, was my introduction to the field when I was promoted at Loudoun Memorial Hospital and given responsibility for inservice education. This service was a one-person department, just me, and I had many questions about how to go about this work. Tobin's book and the ANA Guidelines for Staff Development were my primary sources of information. Colleagues in other hospitals were also helpful as I prepared myself for this role while simultaneously doing it. These served me well and it now my desire to give something back to staff development. This book represents my 15 years of experience in staff development as well as the experience of others specialists and program administrators from around the country, a sum total of more than 75 years of experience! It is written for the new staff development specialist and program manager.

Many people have influenced my thinking about nursing staff development. Trish Stream was the first specialist to help me understand what staff development was all about when I was a novice in 1976. Dorothy del Bueno challenged me to be clear about the role of staff development in organizations. Belinda Puetz gave me opportunities and encouragement to write. My colleagues, who have contributed to this text, helped me think of staff development in many different ways. Other colleagues throughout this country have shared their thoughtful reflections about this work through publishing and presenting seminars—they have also inspired me to continue this work and enjoy it as well. Participants in workshops and seminars have helped me validate and confirm ideas about staff development—to them I am also grateful for their staunch support.

My studies at Virginia Tech and more recently at George Mason University have also caused me to think about my work. In particular, Marcie Boucouvalas taught me how to be an adult educator. The nursing faculty at George Mason University and Dean Rita Carty helped me recognize this field as a nursing specialty and energized my nursehood. And of course, Sister Jude, my eleventh grade English composition teacher at St. Mary's in Elizabeth, New Jersey taught me that to begin to write, one must put one's pen to the paper and begin! With today's technology, to begin to write means fingers to keyboard.

My colleagues at Greater Southeast Community Hospital must also be acknowledged. Words alone will not communicate the deep feelings I have about so many special people in this organization. Special thanks must be extended to Nell Bratcher for allowing me the autonomy and flexibility so essential to the completion of this work; to my Executive Council colleagues who have no problem challenging my ideas while communicating respect for my work. To the head nurses and other managers for their enthusiasm and unflagging support. Finally, to Barb, Bev, Freddie, Bill, Kay, Donna, Sheila and Sherry—thank you for your sustenance and support which was demonstrated every day as you put staff development principles to work. And a special note of gratitude to Phyllis Miller for running the department so smoothly while I attended to this volume. The deep commitment of this group to the practice of nursing staff development through several extraordinarily stressful years is genuinely appreciated.

Special thanks are also extended to Diana Intenzo, Doris Wray, and Lori Bainbridge of J.B. Lippincott for their support and encouragement throughout this endeavor. And a sincere expression of gratitude is given to Nancy Berliner for her editorial and production diligence. More appreciated (and fun to explore) were her musings about literary challenges. Thanks for the insights!

To Shannon, my daughter, who is maturing into a lovely young woman. Thank you for being yourself and standing up for your first amendment rights. To my sister Jane—thank you for validating my beliefs about nursing through your own expert nursing experiences. Lastly, to Mike, my partner, my lover and friend, words cannot express my deep sentiment for this man. His happiness, insights, support and endurance caused me to discover joy in everyday living. What I have learned from Mike is immeasurable and my thanks are enormous.

Contents

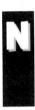

chapter 1

Nursing Staff Development: An Emerging Field of Nursing Practice

Karen J. Kelly

Nursing staff development has a long and rich tradition. This tradition has provided a solid foundation for the continuing evolution of this field of practice. As the practice of this specialty continues to unfold, it is appropriate to begin to define the field as it currently exists. In turn, efforts to define the field will serve future generations of staff development specialists as they continue to refine and develop the field and their practice. This chapter explores the continuing maturation of staff development and provides background about its history and origins. In addition, a variety of issues and agenda items for continued progression are examined. Finally, suggestions for constructing future staff development services are scrutinized. New and experienced staff development specialists will benefit from a review of this chapter. That review will help all specialists consider the state of the art and science of nursing staff development and come to a consensus about future advancements within the field.

Developing Nature of the Field. It is important to note the developing character of this and any specialized field of practice. Without the acknowledgment of this evolutionary and developmental state, the field will not continue to emerge as a viable and necessary component of nursing practice in health care organizations.

In 1990, organizations budgeted $45.5 billion for the continuing development of their employees,[1] $1.1 million more than 1989. A portion of this resource is dedicated to the continuing development of nursing personnel. The field of nursing staff development is responsible for using these resources judiciously in programs specifically designed to assess, maintain, and develop the competencies of staff as defined in job

1

and performance expectations of the organization. Since more than 72% of the budgeted dollars goes toward the salaries of staff development specialist and support personnel, the practices and procedures used by these specialists are the most significant feature of this work. The manner in which each staff development specialist goes about this task varies. However, over time, consistent practices have emerged that have been successful. Grounded theory tells us we can look to our past as well as to current practice to define our future. A rich tradition exists within staff development. This tradition will be used to define our present practice and form our future.

The Tradition

Hospitals and other health care agencies have organized opportunities for nurses to develop their expertise since the time of Nightingale. Her often quoted statement, "Let us never consider ourselves finished nurses," set the stage for the expectation of continued development as a professional practice standard. In 1928, Pfefferkorn[2] discussed issues related to improvement of the nurse in service. Hospitals assigned "inservice education" responsibilities to senior nurses and organized orientation opportunities and classes for the nurse "in service." Thus, the term "inservice education" was used for many years to describe this work.

Few papers and books were written to help nurses learn how to provide staff development. Nurses in hospital-based schools of nursing often served in the dual capacity of teaching student and graduate nurses. It was unusual for a nurse to be assigned solely to the continuing development of nurses in service. In the early sixties, the role began to emerge as nursing became more complex. Senior nurses, sometimes those who could no longer manage the strenuous duties associated with direct care, were assigned to a role called "inservice education." Few resources were available to help these nurses function within this assignment. Staff development nurses had to rely on their own innate ability to identify learning needs of nurses and define methods to meet those needs.

These experienced nurses used a problem-solving approach, intrinsic to the nursing process, as a framework to help organize this work. Learning needs were assessed; educational activities were planned, implemented, and evaluated; and practice was assessed again for improvement and for continued learning needs.

Nurses also continued to learn from each other or on their own. Modeling, mentoring, and preceptoring occurred as nurses were identified by these inservice education nurses to help orient and develop graduate nurses and nurses assigned to new clinical practice areas. Some nurses were more helpful than others, but despite the seeming informality and lack of an organized program, nurses learned new skills and maintained their competence. Most importantly, nursing care continued to be delivered and patients got well or were helped to die peacefully.

Many nurses were assigned or "promoted" to staff development positions because of their good clinical skills. However, limited coursework and few support systems existed to help in this transition from a clinical to management position. In 1974, Tobin, Yoder-Wise, and Hull made a significant contribution to the field with their first edition of the text, *The Process of Staff Development: Components for Change*. This text and the later edition, published in 1979,[3] defined the field of practice until the early eighties.

The American Nurses Association, through the work of the Ad Hoc Committee for Staff Development, of the Council on Continuing Education in Nursing, also published a pamphlet titled *Guidelines for Staff Development* in 1976.[4] This significant contribution to the field was guided by Dorothy Coye, another pioneer in the staff development field, and still serves today as a standard of staff development practice. Nurses who engaged in this field of practice used these two references as primary sources to help organize and deliver staff development services.

Regulatory bodies began to recognize the need for an organized staff development program. In 1978, the Joint Commission on Accreditation of Hospitals (JCAH), as it was then known, required that a position be established for overseeing and coordinating staff development activities such as orientation and inservice education. Many health departments responsible for licensing health care organizations also reviewed staff development activities to help determine if organizations were meeting selected standards and criteria.

Staff development specialists often turned to other fields such as adult education, human resource development, instructional technology, and organization development for help with designing staff development programs. While these activities were practical and rational, they required neophyte staff development nurses to adapt this information to the unique setting of staff development in the health care organization.

Staff development nurses sought out staff development nurses in other organizations and created formal and informal networks, groups, and organizations to help each other learn and adapt to this emerging role. As more nurses began to identify with the staff development term, the need to develop this field of practice became increasingly recognized.

The eighties brought several significant contributions to the development of the field including

- Publication of several texts specific to nursing staff development
- Publication of the *Journal of Nursing Staff Development*
- Recognition of the specialty by the addition of the words "staff development" to the American Nurses' Association's Council on Continuing Education and Staff Development
- Formation of the National Nursing Staff Development Organization (NNSDO)

Nurses now seek out positions in staff development and look for graduate programs to help them prepare for this role. Indeed, several of the first tasks of the newly formed National Nursing Staff Development Organization (NNSDO) were to

- Identify graduate programs that included curricula that would enhance the practice skills of the staff development specialist.
- Explore the feasibility of a certification process for staff development specialist.
- Provide continuing education and networking opportunities for nurses engaged in this field.

Experienced practitioners in this field generally agree that a graduate degree in nursing or adult education is appropriate for this field of practice, yet few graduate programs exist to specifically prepare nurses for this role. Existing programs are often modified and adapted to assist nurses who request graduate preparation for this work.

Despite this lack of a formally defined mechanism to prepare practitioners, the nursing staff development field has flourished and expanded. The practice of responding to the needs of nurses for continued competency development has laid fallow ground for continued growth in this field. Nurses who have experienced or understand this history will find it helpful to plan the future of nursing staff development in health care organizations. This tradition provides a rich history that serves to ground this evolving field. Indeed, it is a testimonial to the profession that nurses have continually sought out developmental activities that will improve their ability to care for their patients.

The Present

As a field of nursing practice, staff development is dynamic, diverse, and developing. Significant changes in the health care delivery systems have caused organizations to restructure. Changing demographics, new technology, and scarce resources have caused health care providers to rethink and retool the systems for delivering services. Nursing care delivery systems have been restructured to meet the changing needs of consumers. Appropriately, staff development activities have evolved and departments have restructured to meet the changing needs of today's health care organizations.

Staff development is practiced in a variety of settings. Most commonly, organized staff development activities will be provided in hospitals; understandably so, since most nurses can still be found working in hospitals. Long-term care settings also engage in a significant amount of staff development activities. As more health care is delivered by nurses in alternative settings such as free-standing clinics, surgicenters, and urgicenters, staff development services will also be needed by nurses in these unique settings.

Despite the commonality of hospital-based staff development practice, staff development departments are organized in a variety of ways. Nursing staff development departments are frequently organized within the nursing department. At times, the department or function can also be found within a human resource development department, within a personnel department, within a hospital-wide training or education department or elsewhere within the organization.

There are inherent advantages and disadvantages of each organizational model for nursing staff development. Some advantages of locating the nursing staff development program within a hospital-wide education department include the perception that limited resources may be used more efficiently. In fact, what often occurs is the expectation that the nursing staff development specialist provide a wide range of services to all departments. This approach dilutes the effectiveness of the nursing component of the staff development program, as the specialist will be unable to attend to the specific and unique needs of nurses. Furthermore, the specialist will need additional personal development to learn about the different needs of other health care professionals and support personnel.

Another often touted advantage of hospital-wide education departments includes the perception that there will be less duplication of services. In fact, it is often the staff development specialists who is simply assigned to additional programs and departments and held responsible for providing services to various departments with dissimilar needs. The specialist is expected to provide basic educational services, often those required by regulatory bodies, to many departments primarily to meet specific requirements. But without attention to the *purpose* of required programs and the specific needs of the learners, the skills of the nursing staff development specialist are underused. This is not to say that nursing staff development specialists are unable to perform these assignments and duties. Indeed, it is often the outstanding past performance that is awarded with these additional assignments. The issue is the use of the specialist in this limited role.

The argument for identifying these services as *nursing* staff development services is rooted in the fact that the specialists providing these services are nurses first. It is this characteristic that underpins the entire approach to nursing staff development and causes nurses to pursue this career path. If nursing is defined as the diagnosis and treatment of actual and potential responses to health care problems, then the role of the nursing staff development specialist is to assist the nurse in developing skills related to nursing.

The commitment of nurses to help people become independent and cope with their health is the essence of nursing practice. The continuing development of nurses as they attempt "to achieve the right level of involvement with a patient"[5] is the specific assignment of the nursing staff development specialist. To attenuate that assignment with responsibilities to other departments is to weaken the effectiveness of the specialist.

It is not inappropriate to assign nurses to the staff development responsibilities of departments other than that of nursing. Indeed, with the tradition of effectiveness and efficiency in the field of staff development, it may be a sound administrative decision. However, these individuals should be titled differently. The titles should reflect their specific assignment and should not confuse consumers of services by adding words, such as nursing, that do not reflect the assignment to other than nursing departments. If, however, a nurse is expected to assess, maintain, and develop nursing competencies within an organization, then the nurse must be uniquely identified as a *nursing* staff development specialist and allowed to spend the majority of time with nurses.

Any organization's approach to the development of its human resources should include clearly communicated expectations by the hospital administration about the role of staff development professionals and the scope of responsibilities assigned to it. In this regard, the recruitment and retention of knowledgeable workers, such as nursing staff development specialists, should include the recognition that some nurses choose to fulfill their career aspirations through a nursing staff development role. Others may choose roles that are not directly related to nursing service. With the myriad talents and creativity of nurses and health care professionals available to the health care industry, all should be able to find fulfillment and satisfaction in the many roles needed to continue to improve the services provided by health care organizations.

To be most effective and able to influence the improvement of nursing practice, nursing staff development departments or programs should be organized within the nursing department. The leader of the department should hold an advanced degree in nursing or adult education and should answer directly to the top executive in nursing. In large organizations, the leader of the staff development department should be in a line position and hold equal title and rank to the operational leaders of the various divisions within the department of nursing. Only within such a structure can the staff development leader have access to the information and participate in essential nursing practice decisions. This information is vital to the formation of a staff development program that is responsive to the changing practice expectations of the organization's nurse leaders.

An emerging model for nursing staff development is the consultative approach. Ulschak and SnowAntle[6] believe this approach improves costs and services and fosters collaboration and cooperation. Assuming that an organization is willing to forego traditional "turf" issues, this model is a powerful organizational development tactic that can enhance organizational effectiveness. With more than eight million health care workers and two million nurses, the competence of all workers can be enhanced through improved collaboration and cooperation skills.

Also of note is the role of staff development within career development and promotion programs. Often called "clinical ladder programs," staff development specialists are expected to participate in the design, implementation, and administration of these programs. This is a natural and logical role for the specialist. These programs use the staff development process to enhance career options for professional nurses. They often use skill acquisition and recognition strategies to reward and engage nurses in their continuing development. Staff development specialists should be intimately involved with career development and promotion programs. A detailed discussion of these programs can be found in Chapter 9.

As any practice field matures, its practitioners will begin to identify a body of knowledge, the best practices, and the way of knowing about the field. Sovie[7] described several stages of professional career development in nursing that have applicability to staff development. She indicated there were three stages: (a) professional identification in which individuals become oriented toward the field, (b) professional maturation in which the potential for development and expansion of competencies is recognized, and (c) professional mastery in which the self-actualization of the potential is realized. At present, many staff development specialists are in the stage of professional maturation. As the field of nursing staff development continues to be defined by practitioners and others, nurses will readily recognize the essential contribution of staff development activities to the professional development of individual nurses and nursing as a whole within organizations.

What Is Nursing Staff Development Today?

Accepted definitions of nursing staff development generally describe it as a process that includes both formal and informal learning activities that relate to the employee's role expectations within organizations. These learning activities can take place within or outside the agency.[3] This process definition is expanded to include three phases—input, process, and output—and identifies these phases as essential to the overall goal of changing behavior.

The American Nurses' Association (ANA) has defined staff development as a term that includes both formal and informal learning opportunities to assist individuals to perform competently in fulfillment of role expectations within a specific agency.[4] The ANA further indicates that resources both within and outside the agency are used to facilitate the process.

The current emphasis of efficiency, quality, and effectiveness causes new definitions of staff development to be forwarded. Staff development can also be described as the organization of prescribed developmental activities that assist the organization in reaching defined goals through the assessment, maintenance, and development of nursing competencies. Key concepts in this definition include the role of nursing staff development in the achievement of organizational goals. All staff development activities should be linked, in some way, to organizational goals. Other key concepts include the activities of assessing, maintaining, or developing nursing competencies. Activities must be related to the knowledge and skill related to performance expectations. To relate staff development activities to performance expectations requires the assessment of competencies in order to plan for continued development of staff. Some skills and knowledge of nurses will require maintenance activities and others will need to be developed to respond to changing health care needs, changing technologies, and changing nursing practice patterns.

This definition of nursing staff development is grounded in education *and* the needs of organizations for continued response to changing health care technologies and health care needs of communities of patients. In addition, the future will also require staff development specialists to help nurses make increasingly sophisticated judgments about which patients receive what kind of care, under what circumstances, and with what expected outcomes.

The issue of staff development as a noun, verb, or adjective is of concern as the field attempts to define itself. Specifically, the misuse of the component of staff development called "inservice education" causes confusion. When acceptable parlance includes the "inservicing of staff" and nurses who have "been inserviced," bewilderment results. Clear, concise, and accepted use of terms is essential to the field, and the appropriate use of these terms by staff development specialists is a hallmark of professional practice.

What Will Staff Development Be in the Future

The future of nursing staff development rests with its practitioners. Through research, publications, thoughtful discussions and debates, and seminars and conferences, the field will continue to evolve. Many nurses have raised superb questions and issues to help staff development specialists consider how to best achieve their goals within their specific work settings.

O'Connor's Issues

O'Connor[8] addressed nine issues in her text that must be addressed by staff development specialists. While also addressing issues for the nurse engaged in continuing education practice, only those related to nursing staff development will be discussed here. The issues consisted of the following questions:

1. Who is responsible for staff development? And who benefits?
2. How can participation in staff development activities be promoted?
3. What should be the content of staff development?
4. How can adult learning principles be applied to the design of staff development offerings?
5. How can the educator assure that staff development offerings are relevant, with applicability to the professional lives of participants?
6. What are the best teaching strategies for staff development?
7. What measures should be used to demonstrate the effectiveness of the staff development program?
8. How can the staff development program most efficiently utilize limited resources?
9. How can quality in staff development programming be ensured?
10. Does staff development make a difference?

These questions provide a sound basis for the design of a staff development program within an organization. The answers to these questions are emerging and many have definitive responses. This book, representative of nursing staff development practice in a variety of settings by experienced specialists, provides many guidelines to help the neophyte specialist answer these questions. The questions cited above can provide the basis of the first step toward designing a comprehensive nursing staff development program for a health care organization. The first step is the organizational needs assessment as discussed in Chapter 5.

Bille's Systems Approach

Bille[9] also developed a systems approach to nursing staff development. He said staff development is an integral component of every organization and expanded the list of components advocated by Tobin. Bille indicated that staff development provides the following learning opportunities for nursing personnel:

- **Induction education:** to introduce new employees to the specific work setting.
- **Remedial education:** to fill in the gaps left by the nursing education program; and to allow re-entry into practice after years of not working.
- **Inservice education:** to increase competence in a specific area of practice; to keep abreast of technological changes and new procedures and new products; and to adapt to changes within the organization.
- **Continuing education:** to enhance the professional knowledge base; to facilitate practice toward higher levels of practice; and to improve health care delivery.

Bille further posits that staff development, as only one component of the total organization, does not exist in a vacuum, nor can it solve all the ills of the organization. In looking at staff development within the organization, Bille advocates using a systems approach which looks at all parts and structures in an organization and the way they relate to organizational goals or outcomes. He further defined three basic components of staff development within a basic systems approach to job performance:

- **Inputs:** entry staff behavior, level of education, and prior experience
- **Throughputs:** orientation, policies, procedures, and managerial direction
- **Outputs:** the final staff behavior and quality patient care

This approach to portraying how nursing staff development fits into the large scheme of organizational behavior and development serves as a sound basis to assist the staff development specialist with program planning and design decisions.

Role Definition

Staff development specialists have continued to define the role of staff development within health care organizations based on their experiences and expertise. Using available texts and references, each attempts to make some sense out of the expectations of organization for staff development services. Singleton and Nail[10] suggested the following key activities to enhance the position of the staff development department:

1. Study the goals of the hospital, both short term and long range.
2. Conduct an assessment of the department.
3. Examine the literature and talk with nurses in key positions to get their perceptions and advice on current and future learning needs of staff.
4. Talk to physicians who use the facility.
5. In conjunction with nursing administration, determine whether first line and middle managers are performing at their peak capacity.

6. Develop an effective learning needs assessment plan.
7. Try to determine opportunities to present information to groups at a regular gathering.
8. Select teaching strategies that are flexible, creative, and cost-effective.
9. Use preceptors in orientation and other programs.
10. Find people in the organization who might be ready resource people who can teach for the department.
11. Establish a network with other staff development departments in other hospitals.
12. Determine whether your department or the network can become income-producing.
13. Contact the continuing education departments at local universities and examine their services.
14. Establish small research projects that will allow systematic data collection to determine impact of staff development activities on patient care.

The use of these steps in the formulation or revision of a nursing staff development program will expedite the process of establishing a viable and contributing service to the organization.

Others have encouraged the use of a position charter and key objective approach to the management and delivery of staff development services.[11] The advantages of this approach include a strategic method that organizes and prioritizes departmental goals and demonstrates outcomes valued by the organization. The position charter, similar to a departmental philosophy, specifies the ongoing commitments, accountabilities, and standards of the service. Goals and objectives are derived directly from this charter. The use of a position charter will also facilitate the understanding of staff development's purpose and service within the health care organization.

Dorothy del Bueno also addressed issues in her key article titled "Critical Times, Critical Issues."[12] She identified four key elements that should be emphasized and clarified:

- **Value:** The value of the staff development department must be perceived by management as both groups work collaboratively to differentiate between system and education problems, and as staff development specialists define the limitations, probabilities, and costs of traditional educational interventions.
- **Focus and mission:** The orientation of staff development must correspond to the organization's mission and goals. The acquisition of new skills by employees, in order that they may provide new services or product lines, is an essential ingredient of the staff development program.
- **Organization:** The administrative structure of the staff development department will create benefits as well as costs to the organization. Centralization or decentralization are two common but dichotomous approaches, with the advantages of one creating the disadvantages of the other. The most important component of any structure is that

it has a direct line and reporting relationship to those who have the authority and power to allocate resources.
- **Cost or revenue:** Identified by del Bueno as a philosophical as well as a financial issue, the cost or revenue issue is one that will be resolved as organizations clarify their commitment to employee development. Staff development specialists should consider the costs associated with the development of nurses to be an investment, and demonstrate the resulting benefits of increased productivity and reduction of time required to achieve competent performance.

These issues and others will guide the agenda for the future of nursing staff development programs in health care organizations.

Our Future Agenda

Our first agenda is to come to an agreement and common understanding about the name of this kind of nursing. Some names of departments in health care agencies with the major function defined as staff development include

- Nursing Staff Development
- Nursing Education
- Professional Development
- Education and Training
- Nursing Resources
- Nursing Education Services

If the nursing department has a research program, it is not uncommon to find the title reflective of this as well, i.e., Nursing Education and Research. It is also common to find changing titles without significant change in service. At other times, new services are added to existing services and new titles are forwarded to reflect the new service or structure. While departments must be responsive to changes in organizational structure and goals, the frequent changes in title cause confusion among consumers of staff development services.

Communicating the services available through a department is a continuing challenge, particularly as so many traditional health care services are transforming to meet changing needs. Title changes of staff development departments often come about as a result of perceived discontent with current services. Simply retitling and making minor shifts of personnel will not accomplish significant change in services. Nurse administrators often have expectations that are not being met through available services. These expectations may seem irrational or unrealistic to the staff development specialist. Regardless of these feelings, there is a need to address these failed expectations. Staff development specialists must help nurse administrators understand the field, what is possible, and what resources are needed to meet additional expectations. The chief nursing executive is the primary customer of staff development services and sets expectations for practice through the established management network. Staff development specialists must establish substantial working relationships with management. To achieve the goals of improved practice through continuing development, it is the role of the staff development specialist to collaborate with these decision makers and teach, as needed, how these services will help the organization achieve goals.

First Agenda: Naming the Field

A core activity of this service is the continuing development of the staff of the organization. While some hospitals have a hospital-wide education department, others have two, and sometimes several, education departments. Each is structured differently and often a different mission serves as a basis for the service. Due to the rich and successful tradition of nursing staff development, these programs are often directed by nurses and have emerged from a nursing inservice education program. Sometimes considered a more efficient use of limited resources, these departments may be given significantly more responsibility than is possible to meet.

However, successful programs in which nursing staff development is a program within an organization-wide education program do exist. The success of the program is often directly linked to the close bonds maintained between the department and administration for all areas. In these cases, the administrator of the department must access top administration on a regular basis and should probably be a member of the executive decision-making group.

The choice for most nurses engaged in nursing staff development is to remain within the nursing department. This is understandable as most nurses were clinical nurses before entering the new role of staff development specialist. The work of these nurses is most often with nurses. This work is more effectively accomplished if the nursing staff development program is located within nursing.

A distinct name, such as "nursing staff development," will contribute to a more common understanding among nurses about the role and capacity of staff development specialists. In addition, the specialist will also be recognized readily and used efficiently within the expectations of the organization. Most importantly, the use of a common term will advance the conceptual understanding of this field by the consumers of the services provided by staff development specialists.

Second Agenda Item: Communicating the Role

A second agenda includes the communication of the role of the staff development specialist. Regardless of the title, the nurses providing staff development are responsible for defining their role and communicating it to the organization. This can be done in a variety of ways, including, but not limited to, verbal clarification, written verification and amplification, and actions that support the operational effectiveness of the role.

Similar but distinct roles must also be differentiated. The role of clinical specialist is a complementary one to staff development but it is not the same.

The most significant difference is the focus of the roles: the clinical specialist is prepared to solve difficult patient and nursing care problems and serve as a consultant to nurses, and the skills of the staff development specialist are program planning and design for assessing, maintaining, and developing competencies.

Preparation for this work must also be defined to help future practitioners prepare for the role. Future staff development specialists will also be managers of change, synergy generators, paradigm creators and master teachers. To prepare for this role, coursework, academic preparation, and experiences must be defined.

Third Agenda Item: Defining the Role

The third agenda item is the continued definition of the field. What it includes and what it does not. Tobin defined the components of the field as orientation, inservice education, continuing education, leadership development, skills training, and incidental learning. Others have added components such as competency assessment, clinical affiliations, patient education, career counseling, and health and wellness education. Central to any staff development program is the orientation and continuing development of nursing staff.

Many resources are used to help operate a staff development program in a health care organization. Arguments can be made to define the field as education, training, or human resource development. These theories are used to design and operate the nursing staff development program. But the substance of this field of practice is nursing. Practitioners are individuals who were nurses first. These nurses bring to this field a unique nursing perspective that helps define the strategies and methods for continued improvement in nursing services and nursing competencies. The role must be defined within a nursing framework.

Distinct and Different

Many terms can be used to title the field as observed earlier but nursing staff development seems to be the most common denominator. However, feelings related to the worthiness of some components must be settled. For example, because the American Nurses' Association has a mechanism to approve learning activities that meet specified continuing education criteria (and as such are called continuing education), there seems to be sense that inservice education is less good than continuing education.

Despite the fact that most inservice education activities are of short duration, the planning and design features are the same as any learning activity, regardless of the adjective used to define the education. Necessary, perhaps in the future, will be a mechanism for a rational and reasonable accreditation process of the staff development program. This process must provide some value to the professionals within the field. It must also be based on accepted standards that have yielded measurable outcomes.

It is time to search out terms that are explicit and communicate the type of education that is offered in a comprehensive staff development program. These terms must be equally valued and acknowledged by all nurses.

Quality assurance mechanisms, as discussed above and similar to the ANA accreditation mechanism for continuing education should also be available for staff development professionals for an evaluation of the comprehensive staff development program. It is only through these types of activities that we will benefit and develop staff development programs that are responsive to health care organizations, patients, and nurses.

Fourth Agenda Item: Meeting Future Needs

A fourth, but by no means final, agenda item for the future is the organization of staff development programs to meet future needs. Puetz[13] presented a report of the American Society for Training and Development (ASTD) titled *Workplace Basics*. This report discusses thirteen essential skills needed in the workplace. Seven have direct relevance for staff development and include

- Knowing how to learn
- Listening
- Speaking
- Creative thinking
- Problem solving
- Organizational effectiveness
- Leadership

These basic skills will need to be integrated into staff development programs as specialists continue to prepare nurses for the challenges of providing care in a constrained health care economy with rapid knowledge obsolescence. Staff development specialists will serve as catalysts for acquiring these and other skills.

The future is dependent on the evolving competencies of the staff development specialists of today. Challenge and opportunity will help this work.

Megatrends and Staff Development

Naisbett[14] identified a variety of trends and predicted these trends would significantly alter our lifestyles and work. This work has been used frequently as a framework for more specific predictions in selected fields. Naisbett and Elkins[15] applied the framework to hospitals and Brunt[16] subsequently applied it to nursing staff development. There are a variety of issues for the staff development specialist to consider within this framework:

1. Increasing emphasis on the continuing development of the professional to meet the changing needs of society (information society).
2. The need to learn how to respond to the continually changing and increasing technology, yet maintain the essence of nursing (high tech, high touch).

3. A variety of options available to professionals to maintain competence (multiple option).
4. The need for mechanisms to help people stay well and continue to learn (self-help).
5. The development of organizations and structures that can respond quickly and competently to new needs (networks).
6. The look to the long-term effects of staff development interventions (long term).
7. The need to create opportunities for learners to participate in the design and implementation of developmental activities (participatory democracy).
8. The use of a variety of resources to assist with the staff development program (decentralization).
9. The economic condition of the health care environment, the constraints and controls currently in place and the effect of new coalitions and alliances (global economy).
10. The need to provide staff development programs in areas of rapid growth as new health care services and initiatives are offered (north to south).

In later work, titled *Megatrends 2000,* Naisbett and Aburdene[17] again analyze trends and predict new initiatives. Included are the global economic boom of the 1990s; the renaissance of the arts; the emergence of free-market socialism, global lifestyles, and cultural nationalism; the privatization of the welfare state; the rise of the Pacific Rim; women in leadership; the age of biology; the religious revival of third millennium; and the triumph of the individual. Most relevant to nursing staff development are the issues related to developing leadership for change and helping women unlearn old authoritarian behavior to run departments. New leadership methods will require people to learn to coach, inspire, and gain people's commitment (p. 217). In addition, Naisbett states "the dominant principle of the organization has shifted, from management in order to control an enterprise to leadership in order to bring out the best in people and to respond quickly to change" (p. 218).

Women will have a dominant role in all future initiatives as they have reached a critical mass in virtually all professions. The human spirit will be celebrated in the future. Nursing's vast knowledge of helping people with the experience of coping with stress and illness will play a significant role as these trends are realized. In addition, since nursing continues to be dominated by women, and with it's emergence as the profession with the commitment for caring for all individuals in need of health care, a clear role for nursing staff development programs emerges for the future. This role will focus on helping nurses realize and achieve new levels of caring using technology and human spirit to guide the healing and coping processes.

Future trends in health care education were also collected and analyzed by Ulschak and SnowAntle.[18] In their Delphi study, they found fifteen trends related to the shortage of providers, financial stability, management and supervisory training, the need for flexibility and creativity, effective use of resources, and a focus on retention. Also service orientation, aging population, need for return on investment for education, increased acuity of patients, uninsured and indigent patients, need to focus on total organizational development, technological advancements, and the continued norm of rapid change were included in the list of prioritized trends in health care education. The analysis of this list led to five recommendations including the following needs:

1. To plan for a future where there will be a shortage of health care professionals.
2. To plan for ongoing turbulence.
3. To approach educating as a business with a clear mission and objectives that will make a difference in the life of the organization.
4. To share key trends with top administration and explore ways education can assist with development.
5. To attend to personal needs to avoid burnout and manage work to maintain optimal energy.

In other work, Ulschak[19] advocated the adoption of new thoughts about change in the future. To create the future of health care education and respond to changes, he uses a metaphor from an Akaido exercise: to take as a given that staff development will be knocked off center, and thus maintain as a goal the ability to recenter as quickly as possible. Ulschak believes that staff development specialists have been knocked off balance by changes in health care delivery brought about by changes in the financing of health care. He advises the maintenance of an ongoing goal for staff development of learning to refocus and recenter, with the expectation that being knocked off balance is an ongoing process.

Defining Roles in the Future

The role of staff development within organizations will evolve as the roles of health care organizations and individual providers emerge. The continuing need to respond to change mitigates strongly for the robustness of this field. Staff development specialists will need to acquire and use characteristics that will help them thrive. These characteristics have been identified and are discussed below.

Future Characteristics of Staff Development Specialists

Stream and Herring[20] studied the characteristics of successful staff development specialists and found three clusters of behavioral characteristics which seemed important in making staff development specialists successful in what they do. The clusters are identified as the examiner, the collaborator, and the specialist. The characteristics of each are as follows:

- **The examiner:** Performs literature review to gather data; attempts to identify all available options and will keep researching and thinking to identify these; prefers to work alone; likes to deal with complex issues—the bigger the challenge, the better; questions fundamental

assumptions, such as "Why do we have to start orientation on Monday?"; is cautious.
- **The collaborator:** Consistently consults colleagues; believes in group process; emphasizes role complementarity; enjoys and is good at mentoring; accepts status quo to "keep the peace"—doesn't like to rock the boat.
- **The specialist:** Reflects on own past experiences when making decisions; acts decisively and seizes opportunities; acts autonomously; appears self-confident in field of specialty; prefers "hands-on" management style—does it rather than delegates it.

Each of these clusters of characteristics has advantages and disadvantages. For example, the examiner knows the literature but may spend too much time analyzing, the collaborator has a strong network of colleagues but may be overly concerned about how others perceive them which may interfere with appropriate decision making, and the specialist can make quick decisions but these decisions may be premature.

Stream and Herrin indicate that successful staff development specialists are aware of their own characteristics, as well as those of others, and can comfortably draw on different behaviors as indicated. In other words, use the examiner approach to analysis in some situations and the quick decisiveness of the specialist in others. These investigators also provide advice about enhancing each cluster of characteristics. For example, to enhance the skills of the *examiner,* the following is suggested:

- Read more.
- Use formal problem solving processes, such as force field analysis.
- Break down complex problems into workable units, develop PERT and GANT charts.
- Persevere in tasks.
- Train to be assertive.
- Ask why.

The following recommendations are made to enhance *collaborator* skills:

- Surround yourself with competence, hire people to complement limitations.
- Trust subordinates, allow freedom to do "own thing."
- Reward good performance.
- Engage in mentor/mentee relationships.
- Join organizations for networking such as ASHET, NNSDO, ASTD, and other specialty or local groups.
- Learn to accept compliments.

To enhance the role of the *specialist,* the following advice is provided by Stream and Herring:

- Engage in positive self-talk.
- Take a self-inventory of skills.
- Define your expertise and turf.

- Publicize your skills.
- Trust your own judgments.
- Think through worst case scenarios, e.g., what would be the worst thing that would happen if this new strategy were tried?

These clusters of characteristics have been tested and validated with an instrument developed by the investigators and have proven to be useful to help staff development specialists learn about how they presently go about their work. Specialists can learn much through self-inventories and should use them to help understand how to position themselves and their work for success within the organization.

The Varied Roles

Like the field of staff development practice, the role of the specialist is varied and ill-defined. Job descriptions and performance expectations help interpret organizational expectations for the individual in the role. Samples of performance expectations are provided in Chapter 3 along with additional information about how to develop the staff development role within the organization. Despite efforts to address all parameters and elements of the role of the staff development specialist, the descriptions rarely define the full range of competencies often expected of the staff development specialist. The elementary reason for this may be simply the need for a role that is broadly and flexibly defined in order to allow the specialist the requisite freedom to redefine the role in response to new and ongoing organizational initiatives.

This may be frustrating for some staff development specialists who prefer structure and a predictable work environment. Role definition efforts are worthwhile, if for no other reason than the process causes the specialist to think through the most important components of the role as it is currently defined or implemented. The role of the nursing staff development specialist in health care is a complex, varied, and changing one and includes many components. Structures, processes, and research that analyze these elements will help specialists understand more about role expectations.

The Delphi study conducted by the American Society of Training and Development (ASTD) is a helpful attempt to begin to identify these many components and roles. Though representative of the "trainer" role throughout all industries, application can be made to the staff development role. McLagan[21] explained this study and said "there will clearly be great economic and personal value in being able to optimize the performance of individuals, teams and entire organizations" in the future (p. 51). She listed eleven key outputs by role:

1. Administrator
2. Evaluator
3. HRD manager
4. HRD materials developer
5. Individual career-development advisor
6. Instructor or facilitator
7. Marketer
8. Needs analyst

9. Organization change agent
10. Program designer
11. Researcher

McLagan further listed thirty-five competencies organized into four dimensions: technical, business, interpersonal, and intellectual. Examples of technical competencies are adult learning understanding, career-development skill, competency-identification skill, computer competence, objectives preparation skill, performance observation skill, electronic systems skill, facilities skill, subject matter skill, and training and development understanding.

A portion of the business competencies listed includes business understanding, cost-benefit analysis skill, delegation skill, industry understanding, organization behavior understanding, organization development theories and techniques, and project and record management skills.

Some examples of interpersonal competencies uncovered in the ASTD study were skills related to coaching, feedback, group process, negotiation, presentations, questioning, relationship-building, and writing. Regarding intellectual competencies, the following were listed: data reduction skill, information search skill, intellectual versatility, model-building skill, observing skill, self-knowledge, and visioning skill.

These competencies may seem daunting and perhaps even not achievable. Knowledge about the competencies is the beginning of acquiring the skills needed for the future. This study serves as a useful model to challenge staff development specialists in their continuing development and role definition. Careful consideration of these sample competencies will help specialists continue to evolve as sophisticated providers of staff development services. The shifts in practice in health care, nursing, and staff development require shifts in practice patterns. These practice patterns can be explored and documented as an integral part of performance standard documents when a framework such as this is used to discover how specialists are currently spending their time and how they should spend their time in the future.

The most meaningful contribution the staff development specialist can make to the competencies of nurses is the ability to learn how to learn. While this concept is not well understood, it is known that people learn in a variety of ways and have preferred learning styles. In pursuing new knowledge or skills, individuals will seek out experiences and engage in their learning in ways that are personal and meaningful. People can be helped to think about how they think. Termed "metacognition" by cognitive scientists, the process of how people think can be expanded to how they go about acquiring new knowledge. If the staff development specialist can simply raise the awareness of learning as something that *is done,* rather than something that is done *to people,* then progress can be made toward this goal.

The changes in health care mitigate for changes in roles. The role of the staff development specialist will not remain the same. Gundlach[22] defined three role shifts that have application to the staff development specialist:

- Reactor to initiator
- "Pair of hands" to collaborator
- Consultant for organizational problem solving to facilitator of organizational learning

The acknowledgement of role shifts as organizations change to respond to new imperatives is inevitable. The successful staff development specialist will seek out new roles and make credible transitions to new expectations.

Naming the Role

Despite the need to advance to new roles in response to organizational change, the need for a consistent title for the nurse who performs within the staff development capacity is evident. Titles of nurses engaged in staff development practice abound. Some samples include:

- Staff Development Specialist
- Staff Development Coordinator
- Education Specialist
- Instructor
- Nurse Educator
- Clinical Educator

It is critical to identify one title to communicate the role and services of staff development. The advantages of one title are

- A common bond among specialists
- Identification of the role by consumers
- Emergence of clearer expectations of the role among various organizations
- Common understanding of services provided by the role
- Opportunity to change perceptions about staff development by upgrading titles, qualifications, and services

This multititled field of practitioners is faced with advantages and disadvantages as a result of these many titles. Disadvantages include the inability of nurses to understand and use resources available to them due to role confusion and failure of the organization to appreciate the contribution of the nurse with a title that sounds powerless and ill-defined. This could lead to the reduction of resources for these services due to vague perceptions about the contribution of individuals with these titles.

It is the responsibility of the nurse in the staff development role, with the assistance of the nurse leader, to define and communicate the services, expectations, and limitations of the role. This is essential to the success of any staff development effort.

The preferred title of the staff development role is specialist and is used throughout this book. The term "specialist" imparts an authority, a mastery and expertise, and an expected level of professionalism; thus its use in this context. Specialists also are dedicated to a particular branch of study and practice. The distinguishing mark of the staff development specialist is the commitment to the continued professional development of *nurses*. In this view, the specialist uses strategies, tools, and skills unique to the field. In addition, the specialist assumes the responsibility to continue to transform and refine the role and the field through systematic inquiry. The title specialist communicates to all consumers these essential components and characteristics. With an understanding of the specialized nature of the field, more nurses will benefit from the distinctive skills of the staff development specialist.

The transition to new titles often provides an opportunity for staff development nurses to clarify and communicate new roles that are responsive to the changing organization. The nurse of today has increasing autonomy. The need to support these nurses in their need for continued development is evident. An individual specifically dedicated to nursing and this development will make a vital contribution to patient care.

Development of the Specialist

Staff development nurses are frequently advanced or placed in these roles based on strong clinical skills and a desire to teach. As mentioned earlier, some nurses are specifically seeking out roles in this specialized field of practice. Any nurse entering this field should recognize the need for the accumulation of a variety of new experiences and learnings in areas different from clinical practice. Though a development model for the new staff development specialist is addressed later in Chapter 3, the Dreyfus[23] model of skill acquisition is a useful one to help a novice in any new field understand the characteristic development of expertise.

This model has been used extensively by Patricia Benner[24] in her efforts to uncover nursing knowledge embedded in practice. The Dreyfus[23] model of skill acquisition defines a series of stages or proficiency levels that individuals pass through as they develop expertise in a field. These levels are as follows:

- **Novice:** The individual uses context-free rules to guide own actions and is not able to identify relevant tasks in actual situations.
- **Advanced practitioner:** The person can demonstrate marginally acceptable behavior and have some real-life experience in which recurring aspects are identified and used to make some judgments.
- **Competent:** The individual has acquired several years of experience and creates a framework to establish a perspective and contemplate options to resolve problems.
- **Proficient:** The person perceives situations as wholes, rather than in terms of aspects, and performs based on maxims or a deep understanding of the situation.
- **Expert:** The individual does not rely on rules or guidelines to understand a situation and act appropriately, rather this individual uses immense experience and grasps situations intuitively and acts efficiently in responding to the circumstances.

Also defined in this model is a change in three general aspects of skilled performance. The first is a movement from reliance on abstract principles to concrete experience, which then serves as a paradigm for future practice. The second is the movement of the individual from many bits of data to a relevant and complete whole. The third change is a passage from detached observer to involved performer. The Dreyfus brothers applied and refined this model in their studies of airplane pilots and chess players.

Benner, in her application of this model to nursing, was also able to categorize levels of proficiency *and* uncover nursing knowledge embedded in practice. Clinical judgments and treatment decisions are made by nurses based on knowledge *and* experience. This is an important finding related to the development of knowledge through experience and the consequent use of experience to generate new knowledge.

Application of this model, along with Benner's findings, to staff development is logical and coherent. An entire program of staff development could be generated using this approach. Simpson[25] proposed a progression to peak performance for the new staff development specialist using the Benner framework. Figure 1-1 shows this progression and defines the characteristics commonly found at each level and suggests activities to help the individual advance to the next level.

Simpson identified the characteristics of the staff development specialist within the skill acquisition model posed by Dreyfus. She also identified staff development activities and programs that will assist the acquisition of skill and progression to expertise. Use of this approach by staff development administrators will help the neophyte specialist develop within a supportive and progressive system of learning.

Continuing development of the specialist also requires attention. The professional activities of journal reading and participation in professional association activities and conferences will help. But work is also needed to describe "how the best ones do it." A staff development specialist with more than five to seven years of experience may be equivalent to the expert described by Dreyfus and Benner. The manner in which these experts intuitively go about their work can provide other specialists with a wealth of information. How does the expert staff development specialist see the gestalt of the work needed to respond to the universe of needs identified? The step-by-step linear process alone rarely provides the final "big picture." As data become available about how these thought processes occur, new understandings will emerge and the field of staff development will evolve to new levels of practice.

Empowerment to Meet the Future

Empowerment is another essential component of staff development practice. Macher[26] discussed empowerment within the bureaucracy and listed characteristics of empowered people as

- Technical competence
- Sense of meaning about work
- Ability to exert power and influence
- Ability to make a difference
- Ability to work in good faith

In addition, Macher said empowered people take personal responsibility for the meaningfulness of work, choose to achieve, choose to stand by beliefs, and exemplify empowerment through actions. As the field of nursing staff development comes of age, practitioners will have the courage and the ability to exert influence and contribute to nursing care through the development of competent nurses.

Progression to Peak Performance

Expert

Characteristics
Intuitive grasp of situation—zeros in on problem/action
Achieves mastery of all aspects of situation

Activity
Provides process consultation to individual/groups
Develops systems to manage data
Develops annual plan for development of nurse managers

Intuition

Proficient

Characteristics
Sees situation as a whole process
Performance guided by subtle nuances
Produces events
Adapts plans to presence of variables

Activity
Develops competency-based orientation program
Develops hospital aide training program
Develops curricula
Develops symposium with multiple tracks

Maxims

Competent

Characteristics
Sees actions in terms of long-range plans
Analyzes "aspects" of situation and applies to a plan of action
Uses guidelines to handle variables

Activity
Develops oncology course
Develops a plan to inservice all nursing staff, re: a practice change
Develops self-directed learning program

Aspects

Novice/Advanced Beginner

Characteristics
Need for structure
Need for specific guidelines
"Aspects" to direct action

Activity
Conducts CPR training
Develops slide/tape program
Develops inservice offering
Teaches in hospital aide course

Structure

0 ·····························▶ 18 mo ····················▶ 3 yrs ····················▶ 5–7 yrs ············

Figure 1-1 *Staff development skill acquisition plan. Application of "Benner's Framework Novice-Expert" to development of the Staff Development Specialist. (Source: Mary Simpson, MSN, RN, Director of Nursing Staff Development, Ohio State University Hospital, Columbus, OH.)*

23

Leadership for the Future

The new rules in health care demand staff development specialists who can serve as leaders and transform nursing visions into reality. By paying attention to what is happening today, specialists will know what to do better tomorrow. Bennis[27] distinguishes leadership from management and makes a strong case for the need for leaders to succeed in the future global economy. This model can be applied to the leadership role requisite to success as a staff development specialist.

Leadership characteristics essential for future success include innovation, originality, developmental approach, a focus on people, and the quality of inspiring trust. Also, staff development specialists who will lead in the future will have a long-range perspective, will ask what and why, will have an eye on the horizon, will challenge the status quo, will be their own person, and will do the right things. Future staff development specialists must have a clear idea of what they want to do and the ability to communicate that vision.

Bennis also provides questions to help shape a vision. The following questions can be asked to help shape and color staff development:

- What is unique about the service?
- What values are true priorities for the next year?
- What would create a professional commitment of mind and heart for the staff development specialist over the next five years?
- What does the organization really need that the staff development department can and should provide?
- What does the staff development specialist want the organization to accomplish so that commitment, alignment, and pride is associated with the role and the organization?

Thoughtful answers to these questions will help staff development specialists provide the leadership qualities crucial to the continuing development of the health care organization and the nursing care provided within that organization.

Positioning for Success

Success in staff development is a planned activity. Strategic use of marketing research to position the department will benefit the organization and the department. Seven steps to accomplish a positive position involve:

1. Set or reset a tone of helping.
2. Hook programs and efforts to organizational priorities and imperatives.
3. Achieve and maintain management commitment and support.
4. Reach a critical mass of personnel.
5. Model professional behaviors.
6. Manage the staff development service well.
7. Proactively respond to changes with innovation.
8. Seek answers to the question posed above to create a future for staff development.

Energizing for Continued Contributions

As nurses, it is easy for staff development specialists to fall into the burnout trap. While aware of all the strategies needed to maintain personal health, it is not uncommon to find nurses failing to practice what is preached. To lead vibrant personal and professional lives, it is essential to balance work and play with a healthy lifestyle. Bortz[28] describes a self-efficacy approach in which one maintains competency, mastery, autonomy, and independence as one grows older. This advice has distinct application to the field of nursing staff development. Bortz advocates a lifestyle that includes the following rules to enjoy a long, healthy, active life:

1. Do at least thirty minutes of sustained, rhythmic, vigorous exercise four times a week.
2. Eat like a bushman, returning to fruits, whole grains, vegetables, and lean meats.
3. Get as much sleep and rest as is needed.
4. Maintain a sense of humor and deflect anger.
5. Set goals and accept challenges that force creativity and aliveness.
6. Don't depend on anyone else for personal well-being.
7. Be necessary and responsible.
8. Don't slow down, stick with the mainstream, avoid the shadows.

This prescription does not contain any information unknown to nurses. It does, however, organize a great deal of research into a way of life that will cause staff development specialists to maintain the high energy levels necessary to contribute to this important field of practice. Through many seemingly small, every day activities, the energized specialist will advance the practice of nursing.

Summary

This chapter has provided a basis for understanding the field of practice currently called nursing staff development. Historical perspectives and traditions were discussed. The present state of the art and science of nursing staff development was also examined and the evolving nature of the field was explored. Definitions of common terms, roles, and processes were inspected. A model to assist the novice staff development specialist was proposed to assist with skill acquisition in the new role. Finally, to set the tone for the continued maturation of nursing staff development, an agenda for the future was proposed and discussed in detail.

References

1. Geber, B. (1990). Industry report: Budget barely budge. *Training, 27*(10), 39–47.
2. Pfefferkorn, B. (1928). Improvement of the nurse in service: An historical review. *American Journal of Nursing, 28,* 700.

3. Tobin, H. M., Yoder-Wise, P. S., Hull, P. K. (1979). *The process of nursing staff development: Components for change* (2nd ed.). St. Louis: Mosby.
4. American Nurses' Association (1979). *Guidelines for nursing staff development.* Kansas City: Author.
5. Mallison, M. B. (1990). Swimming in overstatement. *American Journal of Nursing, 90*(8), 7.
6. Ulschak, F. L., & SnowAntle, S. M. (1990). *Consultation skills for health care professionals.* San Francisco: Jossey-Bass.
7. Sovie, M. (1983). Fostering professional nursing careers in hospitals: The role of nursing staff development (Part 2). *Nurse Educator, 8*(1), 15–18.
8. O'Connor, A. B. (1986). *Nursing staff development and continuing education.* Boston: Little, Brown.
9. Bille, D. A. (1982). *Staff development: A systems approach.* Thorofare, NJ: Slack.
10. Singleton, E. K., & Nail F. C. (1985). Defining the role of staff development in acute care hospitals. *Journal of Nursing Staff Development, 1*(1), 21–25.
11. Habel, M. (1986). A management blueprint for nursing staff development. *Journal of Nursing Staff Development, 2*(4), 134–137.
12. del Bueno, D. (1986). Nursing staff development: Critical times, critical issues. *Journal of Nursing Staff Development, 2*(3), 94–97.
13. Puetz, B. (1989). Preparing tomorrow's workers today. Editorial. *Journal of Nursing Staff Development, 5*(5), 209.
14. Naisbett, J. (1982). *Megatrends.* New York: Warner.
15. Naisbett, J., & Elkins, J. (1983). The hospital and megatrends—Part 1. *Hospital Forum, 26*(9), 9–12, 17.
16. Brunt, B. A. (1988). Continuing education and megatrends. *Journal of Nursing Staff Development, 4*(4), 174–178.
17. Naisbett, J., & Aburdene, P. (1990). *Megatrends 2000: Ten new directions for the 1990s.* New York: Morrow.
18. Ulschak, F. L., & SnowAntle, S. (1990). A glance at the future: A Delphi study of trends affecting health care education. *Journal of Healthcare Education and Training, 5*(1), 3–6.
19. Ulschak, F. L. (1988). *Creating the future of health care education.* Chicago: American Hospital Association.
20. Stream, P. A., & Herring, R. M. (1990). Characteristics of successful staff development specialists. Personal communication, August 10, 1990.
21. McLagan, P. (1989). Models for HRD practice. *Training and Development Journal, 43*(9), 49–59.
22. Gundlach, A. (1990). Change begets change: Emerging role of the human resources development practitioner. *Journal of Healthcare Education and Training, 5*(1), 7–10.
23. Dreyfus, H. L., & Dreyfus, S. E. (1986). *Mind over machine.* New York: Macmillan.
24. Benner, P. (1984). *From novice to expert: Excellence and power in clinical nursing practice.* Menlo Park, California: Addison-Wesley.
25. Simpson, Mary (1990). Development of the staff development specialist: From orientation to peak performance. Paper presented at Nursing Staff Development '90, sponsored by Medical College of Pennsylvania Nursing Continuing Education Program, Orlando, Florida, February 14, 1990.
26. Macher, K. (1988). Empowerment within the bureaucracy. *Training and Development Journal, 42*(9), 41–55.
27. Bennis, W. (1990). *Managing the dream: Leadership in the 21st century.* *Training, 27*(5), 43–48.
28. Bortz, W. (1990). *We live too short and die too long.* New York: Bantam.

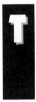

chapter **2**

Theoretical Frameworks: Describing Nursing Staff Development

Karen J. Kelly

Nursing staff development as a field of practice has progressed in the past two decades. Nurses who choose this specialty often bring to it a knowledge of theory development as it is utilized in nursing and other disciplines. When these nurses apply this knowledge to nursing staff development, new understandings of the practice emerge. This chapter is written to help the new staff development specialist understand the theoretical basis of this field. No single theory is purported to be better than any other. As this field of practice continues to evolve, new theories will be proposed. Diverse views and discussions that accompany those theories will strengthen the field of practice. New theories will likely blend concepts and constructs from a variety of sources. One model for nursing staff development is proposed to promote understanding.

Developing Theory for Staff Development

Epistemology is the study of what we know. Schultz and Meleis[1] describe nursing epistemology as the study of the origins of nursing knowledge, its structure and methods, the patterns of knowing of its members, and the criteria for validating its knowledge claims. These ideas can be applied to nursing staff development to help understand the field and to continue to cultivate the practice. Questions to guide inquiry about nursing staff development are

- What are the origins of nursing staff development knowledge?
- What is the structure of nursing staff development and what are the methods?

27

- What are the patterns of knowing used by staff development specialists?
- What criteria are or shall be used to validate this knowledge as it emerges?

To begin this inquiry, we must first recognize that there are many "ways of knowing." Chinn and Jacobs,[2] citing the work of Carper and others, described patterns of knowing that assist us in understanding how we formulate what we know about nursing. These patterns include

- **Empirics:** the traditional scientific approach where reality is viewed as an objective phenomenon that can be reduced and verified by multiple observers
- **Ethics:** what ought to be done
- **Personal knowledge:** that which concerns inner experiences and becoming a whole, aware self
- **Esthetics:** the art of nursing, that is, the comprehension of meaning in a singular, particular, subjective expression including imagined possibilities

In the late 1950s, nurses used the classic scientific approach to develop scientific theory for nursing. This approach reduced broad problems to manageable questions from which hypotheses could be formed and tested, and ultimately generate results and findings that would contribute to the search for truth about nursing. A time-honored approach, this conventional method contributed to nursing knowledge.

However, this approach did not satisfy nurses, as it was unable to capture the fullness of knowing and the knowledge that emerges from each nursing experience. The nursing experience with patients also generated knowledge about care.

Carper's work describing patterns of knowing in nursing has expanded our knowledge. The significant contribution of Benner,[3] in which the personal experiences of expert nurses were collected and analyzed to develop new knowledge about nursing, has increased our knowledge. The work of these nurse researchers and many others has left fallow ground for continued inquiry in nursing and nursing staff development. Through continued inquiry, we will gain knowledge and the ability to explain the process of nursing staff development.

Evolution of a Theory for Nursing Staff Development

What is nursing staff development? If one looks to the rich tradition of this field, to a time when it was called "inservice education," literature can be found describing its history as early as 1928.[4] Nursing staff development specialists have always been concerned with competency improvement of nurses in service, rather than nurses in pre-service education. Hence, the earlier identification of the practice as inservice education was common. As nursing continued to evolve and preparation of nurses moved to academic settings, the field of nursing staff development has evolved. No longer were faculty of hospital-based schools of nursing available to assist in the continuing development of nurses in service. Yet, nurses knew that continued learning was an integral part of their professional lives. In the late sixties, nurses were identified in organizations and given the assignment of organizing learning activities to help nurses in service maintain their competency.

Tobin, Yoder-Wise, and Hull[5] were among the first to propose an organizing framework for nursing staff development. Described as a process, their landmark book gave definition to the field of practice. Staff development was described as a process that includes both formal and informal learning activities that relate to the employee's role expectations and that takes place within or outside the profession. Tobin and others also identified three major components of staff development: orientation, inservice education, and continuing education.

Professional practice issues related to new skills, expanding responsibilities, and increasing autonomy have caused the role of staff development in organizations to change. In addition, the role of universities in the continuing education of nurses has had effect on the continuing evolution of staff development.

Others[6-8] have also described nursing staff development. These contributions have helped practitioners understand and improve their work. Knowledge of nursing staff development work is developing and new theories will emerge. These new theories will blend rich traditions and current methods into new models for nursing staff development practice. Future knowledge regarding staff development will harmonize theories from a variety of sources including those referenced above.

Theoretical concepts used in nursing staff development are drawn from a variety of disciplines. The following theories are commonly cited:

- Adult learning
- Adult education
- Change theory
- Human resource development
- Nursing
- Organization development
- Systems

Staff development specialists are challenged to build theories specific to this field of practice. Theory development may seem like a daunting task. A simplistic but helpful way to think of theory is merely as a way of viewing the world. How one views the world is influenced by many factors. Elements such as beliefs, values, culture, and experience all blend to formulate a personal view of the world. This personal view of the world can be viewed as a personal theory about how one should exist in the world.

Consider this line of thought for nursing staff development practice. What is your personal view of nursing staff development? What words would you use to begin to describe it? Think about how your background in nursing has influenced this view. Consider the effect of your upbringing, values, and cultural practices on your staff development "theory." These are the beginning questions that one asks and answers to develop a theory. The crucial factor is *thinking*. Thinking associated with ideas, concepts, and theories is central to any theory development effort. Serious analytical thinking about the continuing evolution of nursing staff development knowledge is critical to the growth of the field. Eventually, staff development theory will have to answer questions related to the evaluation and criteria used to examine the worth of any theory.

Meleis[9] describes the development of the discipline of nursing as a convolutionary process or one that is a complex, twisting, winding form or design. She cites a pattern of progress depicting nursing's accomplishments, and the inherent practice of careful critique of what has been accomplished and what is yet to be accomplished. This eloquent analysis of the discipline of nursing can be applied to nursing staff development. Consider the complex forms and structures of nursing staff development programs in health care organizations. Think about the progress made during periods of plenty and the deletion of services during economic duress. Contemplate the accomplishments and contributions of nursing staff development specialists to patient care. It becomes evident that nursing staff development is following a similar pattern of development as a discipline.

As specialists continue to attempt to develop a "world view" of their practice, the field will evolve and at times be revolutionized. Dorothy del Bueno's continuing work with competency development and evaluation made a significant contribution to the field and revolutionized it in the late seventies. Other authors have written about staff development practice in a variety of journals, from "how to" articles to comprehensive program planning and evaluation models. This is the beginning work of a discipline. Continuing work will involve research to support many of the beliefs, theoretical frameworks, systems and processes already in use.

Meleis[9] proposes a strategy for theory development in nursing that has application to staff development. This process includes stages that occur in theory development, but not necessarily in a particular order. The first stage of the process begins with the practice situation in which observations of a phenomenon occur. A phenomenon is an event, an incident, an occurrence or a curiosity—something that attracts the observer. The next stage includes beginning efforts to define, describe, or delineate the phenomenon. Within nursing staff development, a common phenomenon is the acquisition of new knowledge and skills through planned learning activities. How does this competency development phenomenon occur? How does it compare and contrast to what happens in other learning activities, such as formal academic classes. Meleis suggests that another stage is the formation of analogies and labels, which communicate the interpretation of the phenomena.

Somewhere through this theory development process, Meleis indicates, a concept emerges. Concepts are organized perceptions that have been labeled. As concept definitions emerge, propositions are advanced as tentative statements about the phenomenon under scrutiny. Explicit and implicit assumptions are analyzed throughout the process.

Key mental activities that must occur during all stages of theory development include questioning, reflecting, studying, appraising, thinking, writing, altering, and modifying. Finally, Meleis also cites intuition as one of the most significant tools for theory development. Nurses who choose to engage in theory development for staff development will find the process challenging and rewarding. The experience of nurses who specialize in nursing staff development will be the primary source of theory development for this field.

A Beginning Attempt

One definition has been proposed in an effort to describe staff development and contrast it to other programs for nurses:[10]

> A field of nursing practice that describes the organized program and process assigned the responsibility for assessing, maintaining, and developing nurses' competence, as defined by the employing agency; most often using learning activities such as orientation, inservice education, continuing education, leadership development, and skills training; and most often occurring within health care organizations and agencies.

This definition draws on traditional definitions and current experience and uses a label that has been assigned to this work for more than fifteen years. While the phenomenon of nursing staff development is not completely understood, certain concepts are emerging. For example, a standard program concept is one in which the staff development program includes such activities as orientation, the use of preceptors, the management of new graduate nurses, and new product orientation. The satisfaction of nurses and subsequent retention of staff is a concept frequently integrated into staff development programs.

Another emerging concept is the interrelated role of staff development specialists and nurse managers. The concept of linkages, that is, the importance of linking to organizational goals and priorities for program planning, is another concept that is surfacing. Finally, the concept of competency development through processes designed to assess, maintain, and develop the abilities of nurses as they practice nursing is dawning. These concepts are interwoven throughout this book and provide a wealth of information about the experience of staff development to the new specialist and program manager.

A schematic of nursing staff development which incorporates these ideas is shown in Figure 2-1. This diagram identifies the primary processes used in nursing staff development. They are defined as:

- **Assessing competence:** those processes and programs designed measure and evaluate the competence of nurses in relation to expected performance standards
- **Maintaining competence:** those processes and programs designed to conserve, preserve, support and sustain the competence of nurses in relation to organizational expectations
- **Developing competence:** those processes and programs designed to cultivate, generate, and extend the competence of nurses related to expectations and performance standards new to the individual or new to the organization

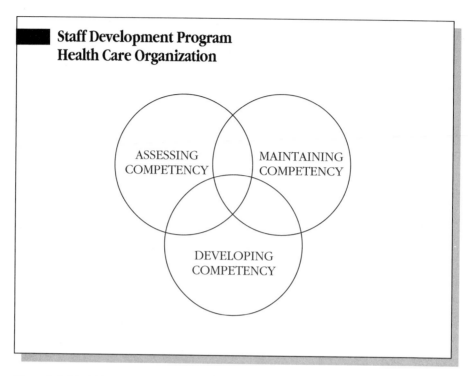

Figure 2-1 *Model for nursing staff development.*

The illustration also shows these processes and programs as interrelated. In the experience of staff development, programs may be designed to accomplish several processes. The schematic also places these processes against a program background as the nursing staff development program may include processes or assignments not clearly associated with the above three processes. Many of these unknown processes are related to an organization history and tradition. For example, does the organization place a research component within the staff development program? The organization often decides these elements. Finally, Figure 2-1 shows the staff development program within the box of a health care organization. As the definition has proposed, nursing staff development occurs within and is funded by health care organizations and agencies. This beginning work is an effort to illustrate nursing staff development as it exists in many organizations.

Staff development in health care organizations may be organized as a program or a department. Is one structure better than another? Many approaches work, some do not. But what works best? Are there certain procedures and methods that are more efficient than others? These questions and many others need to be answered through systematic research and evaluation of staff development practices.

Summary

Using methods described by Benner and others, the study of "how the best ones do it" will make a significant contribution. Future definitions will more adroitly merge concepts from adult and lifelong learning theories; human resource development theory; and the theories of change, systems, and organization development. This blending of knowledge from various sources will strengthen staff development practice and make this knowledge relevant to the complex reality of staff development within health care organizations. It will also affirm the value of the diverse background, experience, academic preparation, and beliefs of staff development specialists.

References

1. Schultz, P. R., & Meleis, A. I. (1988). Nursing epistemology: Traditions, insights, questions. *Image, 20*(4), 217–221.
2. Chinn, P. L., & Jacobs, M. K. (1987). *Theory and nursing: A systematic approach.* St. Louis: Mosby.
3. Benner, P. (1984). *Novice to expert: Excellence and power in clinical nursing practice.* Menlo Park: Addison-Wesley.
4. Pfefferkorn, B. (1928). Improvement of the nurse in service: An historical review. *American Journal of Nursing, 28*(11), 700.
5. Tobin, H., Yoder-Wise, P., & Hull. P. (1979). *The process of nursing staff development: Components for change.* St. Louis: Mosby.
6. Coye, D. (1976). *Guidelines for staff development.* Kansas City, MO: The American Nurses' Association.
7. Bille, D. A. (1982). *Nursing staff development: A systems approach.* Thorofare, NJ: Slack.
8. O'Connor, A. B. (1986). *Nursing staff development and continuing education.* Boston: Little, Brown.
9. Meleis, A. I. (1985). *Theoretical nursing: Development and progress.* Philadelphia: Lippincott.
10. Kelly, K. J. (1990, April). Reveries, renewals and reformation: Nursing staff development in the future. Paper presented at the Staff Development '90 conference sponsored by the Medical College of Pennsylvania Continuing Nursing Education, Philadelphia, PA.

Chapter 3

Staff Development in the Nursing Service Organization: Modeling for Success

Francie J. Wolgin

The staff development department or program can exist within or out-side the nursing service department. The varied structures within today's health care organizations preclude attempts to describe a typi-cal structure and relationship of nursing staff development and the nursing service organization. In some organizations, the staff develop-ment program is identified within a hospital-wide department. It may be a separate section within the hospital-wide education department with its own nurse leader, or it may be integrated within the depart-ment with all the nursing staff development specialists answering to a department head who may or may not be a nurse. In yet other organi-zations, the staff development department may be a separate, identified unit within the nursing service division that holds the same rank and status as all other units. In a third type of organization, the nursing staff development program may be managed by a nurse who heads other efforts as well, such as quality management, nursing recruitment, and infection control.

New structures are proliferative in health care organizations. Within many traditional departments, new services are requiring unique and different approaches to providing the best service efficiently. In turn, these changes have had an effect on the structure and services provided by the staff development department and its personnel. Names of departments vary and sometimes change when new services are added. Sometimes, the name of the department does not communicate the service at all. In addition, the title given to staff development special-ists ranges from coordinator to manager to instructor to educator to clinician. These titles may be understood by some individuals within some organizations. However, it is doubtful that nurses, who work in many hospitals and health care organizations, can identify the staff development specialist by a single universal title. Despite this, nursing staff development services are delivered at a highly productive rate.

Despite the variances in structure of the staff development program or department, in the titles of the personnel, or in the department's location within the health care organization, certain components are common. This chapter describes those components and provides guidelines to help the new or experienced staff development specialist consider related but separate elements of a nursing staff development program. Whether this program is delivered by an individual or a cadre of specialists depends on the resources and goals of the health care organization. The features described here are necessary for a sound and complete staff development program and can be considered by the new staff development specialist building a new program. An experienced staff development specialist can also use this chapter to appraise a program and imagine alternative ways to develop the existing program.

Getting Started

As a new staff development specialist, recall how it felt to be a new graduate nurse or an experienced nurse in a new specialty. The feelings of awe and inadequacy are common in any new role. Benner's[1] description of skill acquisition in nursing has become a classic. Using the Dreyfus[2] model, Benner uncovered knowledge embedded in practice in her study of the competency of nurses in various roles and in various specialties. She described five levels—novice, advanced beginner, competent, proficient, and expert. Using vivid exemplars to illustrate actual nursing practices, it became clear that nurses do proceed through a logical series of skill acquisition phases that change and develop with experience and knowledge.

The Dreyfus and Benner models can be used to help the novice staff development specialist understand how to proceed through a logical developmental pattern as well. Simpson[3] has modified Benner's work and applied it to nursing staff development. Discussed in Chapter 1, the suggested developmental activities will help the staff development specialist learn requisite skills in a logical way.

Many staff development specialists feel frustration when they are not consulted on changes within the organization that will have a direct or indirect effect on the nursing staff development department. For example, the staff development specialist may hear in a meeting that ten new nursing assistants (or extenders of some sort) have been hired and are scheduled to start work in two weeks. In this situation, the institution has failed to consider the resources needed to organize an orientation program, and the competency assessment process that will have to be implemented for these new nursing personnel. In another scenario, the staff development specialist hears during lunch that the nurses on the oncology unit will be giving the chemotherapy in the future. Again, no one has considered the need for nursing education related to this new competency expectation. Or if it was considered, the expectation was that the "class" can be put together in a day or two and all the nurses will attend willingly. This somewhat common occurrence can be managed by the staff development specialist who uncovers the organization's goals, priorities, and imperatives and discovers ways to link to them.

Linking to the Organization's Priorities

The successful staff development specialist will spend effort and energy finding out about the organization's goals. There is no easy recipe to organize this effort but information about organizational goals is helpful.

Organizational goals serve a variety of purposes. Goals assist in the task of carving out a specific arena of activity and in mobilizing legitimacy and support from the environment. Goals can serve as a source of identification and motivation for participation within an organization. Hodge and Anthony[4] suggest that in most medical or hospital organizations, goals emerge from a continual bargaining process among shifting coalitions of the more powerful participants. Coalitions are formed and reformed through the use of side payments—one group backing another and in return, receiving support for its demands or identified agenda. The allocation of scarce resources, in the form of money, space, or positions, becomes a determining factor in which goals can be truly implemented and accomplished.

Goals are also established in other ways including

- The use of an entrepreneurial model in which the top management or owners of the health care agency set the goals
- Consensus building of all or selected participants within the organization
- The use of patient-centered goals in which organizational efficiency, medical excellence, social purpose, and the well being of the patient define the goal setting and achievement measurement processes

In most organizations, a combination of all the above mentioned approaches is used to varying degrees. In some hospitals, individual departments are expected to identify departmental goals, which, in turn, are used to develop overall division goals and then hospital goals—a bottom-up approach. Many organizations today use a top-down approach. Due to changes in the health care economy and to reimbursement issues, many organizations must set the goals based on the most efficient projected use of increasingly limited resources. This, in turn, causes many patient-centered goals to be considered carefully against the test of financial viability. Decisions are made to limit or not to offer some health care services due to the potential lack of profitability or simply to the lack of financial resources.

Despite these limitations, organizations and departments within the health care organization generate a set of goals to be accomplished within an identified time frame. The staff development specialist should investigate who sets goals and how they are set, and determine how to influence this process. With careful questioning, listening, and networking, data useful to the development of appropriate educational programming can be uncovered.

Influencing this process usually takes the form of suggestions, advice, and counsel regarding the necessary preparation of staff with knowledge and skills to meet new competency expectations. For example, if the goal is to expand the chemotherapy services provided by nurses, it is also necessary to expand their skills and knowledge in this area through the staff development process. The staff development specialist who connects with the department head of the oncology unit and establishes a service-oriented working relationship will uncover this goal early in the planning stages. Eventually, the staff development process is considered as an integral part of any goal. Most department heads and administrators learn about the need for staff development support for goals through trial and error or through the effort of staff development specialists. Part of the role of the staff development specialist includes the responsibility to help managers and staff understand the role.

Priority Goals for Staff Development

The priority of staff development goals is influenced by the expectation of the specific institution. Frequently, goals related to quality care, nursing excellence, and staff education are delineated. Staff development specialists can readily identify those areas that educational activities will directly influence or which will support goal accomplishment for the organization or nursing division. Nursing staff development goals are usually grounded in the goals of the nursing division and are set in priority accordingly. Specific staff development objectives can be written to reflect those activities that lead to goal accomplishment. For example, a nursing division goal may read: "Resolve all deficiencies cited by JCAHO by September 30." Objectives for staff development may then be listed as

- Sponsor bimonthly annual review days to enable nursing employees to meet JCAHO requirements for safety, infection control and CPR review.
- Demonstrate changes in nursing practice or patient outcomes resulting from specific educational offerings.
- Provide quarterly reports for nursing department heads, listing employee activity in required education programs.

A second example relates to "guest relations" training. It is not uncommon for health care organizations to engage in efforts to improve the relationship among all providers and patients. This effort usually includes expectations about education and training programs to change undesirable behavior. While there is some question regarding the effectiveness of these training efforts to change behavior in this area, many hospitals have adopted guest relations improvement goals and staff development personnel should define education objectives in concert with these expectations.

The key to success in linking to the organization's goals, priorities and imperatives is to assure that the activities of the staff development program are in line with those expected and valued by the organization. The value of the staff development effort is enhanced when the quarterly or annual goal evaluation reflects specific activities resulting in or demonstrating goal accomplishment.

Organizational Imperatives and Goal Setting

The following list of activities can be used as a guide when developing staff development department goals.

1. Review existing goals for the organization, the nursing division, and the staff development program. Review related department goals such as human resource development or personnel department goals.
2. Recognize or identify how the current goals will be formulated and remember that new administration or significant change in your existing structure will influence this process.
3. Offer suggestions to key administrators regarding the goals of the organization and relate how the staff development department program can support those goals.
4. Write staff development goals using the same format as the central goals, particularly identifying staff development activities that will support identified goals. All personnel should be involved in this process for consensus building and commitment to goal accomplishment.
5. Share a final draft of the nursing staff development goals with the Vice President of Nursing and follow suggestions to modify the document if necessary.
6. Accept that changes in organizational priorities will cause some changes in the staff development goals, either additions or delays due to fiscal, personnel, or other restraints.
7. Celebrate goal accomplishments and energize for the next round of goal-setting activities.
8. Prepare to negotiate goals and challenges within a framework of a reasonable and rational workload, replacing some goals with new ones or adding goals as additional resources are made available.

Developing a Staff Development Philosophy

A philosophy is the expression of the attitudes, values, and beliefs of a group of people, a department, or an organization. The philosophy can be based on one or more theories of nursing. In many facilities, rather than embracing one particular theory, an eclectic mixture of common beliefs and values are merged to reflect the organization's philosophy.

Philosophy development is a time-consuming, yet rewarding process. The interaction among involved individuals as they thrash out the content of the document is often a greater achievement than the philosophy document itself.[5]

A philosophy serves to provide new employees, accrediting agencies, and others within the health care institution with a descriptive statement of values and beliefs. Philosophy statements should be consistent with actual practice within the setting. These statements serve as an operational belief system for the staff development specialist.

Need for Congruence

The staff development program personnel and department leader develop a staff development philosophy that is congruent with the organizational and nursing division philosophy. Building on the belief system stated in the nursing philosophy regarding the commitment to developing staff, providing education, and expanding nursing knowledge or research, the staff development specialist constructs a philosophy that guides the staff development program. Statements about learning theory and adult development are typically included. In addition, statements about nursing and staff competency are also detailed. Chart 3-1 illustrates a philosophy statement of a staff development program in a large urban university hospital.

Congruence with the Organization

A philosophy encompasses a system of beliefs under which the staff development specialist operates. The staff development department's philosophy must be consistent with the philosophy of the nursing division and the organization. It is important to recognize the constant state of flux of the health care environment. The astute staff development specialist acknowledges that philosophies are ever-evolving and change as the organization changes.

Turnover in administration or significant changes in health care delivery or reimbursement systems will cause a philosophy to be completely rewritten or at least modified to accommodate new variables. During any philosophy review or rewriting process, value statements of other organizations and divisions should be scrutinized. These philosophies may serve as a guide for the continuing development of the the staff development belief statement. Specifically, the specialist should look for statements regarding the commitment to developing staff, providing education, and expanding nursing knowledge. These areas should be incorporated into the staff development philosophy.

Congruence with Nursing Administration

If the staff development specialist is unable to find statements about the belief system for nursing staff development, it may be necessary to influence nursing administration to explore their value regarding this process. New information may be discovered with an inquiry designed to examine a

hart 3-1
Nursing Staff Development Philosophy

In accordance with the Nursing Department, the Staff Development Department believes the primary function of nursing at this hospital is to provide patient services in a manner conducive to the education of health professionals and supportive of appropriate research activities.

Staff Development accepts responsibility for providing educational programs that effectively meet the learning needs of all nursing service personnel as they relate to performance of assigned duties and increased patient care skills. In order to adequately meet the learning needs of all nursing personnel, we believe that:

• The Staff Development Department plans, implements and evaluates inservice and continuing education offerings in collaboration with nursing administration, the Continuing Education Advisory Committee and nursing service personnel for the improvement of patient care.

• Inservice and continuing education offerings also serve to update personnel on current trends in nursing practice, nursing education and the health needs of the community.

• The Staff Development Department promotes the professional development of individual nursing personnel through educational guidance, promotion of advanced professional study and by participation in educational offerings. The responsibility and obligation to seek professional advancement by participating in staff development programming and sharing knowledge and skills rests with the individual nursing employee.

• Educational offerings encourage coordination and cooperation with other hospital departments and outside related agencies and serve as a means of promoting the development of the nursing community.

Source: University of Cincinnati Hospital, Cincinnati, OH. Reproduced with permission.

group's beliefs about the role of staff development in nursing. Perhaps some administrators believe staff development is a responsibility of the nurse manager or regard the staff development process as unnecessary to goal achievement. Other managers may have expectations that require clarification. Through an inquiry of the beliefs of nurse managers, staff development may identify additional developmental needs.

Philosophy statements about the nursing care delivery system are often found in the overall nursing philosophy. These statements can help the staff development specialist begin a staff development document, particularly if a new care delivery system is in the implementation phase. Since all staff development programming must be consistent with the care delivery system, these statements can serve as an affirmation of the role of the staff development specialist in assessing and maintaining skills of staff in the identified nursing care delivery system.

Agreements may need to be negotiated and new belief systems developed that are congruent among all parties involved with the staff development process. Without this congruence, the staff development specialist will experience frustration and little cooperation with goal achievement.

Unwritten and Informal Belief Systems

In addition to beliefs at variance with the staff development process, managers may also have other values that are not formalized with a written statement. These unwritten philosophies are evident in many ways. For example, a nurse manager may espouse belief in the continuing development of staff, but subsequently decline to provide opportunities for personnel to participate in learning activities. In addition, some philosophy statements are so idealistic that the possibility of acting within the precepts of the belief system are severely limited.

Ideally, the philosophy should reflect realistic and practical values within the organization. Most philosophies do not include implementation strategies. Implementation strategies are usually found in goal and objective statements. However, while goal and objective statements should be congruent with the stated philosophy, there may be occasions in which selected goals are expected by administration. These goals may not specifically be grounded in the philosophy. For example, a philosophy document may not include a statement about the expectation that the staff development department will organize and implement all learning activities required by regulatory and accrediting bodies; yet this "unwritten belief" is held by nursing administration.

There are no right or wrong statements in a philosophy document. It is a dynamic set of statements that reflects a belief system about nursing staff development within a specific organization. The careful crafting of statements will communicate this belief system to the people affected. For example, is the development of staff an organizational, individual, or shared responsibility? If the philosophy statement indicates it is an organizational responsibility, it would follow that staff would be paid to attend educational activities and can expect to be scheduled to attend programs. If, however (and this is more often the case), the organization values professional development and considers it a shared responsibility, then attendance and schedules are usually negotiated between staff and management. In the case in which the organization considers education of staff a value but indicates it is the individual's responsibility to pursue it, the organization will likely have supporting policy statements about participation and payment.

Nurses in some organizations are covered by collective bargaining agreements, which often include a minimum number of paid educational leave hours or days for all staff as part of the contract. This is an effort to guarantee equity for all nurses.

The key to the development or revision of any philosophical statement for a service such as staff development is the orientation toward the values and beliefs of the organization as they relate to the continuing development of nursing personnel.

Service Delivery Mechanisms

The new staff development specialist will find services provided through a variety of mechanisms. These mechanisms include

- Direct provision of services
- Coordination
- Collaboration
- Consultation
- Support

The specialist may find new roles evolving as a result of other organizational expectations. However, the mechanisms defined above serve as a general framework for most staff development services. It is up to the staff development specialist to determine which service delivery mechanism is appropriate to meet a particular staff development need. These judgments are made based on the need, the target audience, and the resources available to meet the need.

Defining Target Audiences

The new staff development specialist may find the number of service clients overwhelming at first. Depending on the size and scope of the organization, the specialist may be responsible for several units, several programs, or the entire staff development service. One way to manage these customers is through a categorization process in which the service delivery mechanism is cross-indexed. Using a loose framework or roles, the specialist can arrange nurses into target audiences. For example, for certain services like orientation, the target audience is obviously new nurses and the service delivery mechanism is primarily the direct provision of services. The specialist will also find it necessary to coordinate selected portions of the orientation program, such as the presentations by other key organizational members. With experience, the staff development specialist will also find a need to collaborate with nurse managers about the orientation program as it continues to evolve.

This target audience categorization process, cross-indexed with the service delivery mechanisms, could also be applied to providing new product training. The first question to answer is, Who needs to know how to use this product? The answer to this question becomes the target audience. The next question to answer is, What is the most efficient and effective service delivery mechanism to help the target audience members use this product? The answer will cause the specialist to choose among several options from available resources. For example, the specialist may

- Directly provide the learning activity needed.
- Coordinate the activity and have the company representative provide the classes.
- Collaborate with nurse managers and plan an activity in which selected staff members are taught about the product and given a training package to teach the remainder of the staff.

A final application of this approach to organizing staff development services is the grouping of selected audiences for ongoing services. For example, nurse managers are a target group which requires leadership development services. The staff development specialist will often collaborate with nursing administration to design the program and may use any of the service delivery mechanisms to meet needs. Clinical nurses serve as another target audience requiring ongoing clinical update services. Assistive personnel such as nursing assistants, medical-surgical technicians, and specialty technicians also comprise a separate target audience. Other nursing personnel such as support or clerical staff also have ongoing staff development needs and make up distinct target audiences.

Once the target audience is identified, the staff development specialist will find it easier to organize the service delivery mechanism. On occasion, it may be determined that the entire nursing division requires a particular service, for example, a safety or infection control update. In this case, the target audience can be organized by clinical unit or by group, and the specialist will most often coordinate the provision of the learning activity with others.

Each of these options is available to the staff development specialist and may be used to assist with the organization and delivery of services to selected target audiences.

Getting and Using Resources

When the staff development specialist is getting started, it will quickly become evident that the requests for services far outweigh the resources available to provide these services. Productivity measures and formulas to determine adequate staff for services are discussed in Chapter 10 in detail, however, several suggestions are included here for the neophyte specialist.

The new staff development specialist should discover early in the experience what expectations exist regarding the provision of ongoing and upcoming programs. This information can be culled from the staff development leader and other managers expecting services. Armed with this information, the specialist should determine who the target audiences are and what service delivery mechanisms may be used to meet identified needs.

The next step is to organize a personal calendar in which planning and implementation activities are recorded. For example, if the staff development specialist will be providing a clinical update topic, the need to prepare for this presentation is evident and should be scheduled. In general, for each hour of presentation, an average of three hours of preparation time is needed to prepare a new topic. Topics familiar to the specialist or previously presented topics require less time—an hour may be adequate.

For those programs that will be coordinated by the staff development specialist, appointments, dates for sessions, announcements, and documentation of the learning activity must be scheduled in the calendar.

Time for conducting needs assessment activities (discussed in Chapter 5) must also be scheduled as well as the evaluation processes (discussed in Chapter 8). The staff development specialist will find the primary resource, time, quickly used up. However, through this scheduling process, the specialist will be able to demonstrate how time will be used and will have data needed to negotiate for additional resources. For example, if a learning deficit is identified that is considered essential to the safety of the organization, the staff development specialist may be required to meet the need in some way, despite an already full calendar.

The savvy specialist will approach nursing administration with several options to meet the need. These options should include several service delivery mechanisms. The key to success with this negotiation is the description of which other services will *not* be provided in order to replace the planned programs with the new program. The options should also include a choice to contract for additional assistance as a special project. Costs should also be projected with this option and several individuals known to be skillful in the needed area may also be identified. If this option is chosen by nursing administration, the staff development specialist will still need to oversee the project and take responsibility for the outcomes. If another option is selected, other programs may simply be delayed and rescheduled; some programs may simply be cancelled in order to meet the current priority need.

Through the development of a strong network of nurses and managers and astute observations at meetings, the staff development specialist may find out early about future needs. The ability to respond quickly and appropriately to organizational imperatives and priorities is a valued characteristic that will serve the staff development specialist well.

Health care organizations have a wealth of human resources. Most are in the health care field because of a desire to do good. This very characteristic is the asset the staff development specialist can use to expand resources. In addition, the ability to teach is a valued professional characteristic that will cause many nurses to offer help. Others may need support and coaching to overcome feelings of inadequacy in the new role of teacher.

The specialist can set up a system in which neophyte nurse teachers are helped throughout the process of preparing and presenting information. Any system that encourages continued development in this area will expand the resources of the staff development program.

Obtaining support materials and other teaching resources are discussed in Chapter 11. However, the staff development specialist who recognizes and develops the human resources available within the organization to expand the program will be making a significant contribution to the overall development of nursing and the organization.

Staffing to Provide Services

The number of staff development personnel found in health care organizations is as varied as the number of organizations. There is some support for Kelly's proposition that one staff development specialist is appropriate for

every 100 beds in an acute care setting.[6] However, organizations are still operating under a variety of models and theories for staff development services
and therefore no consistent formula for staffing has emerged as yet. In general,
the values held by nursing administration about continuing professional development and the beliefs about the role of the organization with assisting that
development will determine staffing levels for the staff development service.

Qualifications

As the field of staff development has evolved, the qualifications of individuals have changed. Fifteen to twenty years ago, it was common to find
nurses assigned to "inservice education" as a recognition of good service.
These nurses had often made a significant contribution to nursing, had years
of experience, and may have been offered the position as a less stressful role
during their final years in nursing. In some cases, managers seeking less
stressful positions gravitated to this field. Unfortunately, even though these
individuals were not the majority of staff development directors or specialists,
this image is still present in minds of many nurses.

In the publication of the American Nurses' Association (ANA) titled
Standards for Nursing Staff Development,[7] criteria are identified for both the
staff development administrator and the educational staff. These standards
were developed with input from a number of staff development educators
throughout the country and are consistent with actual practice. The following
qualifications were specified in this document for the administrator:

> The administrator of a nursing staff development provider unit has a bac-
> calaureate degree in nursing, a relevant graduate degree in nursing or a
> related field and has demonstrated clinical, managerial and educational
> knowledge and skills through progressive experience.

For the staff development specialist, the following qualifications are specified:

> The educational staff have a baccalaureate degree in nursing, with a grad-
> uate degree in nursing or a related field preferred. They have demon-
> strated clinical expertise and have shown interest and ability in providing
> education.

In actual practice, one will find that the expectations or preferences of organizations will vary, and in many cases, be more stringent. In those geographic
or metropolitan areas in which a significant pool of nurses with advanced
degrees exist, additional qualifications may be required. For example, an organization may have the following qualifications listed for the staff development
specialist position: a masters degree in nursing, with advanced preparation
related to the specialty or position requirements, and several years of teaching
experience in a staff development department or academic setting. Some facilities require two to five years of recent clinical or managerial experience, evidence of leadership capabilities, and knowledge of adult learning principles.

Many staff development specialists currently working in the field have
associate degrees or BSNs. Many of these individuals have experience and

developed expertise on the job and are functioning well in their positions. When standards are set or preferences stated, it is usually with the future or the ideal in mind. The best time to recruit a staff development specialist with the desired credentials is often when the position is vacated. Incumbents for the position can be screened for the desired qualifications.

Organizations must abide by personnel screening and hiring laws and the staff development administrator will need to follow these rules when upgrading any position. Concurrent with the upgrading should be a salary review for consistency with academic credentials and performance expectations. Often, if the decision is made to upgrade qualifications for a position, assistance is given to enable those who do not have the basic credentials to attend classes to obtain those credentials.

Few programs exist to help nurses specifically prepare for the staff development role.[8] Nurses interested in this field must often design their own programs of study to assist them in gaining knowledge needed for this field of practice. Graduate programs in nursing are becoming more sensitive to the need for flexibility in curriculum design. The coursework often required for advanced preparation in adult education or human resource development often has more relevance to skill requirements of the staff development specialist. For example, coursework for these programs often includes

- Adult learning theory
- Teaching learning strategies
- Needs assessment methods
- Program development
- Educational evaluation
- Administration of adult education programs
- Organization behavior
- Educational research

Nurses who are able to build their own program of study should include most of the coursework listed above to prepare for a staff development specialist role. Nurses already engaged in the specialist role may seek out this information through formal academic coursework, continuing education opportunities, and personal reading.

The qualifications of nurses in staff development roles in some organizations may also include a doctorate. Depending on the expectations and goals of the organization, nurses with this degree are being sought out to assist with the advancement of nursing practice models. In many large organizations, doctorally prepared nurses are responsible for the nursing research program. The research program may be located within the staff development program or department, or it may be a separate entity.

Regardless of the structure, staff development specialists should participate in research activities within the nursing field. The degree and level of participation is determined by organizational expectations and performance standards. However, as a role model for professional nurses, staff development specialists have a responsibility to demonstrate the use of nursing research in clinical practice. In addition, this responsibility extends to helping nurses learn how to use research findings to improve clinical practice.

Credentialing

Certification in nursing staff development continues to receive the interest of specialists. Certification is defined in the *Study of Credentialing in Nursing: A New Approach*[9] as "a process by which a nongovernmental agency or association certifies that an individual licensed to practice a profession has met certain predetermined standards specified by that profession for specialty practice. Its purpose is to assure various publics that an individual has mastered a body of knowledge and acquired skill in a particular specialty."

Credentialing in nursing has become commonplace. The ANA reports that more than 60,000 nurses are currently certified through the association. Certification through other specialty organizations adds significantly to the total number of certified nurses. Although credentialing denotes maintenance of minimal competence in a field of nursing specialization, the achievement of credentialing is positively viewed within nursing. Some organizations have programs (a) to help nurses prepare for certification exams, (b) to assist with the cost of the exam, and/or (c) reward certification status with bonuses and other awards.

Individuals in staff development have options for credentialing within the field. Most directors or administrators of nursing staff development programs are qualified to use the ANA certification process for Nursing Administration (CNA) or Nursing Administration, Advanced (CNAA). The placement of the staff development director position within the nursing organization will often determine if the nurse can take the CNA or CNAA exam. Qualifications to sit for the CNAA exam include line responsibility and participation in nursing practice decisions. In some cases, the staff development director may choose to take one exam rather than another.

In October, 1992 the ANA will offer the first opportunity for nurses who practice staff development and continuing education to become certified as generalists. The ANA plan also includes a certification exam for staff development specialists to be offered in 1996.

Staff development specialists often qualify for certification in a clinical specialty. Occasionally, practice requirements may be prohibitive, as many staff development positions do not afford the time required to maintain certification for the provision of direct patient care.

The issue of certification for nursing staff development specialists has been addressed.[10] Efforts to develop a mechanism to credential staff development specialists are in progress. The National Nursing Staff Development Organization (NNSDO) has organized a task force to explore the development of a credentialing process. Work is progressing and a variety of credentialing mechanisms will be available in the future for those specialists who choose to pursue it.

Needed Skills

There are a variety of skills needed to function effectively as a staff development specialist. These skills are grounded in an existing knowledge base which is consistently expected of individuals practicing within the field of staff development.[11] Skills related to the roles of nurse, educator, manager, researcher, consultant, liaison, and entrepreneur are all essential to the skillful implementation of the staff development specialist role.

The knowledge base of staff development is fundamentally found in adult learning and human resource development theories, as discussed in Chapter 2. It includes some of the following:

- Adult learning principles
- Adult development issues and principles and the nature of the adult learner
- Assessment of adult learner's needs and development of strategies to effectively meet those needs
- Methods to plan, coordinate, present, and evaluate staff development offerings
- The use of change theory to effect change within the organization
- Systems to retain and motivate nursing personnel
- Negotiation and conflict resolution strategies
- Current trends in health care, nursing, staff development, and continuing education

In addition to the development of a working knowledge of the above areas, the staff development specialist would also benefit from the development of several personal characteristics including:

- High tolerance for change and ambiguity
- Acceptance and respect for individual differences and diversity
- Personal commitment to the accomplishment of organizational goals and objectives
- Flexibility

Developing Desired Characteristics

The staff development specialist who develops the above characteristics will thrive within health care organizations. To develop these characteristics, the specialist may find the use of the following list helpful. Individual organizational expectations will determine which characteristics are most important in a given setting.

1. Recognize the Role of a Service Provider. A difficult concept for some new staff development specialists to grasp is that of the service provider functioning in a staff capacity within the organization. In this capacity, the specialist is expected to provide services without the authority to require that the requested services are consumed. It is helpful to negotiate with nurse managers about expectations about service provision and consumption early in the planning process. The need for this approach becomes more evident when the specialist must provide services that are not part of a program plan, nor are they consistent with the department's planned priorities. And yet, in the service provider role, the specialist must maintain a satisfactory relationship with the nurse manager as consumer of these services. Personal flexibility and a willingness to see and share the "big picture" are useful in these situations.

2. Ask or Determine What Is Expected and Follow Through. It is particularly important to assess and identify what is expected of the staff development specialist role within the organization. While some may respond that the specialist should know what is expected, without a clear agreement about services and programs, the specialist will be operating in a vacuum. Department leaders and nursing administration are key individuals to assist with this process of clarifying expectations. Much energy and time can be wasted working on the wrong projects or providing programs that are not supported by nurse managers.

3. *Be Open to Opportunities.* Opportunities to excel and demonstrate expertise come in many forms. They can be packaged in the form of requests to provide services to others outside your usual area. In many agencies, opportunities include being asked to administratively cover selected areas or assist with staffing on a short-term basis as a cost cutting measure. A common response to such requests is a begrudging acceptance, particularly if the alternative appears to threaten job security. In these cases, it is important to arrange for orientation if the challenge of a new opportunity is accepted. These opportunities provide the staff development specialist with a chance to observe nursing practice in a way not possible in other roles. It may also add to the credibility of the individual who is able to respond to the many and changing needs within the organization. Experiences gained within these opportunities serve as stepping stones to expanded responsibilities and access to resources to meet those responsibilities. Generally, the time to articulate these specific needs for resources in order to meet the challenge of new or different opportunities is when the agreement is made to accept the challenge. Occasionally, needs for additional time, money, or human resources may be held in abeyance until a future time when the need is more likely to be met.

4. *Avoid Isolationism.* While nurses may be unique and unusual individuals, there are other health care professionals within the organization who make valuable contributions. These individuals can be involved with the staff development programs and may provide constructive advice about how to use available systems to improve nursing care delivery. In addition, nurses can certainly participate in programs for all health care professionals. They may benefit from participation with others in programs related to such issues as guest relations, management development, and safety. Benefits may include an expanded appreciation for the common concerns and issues held by many health care colleagues. The staff development specialist may also provide these training programs for a cross section of health care professionals, again, providing an opportunity to demonstrate acquired expertise in presentation skills and adding to the credibility of the department. A significant contribution to the accomplishment of organizational goals may be realized through these activities.

5. *Avoid Counterproductive Behavior.* There is a saying, "Avoid slitting your wrist while swimming with sharks." In some cases, it may be counterproductive to the staff development department's health and longevity to expose weaknesses to others. Some members of the organization may be upset by the staff development department's perceived favorable status. They may be jealous of the department's accomplishments and productivity. In these instances, information that may be used against you should not be provided. Correct your problems and deficits quietly and involve a minimum number of people to carry out the correction plan. Always let administration know, in a proactive way, what the problem is and how the plan for correction is coming along.

6. Identify a Role Model and Support Network. Professional support comes from various sources. Peers and colleagues within and outside the organization, old friends and classmates, mentors, and preceptors. Staff development specialists should consider joining a professional organization that will meet their needs. There are several, each with its own mission and agenda, including:

- **National Nursing Staff Development Organization (NNSDO):** Convened in January, 1990, this is the largest organization dedicated specifically to nursing staff development.
- **Council on Continuing Education and Staff Development (COCE&SD):** This group is sponsored by the American Nurses Association and consists of staff development specialists and continuing education providers from a variety of settings.
- **American Society for Healthcare Education and Training (ASHET):** This association is organized under the auspices of the American Hospital Association and is composed of nurses and other health care professionals in training and education roles, including patient education. State and local chapters exist.
- **American Society for Training and Development (ASTD):** This group consists of training and development professionals across all industries, including health care. Local chapters exist and a special interest groups for health care training and development are accessible.
- **Other local groups:** In many regions, local staff development specialists meet on an ongoing basis. Some of these groups are more formal than others. Many have several decades of tradition and experience. These groups exist specifically to support and nurture the mission and goals of staff development specialists. Some are affiliated with NNSDO and some are not.

A new member of a larger department can identify an individual with a similar style and personality and ask the individual to serve as their role model, resource, and mentor. Experienced staff development administrators arrange for this relationship to begin with the orientation of the new member to the staff development department.

Attending national conferences on a regular basis is another way to meet colleagues who have similar job challenges. Through these interactions, staff development specialists will expand their knowledge base and develop an appreciation for current trends in nursing staff development. Involvement in any of the above organizations will also provide professional development opportunities for the specialist. Most associations are made up of interested volunteers and would welcome the fresh ideas and perspectives of new members.

7. Do Not Believe Education Is the Solution to Every Problem. Veteran staff development specialists are always amused by the number of health care professionals who believe education is the quick fix that will solve all problems. Armed with knowledge about change theory, conflict management, and negotiation skills, the savvy staff development specialist will help the individual (usually a new nurse manager) understand the partnership between staff development and management. Many options exist to handle the myriad problems that occur on a day to day basis. The specialist can help the manager assess the problem, and identify various solutions and implement one. Solutions may be disguised as education, but the agenda is clear. The problem is identified at the beginning of the "educational" activity and new or different performance expectations are discussed. Through a consensus building process, the staff development specialist can use a staff development intervention to assist with problem solving that is likely to yield a more committed and positive response.

In some cases, the staff development specialist must work with the nurse manager and help with role clarification. For example, a head nurse may request a telephone courtesy class for her staff. After some discussion about the observations the head nurse has made that led to the conclusion of a need for a class, the specialist may conclude that the head nurse needs help with setting performance expectations for the staff. After working with the manager on this area, the specialist may or may not conduct the class, depending on the continuing needs of the unit. Using the telephone courtesy request as a conduit, the specialist could design a program that focuses on meeting performance expectations and how each can assist the nurse manager set the desired tone on the nursing unit.

8. Develop and Use Time Management Skills. To be able to focus on the real priorities of any role, time must be available to do so. Even the best intentioned staff development specialists will find themselves "majoring in minors," that is, attending to programs or issues of minor importance to the overall program plan. Learn to identify which items can wait. At times it may be necessary to go to others for assistance with prioritizing. This approach will also give support for *not* doing some items on the "to do" list. As new priorities replace items on the list, other items will and should receive less time and attention. When too many items and programs are being juggled, most, if not all, will suffer. It has been said that to be successful, one must learn how to juggle many balls. The key to success is also to learn which balls are made of glass—and ensure that they will never be dropped.

9. Know When to Ask for Help. This characteristic is closely related to time management and priority setting. The key difference is acknowledging that real help is needed to deal effectively with a situation. Others may be able to shed new light on difficult situations and offer alternatives unknown to the specialist. Helpful others may be able to advocate for a particular solution and help the staff development specialist accomplish a goal.

10. Become Politically Astute. Understanding who the key players are in the organization is imperative. It is good practice for new specialists to cultivate the acquaintance of several individuals who have been with the organization for some time. These individuals can often shed light on selected situations and relate the history of problems and solutions attempted. This background will help the staff development specialist formulate responses that take this history into consideration. Honor those sources and return these favors when possible. Find out about particular events or community groups that the organization expects to be supported. Develop a trusted network of colleagues that stay alert to the unwritten tenets of an organization. Fostering allies and supporters is essential for success.

Develop a positive approach to problem solving and seek to resolve conflict at the level closest to the problem. Problems can often be resolved between two or three involved individuals who make agreements about solutions. It is not necessary to involve many others in most problems, though it may be necessary to inform others of solutions agreed upon by new coalitions.

Treat others with respect and dignity. Walk in others' shoes to see another perspective. While it may be tempting to go for a dramatic or heavy-handed solution to a problem or conflict, the boomerang effect is ever present in politics. Today's enemy may be needed as tomorrow's ally.

11. Develop an Interdisciplinary Philosophy. Some hospitals are developing a hospital-wide or institutional approach to staff development. When opportunities are presented, take advantage of other resources, persons, or departments. There are many services within nursing staff development that may also be appropriate for other departments. Invite them to your programs. Share materials that come through the staff development department. Work out bartering systems, where the staff development specialist teaches CPR for the physical therapy department in exchange for body mechanics classes.

12. Identify Ways to Eliminate Unnecessary Procedures and Paperwork. Staff development specialists are in the unique position to identify alternatives for common nursing practices such as documentation and selected procedures. During orientation, new employees may question why a particular procedure is done a certain way. These questions can serve to open discussions about alternative or new approaches to nursing. Some alternatives may save on costs, others may improve practice and others may not. An exploration of these questions and referral to appropriate committee chairs or individuals is worthwhile.

13. Develop Business, Financial, Marketing, and Management Skills. The health care industry has developed a more business-like approach to the delivery of services. This transition was necessary to ensure the continued ability of organizations to deliver services within an increasingly constrained economic environment. Staff development specialists are expected to provide cost effective programs and demonstrate how these programs contribute to the bottom line. To gain these skills, specialists can read the professional literature, discuss findings among colleagues, try new and innovative approaches, and test new knowledge. In addition, local universities and colleges offer courses for continuing education and academic credit related to these topics. These topics may be taken as electives in formal academic programs.

14. Demonstrate Improvements in Quality That Relate to Staff Development Efforts. The Joint Commission on Accreditation of Healthcare Organizations (JCAHO) requires evidence of patient care outcomes directly tied to educational offerings and activities. Advance planning will help identify which programs are needed as a result of quality monitoring and evaluation. These programs should be carefully followed to monitor change in practice that results from the program plan.

These guidelines will help the new staff development specialist organize a plan to achieve success within the organization. The plan may take several years to complete. All good efforts take time and the place to begin any plan is at the beginning.

Performance Standards for the Specialist

The evaluation of the staff development specialist should include standards which reflect both process and outcome. Assessment of the need, educational objectives, numbers attending, and benefits or results related to the staff development offerings are all important. However, since the staff development specialist's role is interdependent on the ability to effectively work with individuals and groups, process frequently is more important than outcome. A specialist with limited interpersonal skills will be perceived poorly by others in the organization, regardless of how thoroughly the program planning and design tasks are completed.

It is important to have a sufficient number of job performance expectations or standards to adequately reflect the scope of expected tasks, duties, and responsibilities. During the process of reviewing and revising a job description, an important question to ask is, Do the statements reflect the actual work expected and performed? If not, the position description may need a significant rewrite. When revising the staff development specialist's job description, performance standards should be incorporated. Most job descriptions begin with a brief description of the position, followed by the qualification required for the role. The scope of responsibility is described next. This statement is often followed by performance standards which can be categorized in several ways. Chart 3-2 provides an example of such categorization to organize the document:

- Staff teaching and development
- Leadership
- Interpersonal relations/communication skills
- Organization and productivity
- Professional responsibility

An alternative approach is illustrated in Chart 3-3. This method organizes performance standards into the problem solving or nursing process categories:

- Assessment of needs
- Planning, designing, and implementing programs
- Evaluating programs
- Collaboration
- Special projects and committees
- Professional development

There are various ways to organize the job description and performance questionnaire. Other options include a listing of all tasks, duties, and responsibilities which can be rated individually and supported with descriptive examples. Regardless of the format used, the most useful job descriptions are those that accurately reflect expected performance and are used to monitor and evaluate accomplishments on a regular basis.

Staff development specialists are often expected to use the performance standards to develop annual goals that guide their efficiency over a fixed time frame. These goals are useful and become an important aspect of the performance evaluation process for the specialist. Not only do these goals serve as a document of accomplishments, they often also serve as a determinant in salary increases, particularly if the organization has a merit pay component.

Staffing for the Program

A frequent question asked at gatherings of staff development specialists is, How many positions are enough to provide adequate staff development services? Of course the answer is, It depends. Organizations define and use the staff development specialist role differently. Every organization is expected by the JCAHO to have individuals responsible for staff development. How the development program is operated is completely up to the organization. Staff development departments vary in size and scope depending on the positions assigned to the department. They may or may not include

- Staff development specialists
- Patient education specialists
- Enterostomal therapists
- Intravenous therapists
- Diabetes educators
- Clinical specialists or clinicians
- Ancillary personnel educators
- Continuing education coordinators
- BLS/ACLS program coordinators
- Other specialized staff providing some educational service

The scope of service is the only method that can be used to predict the kind of staff needed for the service. Traditionally, individuals have been added to staff development services as the organization perceived a need for an individual specialized in a specialized area. Positions were created to organize services to meet the identified need (and positions were deleted as the perceived need for the services no longer existed). Often positions were assigned to staff development simply because there did not seem to be any other place.

Staff development department administrators attempting to expand services often use the experience of other local staff development departments. This experience is used to build a case for the need for specific services. It is essential that any added services be evaluated against the contribution the service will make to the overall efficiency and effectiveness of the organization.

Clinical Specialists and Staff Development

Confusion exists about the complementary role of the clinical specialist and the staff development specialist. The clinical specialist is specifically prepared through an academic program to manage difficult patient and nursing care problems in an identified specialty. By contrast, the staff development specialist is prepared by academic preparation and experience to help nurs-

Chart 3-2
Performance Standards for Nursing Staff Development: General Categories

Name _____

Rating Scale

1–Inadequate
2–Needs
   Improvement
3–Satisfactory
4–Superior

I: Staff Teaching and Development

1. Understands principles of adult learning and incorporates them into formal and informal teaching activities.   1 2 3 4

2. Actively contributes to the development of unit educational programs by developing or participating in: 1 2 3 4
   a. preceptorship
   b. inservice
   c. courses
   d. learning aids
   e. patient teaching programs
   f. patient care guidelines

3. Recognizes and utilizes opportunities for incidental teaching with staff members (during rounds at the bed side during discussions).   1 2 3 4

4. Initiates and develops continuing education program based on assessment of unit and Nursing Department needs.   1 2 3 4

5. Projects a positive classroom learning environment that motivates creative thinking and learning.   1 2 3 4

II: Leadership

1. Accepts responsibility for being a resource person for designated clinical expertise to the Department of Nursing through: 1 2 3 4
   a. consultation
   b. committee participation
   c. requested personnel counseling

2. Supports and helps interpret Nursing Department and unit goals and changes to personnel.   1 2 3 4

III: Interpersonal Relations/Communication

1. Understands the principles and steps of problem solving and acts as a resource to others in problem identification and resolution.   1 2 3 4

2. Demonstrates respect for the ideas, opinions, and feelings of others.   1 2 3 4
3. Fosters open communication through personal example.   1 2 3 4
4. Gives and accepts appropriate constructive criticism.   1 2 3 4
5. Understands and assumes responsibility for own effect on others.
6. Handles sensitive/confidential information appropriately.   1 2 3 4
7. Utilizes appropriate delegation.   1 2 3 4

IV: Organization and Productivity

1. Sets realistic measurable short- and long-term goals for self-improvement.   1 2 3 4
2. Assumes responsibility for acquiring knowledge or experience to meet goals.   1 2 3 4
3. Seeks feedback on performance from peers and Nursing Unit personnel.   1 2 3 4
4. Uses work time productively; able to prioritize and accomplish tasks on time.   1 2 3 4
5. Products are thorough, accurate, and well-designed.   1 2 3 4

V: Professional Responsibilities

1. Participates and encourages participation of personnel in hospital and community health related activities.   1 2 3 4
2. Promotes optimum public relations for nursing.   1 2 3 4
3. Evidence of continuing nursing professional growth or involvement.   1 2 3 4

Personal Goals:

Goals for designated area/units or department:

Employee Signature	Rater	Title

Chart 3-3
Performance Standards Education Specialist

Major Function I: Assessment of Needs

Collaborates with nursing managers and staff to assess learning needs.
Performance is satisfactory when the education specialist:

1. Develops and utilizes a mechanism for ongoing needs assessment for designated areas.
2. Participates in department-wide needs assessment.
3. Meets with staff and management as necessary to validate needs and assessment of future needs.
4. Responds appropriately to perceived needs with learning activities or other recommendations to assist change.
5. Collaborates with Associate Director, Nursing Education, and Research to prioritize needs based on organizational and departmental goals.

Major Function II: Planning, Designing, and Implementation

Plans and implements educational activities to meet identified learning
needs, utilizing adult education principles.
Performance is satisfactory when the education specialist:

1. Plans learning activities based on needs assessment.
2. Collaborates with selected members of target audience in planning program content.
3. Conducts program planning within appropriate time frame.
4. Functions within the guidelines of Center for Nursing Education Practice Manual.
5. Utilizes adult education principles in conducting programming.

Major Function III: Evaluation

Develops and utilizes appropriate evaluative systems to determine
effectiveness of educational activities.
Performance is satisfactory when the education specialist:

1. Develops and utilizes an appropriate evaluative tool for each educational activity.
2. Provides feedback regarding program evaluation to the learner and other appropriate individuals.
3. Provides feedback regarding participant performance to the participant and immediate supervisor, when appropriate.
4. Revises educational programming based on compiled evaluative data.

Major Function IV: Collaboration

Promotes collaborative relationships among health care professionals. Performance is satisfactory when the education specialist:

1. Assists in the identification of appropriate resource people to promote collaboration.
2. Promotes collaboration among nursing professionals and with other health care disciplines.
3. Works in conjunction with clinical specialists in assessing and meeting the needs of staff.
4. Works in conjunction with other education specialists to establish and maintain standards of educational programming throughout the hospital.

Major Function V: Special Projects and Committees

Participates in committees, task forces, meetings, and activities to assist in the development of staff, ultimately resulting in improved care. Performance is satisfactory when the education specialist:

1. Participates in the development and attainment of goals and objectives for Patient Care Services.
2. Participates as an active member in at least one Patient Care Services/hospital committee.
3. Participates, as an active member, in the Nursing Education and Research Committee.
4. Participates in additional meeting and task force activities as appropriate.

Major Function VI: Professional Development

Participates in activities that promote professional development through education and other activities that enhance the practice of nursing and education. Performance is satisfactory when the education specialist:

1. Attends continuing education offerings and other activities to meet identified learning needs.
2. Collaborates with other education specialists for purposes of seeking validation of professional effectiveness.
3. Develops annual goals and objectives to guide professional performance.
4. Serves as a consultant to health care providers in regard to health care issues.
5. Actively participates in the research program of Patient Care Services Department.

Source: University of Cincinnati Hospital, Cincinnati, OH. Reproduced with permission.

ing personnel assess, maintain, and develop competencies through refined educational program planning and design skills. These roles are complementary. One or both may be found in many organizations. If only one of the roles is identified in a given organization, without the benefit of the complementary role, it is common to find the individual in the role performing the tasks of both. This is unfortunate, as it leads to role confusion for the specialist and the consumers of the specialist's services.

Staff Development Structures

Staff development departments can be organized in different ways and function quite effectively. The primary objective of any organizing structure is effectiveness. Does it work for the organization. The secondary objective is communication. To use any service, clients must understand how to access and use services efficiently. Staff development structure will generally depend on two items, (a) the preference of the organization's leadership, and (b) the ability of staff development leadership to convey an efficient structure to provide needed services.

In some organizations, structure is based on tradition. In others, new structures are created to resolve identified problems related to efficiency and effectiveness. More success will be realized by the staff development specialists who assess the quality of services and communicate a plan to improve services through a different structure. These plans must be marketed carefully to key individuals and explained judiciously to all parties affected by any change in structure. Strategic planning for improved structure may indicate that several small steps toward an overall change may be more readily accepted than a major overhaul of structure and services. Any requests for additional staff to provide services within new structures must be carefully linked to organizational imperatives. It may be more efficient to reassign and realign roles within the department to meet staff development requirements for new services.

Models commonly used to communicate staff development structures are usually described as centralized, decentralized and centralized-decentralized.[12] Though each organization may develop a hybrid of any of these models, effective structures clearly communicate how consumers can access services quickly and efficiently.

Centralized Structures

A centralized department is organized to provide a range of defined services to staff. Staff development specialists report to a director who assigns all programs and tasks. Communication generally flows through the nursing administrator to the director to the specialist. Requests for services follow an established communication pattern. The staff development department is held responsible and accountable for assessing needs, implementing, and evaluating programs. This approach is considered by many nurse leaders to be the most economical and effective for meeting quotas and standards.

Decentralized Structures

A recent trend in health care is to decentralize or flatten the organizational hierarchy. The net effect is designed to eliminate one or more layers of management and encourage decision-making at lower levels. When this need is combined with the need to reduce nursing administration overhead (where many staff development payrolls are located), the decision to decentralize may be in everyone's best interest.

In practice, each clinical nursing area becomes responsible for its own staff development program. Usually, a staff member is designated as the unit educator or preceptor. In many cases, if a centralized staff development department existed before the decentralization decision, the specialists from the centralized department are placed in staff positions responsible to the head nurse or department head. Haggard[13] describes the role of the unit-based resource person as one responsible to provide "follow-up for orientees, inservice new equipment and forms on the unit, update staff on new developments in their area of practice and conduct patient conferences and unit classes." The success or failure of decentralization depends on the ability of the designated individual. If the resource nurse is allowed to function within their assigned capacity and this capacity is communicated and accepted by the staff, the role will work.

In organization where decentralization has not worked, a primary reason is the failure to remove the resource person from the staffing pattern for direct care at established intervals to allow the individual to perform the resource nurse role.

McElroy[14] describes a decentralized model which is incorporated into a professional practice model. The decentralized unit orientation follows a two week central orientation. A staff development coordinator and assistant head nurses worked together to identify a conceptual framework, select topics, develop behavioral objectives, content outlines and a teaching plan. This approach was evaluated after implementation and deemed successful.

Centralized-Decentralized Structures

Modified decentralized departments are those which have the core staff development responsibilities centralized. The remaining staff development specialist positions are linked in a liaison fashion to assigned groups of head nurses and department heads. In this arrangement, specialists continue to report to the staff development leader but also attend unit meetings in the assigned areas. These specialists are expected to establish solid working relationships with their head nurses and staff and assist them with staff development programs. Figure 3-1 illustrates an organizational chart using this approach.

Working Models

Staff development departments are structured in ways that are rational for a particular situation and organization. The modification of any structure is possible. There is no pure form that is more likely to enhance the effectiveness of the staff development program. Rather, the commitment of nursing and staff development administrators toward creating a functional, efficient

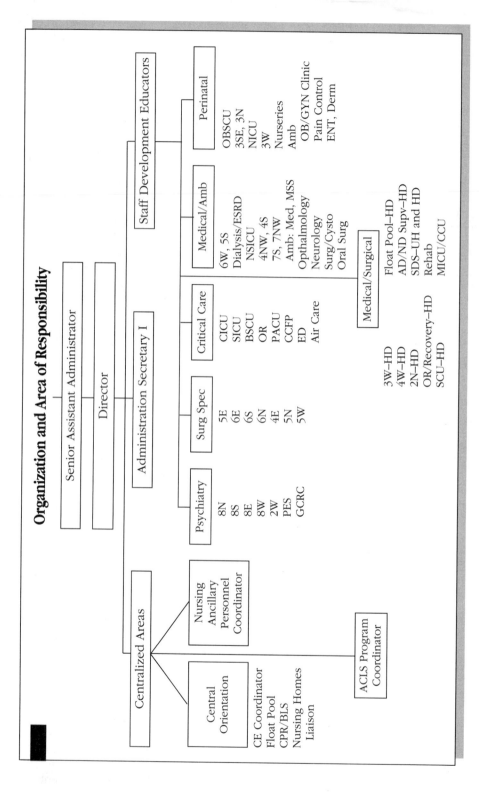

Figure 3-1 *Staff development organizational chart without responsibility for direct clinical services. (Source: University of Cincinnati Hospital, Cincinnati, OH.)*

and effective structure will contribute more to the success of the staff development program than any single structure. Table 3-1 compares and contrasts the most common structural models for nursing staff development.

Position Titles

As previously discussed, the titles of individuals assigned to staff development role are varied and multitudinous. Most of the guidelines in this text are directed toward the individual in a role that is primarily dedicated to providing staff development services. For clarity, the title of staff development specialist was selected and used throughout. It is recognized that the role may be titled in a variety of ways, depending on the size and tradition of a given organization. In addition, the role may include administrative responsibility, particularly in health care organization with less than 100 beds. A list of common assignments to the staff development specialist role are listed and described below. These roles may be combined and executed by one individual or each may be implemented by a single individual.

Director of Nursing Staff Development. This individual provides leadership and direction for the operation of the staff development program; works cooperatively and collaboratively with management; sets and implements departmental policy; assesses and develops nursing competencies related to clinical practice and nursing management; provides leadership for the continuing development of the staff development program; may coordinate research activities; provides consultation; operates school of nursing student placements; may administer clinical ladder/career development programs; maintains membership in nursing executive group that makes decisions related to clinical practice and nursing care delivery systems. Other common titles include Associate Director of Nursing for Staff Development, Assistant Vice-President for Nursing Staff Development, Assistant Administrator for Nursing Education.

Staff Development Specialist. This nurse is responsible for providing all staff development services related to assessing, maintaining, and developing competencies related to performance standards and expectations; uses refined needs assessment strategies, program planning, and design methods and evaluation systems; serves on committees, may provide leadership for selected projects; models professional nursing behaviors. Other titles include staff development educator, coordinator, education specialist, instructor, and clinician.

BLS/ACLS Coordinator. This individual is assigned the responsibility for planning, implementing, and evaluating the courses necessary to help maintain certification or competence with resuscitation techniques; usually uses courses structured by the American Heart Association or the American Red Cross; maintains records to demonstrate competency status of nursing and other personnel for regulatory bodies; maintains all CPR training equipment; reviews actual resuscitations for trends and training needs.

Centralized Orientation Coordinator. This nurse is responsible for coordinating and/or providing core orientation topics for all new nursing employees; plans, teaches, and evaluates the orientation program; may pro-

Table 3-1
Comparison of Common Structural Models for Nursing Staff Development Departments

	Centralized	Decentralized	Modified Decentralized
Accountability	Director and educators report directly to AVP/Admin for Nursing	There may be one or more individuals responsible for CE Coordination and/or hospital orientation; HN/Dept Head may be designated as responsible for education	Director is reporting to Administrator or Asst Admin; Staff Development Educators report and are responsible to Staff Development Director; specific liaison relationships are established with other Asst Administrators
Orientation	Classes and program are held in a central location for all new personnel	Orientation of new personnel becomes HN/Dept Head responsibility; usually delegated to AHN/nurse clinician/unit educator	Core orientation classes are taught in a centralized monthly or bimonthly format; preceptors are used for unit orientation
Inservices	All inservices are coordinated, planned, taught, and evaluated centrally	Units responsible for own inservices	Inservices affecting entire facilities are offered centrally; unit-specific inservices are arranged by designated educator from SD

Continuing Education	CE Coordinator is part of the central SD or Human Resources Dept.	CE Coordinator single position or small dept within nursing or hospital-wide in Human Resources; no direct unit relationship; not available in some organizations	Continuing Education is a part of the centralized services of the SD Dept
Committees	SD members participate on key hospital and nursing committees	Individual clinicians may be requested to serve on committees; excluded from most	Committee participation shared among dept. members; active involvement in all key committees
Resource Consultation	SD Dept contacted and used extensively by a variety of nursing and hospital staff	Known individuals may be highly used by staff in their speciality area; less effectively used by others outside their area	Individual educators are contacted for their area of expertise; centralized members field and refer specific requests to speciality persons within SD or Consultation Dept
Required Specialty Courses: CPR, ACLS, IV Certification, etc.	All are offered within the department; follow-up done or provided as needed	Unit educator may do CPR review for staff or arrange for outside provider to do individual staff	All speciality courses are offered as part of the centralized function of SD; open to all staff needing specific training or certification; managers schedule staff to attend or individuals self-select to come

vide other staff development services; may provide preceptor and new graduate training programs.

Ancillary Personnel Trainer. This person is responsible for coordinating or providing orientation and ongoing staff development services for assistive personnel in nursing, such as nursing assistants, medical-surgical technicians, specialty technicians, unit secretaries, unit managers, escorts, and other assistive personnel.

Secretary/Administrative Assistant. This individual is responsible for managing the support services needed to operate the staff development program; processes paperwork, keeps records, maintains registration lists, maintains the program record keeping system; may develop and maintain automated systems used to support the staff development program such as transcripts, productivity reports, and data bases.

Developing Effective Relationships

The essence of effectiveness for the staff development specialist is the ability to form working and collaborative relationships with many resources. These relationships will contribute to the expansion of services. Several specific resources are listed below. These represent assets of particular value to the specialist.

Instructors in Other Departments. There are frequently instructors employed by the organization and located in other departments. It is useful to get to know these individuals and find ways to collaborate with them. Explore ways that resources may be shared. Barter and swap services to enhance each other. Collaborate about training equipment purchases and use.

Clinical Specialists. These highly qualified nurses may be located in many services, depending on the scope and size of the total organization. These individuals should be sought out to serve as consultants and faculty in their areas of expertise. Many can be counted on to provide regular segments of a selected course, such as a critical care course.

Other Education Departments. Other hospitals, health departments, long-term care facilities, universities, and local organizations are often willing to explore the possibility of co-sponsorship for selected topics. For example, the state health department may be willing to assist with and co-sponsor a seminar about AIDS. A local group of nurse attorneys may be willing to discuss the possibility of organizing a seminar with the organization that will also benefit their local group. Other hospitals or similar organizations may be willing to form coalitions in which a standard course, dysrhythmia interpretation, for example, is offered at various hospitals or a neutral site. Each organization contributes certain resources in exchange for a number of slots.

Experts. It is common for the staff development specialist to seek an expert to present a topic for the staff. These experts may or may not exist within the facility. Before contacting experts, several decisions must be made. For example, what is the expert expected to present and how much can the organization afford to spend on the expenses of this expert. Clear objectives must be shared with the expert. Expectations of all parties should be clarified. Additional information about contracting with experts may be found in Chapter 5. Experts are often identified through word of mouth. The staff development specialist can cultivate a network of experts by staying alert to comments of staff after attendance at outside programs and encouraging them to bring back names of expert speakers. In addition, the specialist can contact other staff development specialists to find out about experts that may be available in other organizations. Universities and proprietary groups also may be sources of expertise. These sources usually have very specific contracts and should be contacted directly about providing experts and programs within the organization.

Summary

This chapter has presented various topics and strategies to help the new staff development specialist get started in this field. Areas discussed include the importance of linking early to the organization's goals, priorities and imperatives, how to develop and refine a philosophy about nursing staff development, service delivery mechanisms, staffing patterns for the service including qualifications, skills, and desired characteristics. Several staff development department structures and roles are also explored. The remaining chapters discuss in detail each of the steps essential to refinement of a sound staff development program.

References

1. Benner, P. (1984). *From novice to expert: Excellence and power in clinical nursing practice*. Menlo Park, California: Addison-Wesley.
2. Dreyfus, S., & Dreyfus, H. (1985). *Mind over machine. The power of intuition in the age of the computer*. New York: Free Press.
3. Simpson, M. (1990). Development of the staff development specialist: Presented at the Medical College of Pennsylvania Staff Development '90 Conference, February 14, 1990, Orlando, FL.
4. Hodge, B., & Anthony, W. (1982). Organizational theory: An environmental approach. In: Magula, M. *Understanding organizations*. Rockville, MD: Aspen.
5. Stevens, B. (1980). *The nurse as executive*. Wakefield, MA: Nursing Resources.
6. Kelly K. J. (1990). Nursing staff development administration: Evolution of the field. Presented at Staff Development '90, Medical College of Pennsylvania, Philadelphia, PA, April 17, 1990.
7. American Nurses' Association (1990). *Standards for Nursing Staff Development*. Kansas City, MO: The Association.
8. Kelly, K. J., Carty, R. M., & Haskell, C. A. (1988). Preparing nurses for staff development practice: An educational opportunity. *Journal of Nursing Staff Development*, 4(2), 50– 53.
9. American Nurses' Association (1979). *Study of credentialing in nursing: A new approach*. Kansas City, MO: Author.

10. Piemonte, R. V. (1986). Certification of nursing staff development educators. *Journal of Nursing Staff Development, 2*(1), 2–4.
11. O'Connor, A. B. (1986). *Nursing staff development and continuing education.* Boston: Little, Brown.
12. Tobin, H. M., Yoder-Wise, P. S., & Hull, P. K. (1979). *The process of staff development: Components for change.* St. Louis: Mosby.
13. Haggard, A. (1984). Coping: Decentralized staff development. *Journal of Continuing Education in Nursing, 15*(3), 90–92.
14. McElroy, M. J. (1989). Decentralized unit orientation. *Journal of Nursing Staff Development, 5*(2), 84–90.

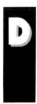

Chapter 4

Designing the Staff Development Program

Susan E. Costello

The primary goal of any staff development program is to assess, main-
tain, and develop the employee's competence to meet the expectations,
standards, and mission of the organization. The institutional focus of
the program is a critical concept to the design of a staff development
program. It is the institution which establishes the goals for the staff
development program. This is facilitated by the program administrator
through assessment activities discussed in Chapter 6.

Some of the expectations or standards established are internal,
that is, they are set by the organization. Job performance standards are
a good example of internally set expectations. Other expectations are
external, that is, set by licensing or accrediting agencies. The manda-
tory use of Universal Precautions illustrates an externally set expecta-
tion. The staff development program must be designed to assist employ-
ees in meeting both types of expectations. Additionally, the program
should assist the employee in developing the professional knowledge
and skill needed to advance within the organization.

Core Curriculum

At its most fundamental level the core curriculum, or basic course
offerings of a staff development program, includes components which will
insure that employees have had the opportunity to gain the knowledge and
skill necessary to perform their jobs. In order to meet this fundamental
requirement, the staff development specialist identifies the basic or minimal

competencies needed by the target populations. Note the use of the term minimal. This is an important concept when designing a core curriculum. It is essential to differentiate the "must know" from the "nice to know." In an ideal world, a core curriculum might include both the must and the nice to know. However, the purpose of the core is to ensure that employees have been provided with the opportunity to learn the "must know" information.

What is the range of knowledge and skills that need to be addressed by the program? Who are the learners? Are they RNs only, RNs and LPNs, all patient care service providers, or are other members of the organization also included? The answers to these vital questions form the foundation of the staff development program curriculum. The content of the core curriculum will be determined by the degree to which the knowledge and skills to be taught vary. For example, the knowledge and skills required in an acute care hospital are significantly more diverse than those required in a long-term care facility.

The degree of specialization within an organization will also affect the range of requisite knowledge and skills. For example, mixed medical-surgical units require a broader range of knowledge and skills than do highly specialized units. The degree of compartmentalization of functions within the organization will also affect the range of knowledge and skills required. If there are many narrowly framed jobs, the requirements will be different than if there are fewer broadly framed jobs.

Basically, defining the population means identifying who the learners will be, the knowledge and skills they bring to the job, and the scope of their jobs. The best sources of this information are the learners themselves and their managers. The primary staff development program consumer is often the nurse manager who is responsible and accountable for the competence of the personnel delivering care to patients. Strong collaborative relationships with nurse managers are crucial to the development of a sound curriculum.

Defining Target Populations

The first step in designing the core curriculum is to define the target populations that the program will serve. In most departments of nursing, the target populations for the staff development program can be divided into three broad categories:

- Direct patient care providers (staff nurses, LPNs, nursing assistants, technicians, etc.)
- Nurses in management and leadership positions (nursing head nurse and clinical coordinators and their assistants)
- Clerical (unit secretaries, patient escorts)

While these three categories are not all inclusive, they do encompass the vast majority of job classifications within a department of nursing. Most job classifications not included within these categories are solo positions (i.e., Quality Assurance Coordinator, Infection Control Practitioner). The knowledge and skill requirements of these specific job classifications are usually not included within the scope of the core staff development program.

Once the target populations have been identified, the next step in designing the core curriculum is to examine the job descriptions of these employees. Each job description will include the major responsibilities of the job, as well as identify the basic education, licensure and/or certification, experience, and special knowledge and skills an applicant needs to possess in order to be considered for the position. For example, the job description of a staff nurse is likely to include statements regarding the use of the nursing process in providing nursing care, the administration of medications, the transcription of orders, the participation in quality assurance activities, the written and verbal communication of information related to patient care, the maintenance of a safe environment, the participation in continuing education, and the assumption of other duties as assigned. The job descriptions of the other direct patient care providers will generally consist of modifications of the responsibilities included in the clinical nurse job descriptions.

In addition to the job descriptions, there are performance standards for each position. Performance standards are more detailed than the job descriptions, and address the ways in which the incumbent will actualize each of the major responsibilities identified in the job description. The performance standards serve as the criteria by which the incumbents' performance is evaluated. These may also be considered the basic competencies of all incumbents within the job classification. Taken together, the job descriptions and the performance standards provide the staff development program specialist with the basic information needed to construct the core curriculum.

Assessing Competencies

The evaluation of competence, or the validation that an employee has sufficient knowledge and skill to carry out the assigned responsibilities, has received a great deal of attention in recent years. The 1991 Joint Commission on Accreditation of Healthcare Organizations (JCAHO)[1] Nursing Care Standards speak directly to the evaluation of competence in Standard 2. This standard states, "All members of the nursing staff are competent to fulfill their assigned responsibilities." Each organization must determine the degree to which they need to validate the competence of their employees. By establishing minimum qualifications for a position, such as licensure or certification, the institution has in fact validated the presence of the competency required for entry into the position. By establishing performance standards that are specific to the area of clinical practice, the institution has defined the competencies required to succeed in the position. The performance standards for a nurse working on a general medical or surgical unit are different from those of a nurse working in an ICU. Figure 4-1 illustrates a portion of a typical job description and associated performance standards. These performance standards form the basis for determining which competencies should be assessed.

There are several approaches to assessing competencies. The first and most commonly used is a written test which determines whether the

Georgetown University Hospital
Performance Evaluation Addendum
Knowledge and Skills

Performance Standards

Department of Nursing Staff
Staff Nurse–ICU
(N4410GI.S64) (page 1 of 4)

Name: _____

	PS	Outstanding	More than Satisfactory	Satisfactory	Less than Satisfactory	Unacceptable	Total Points
A. Assessment and Evaluation							
1. Nursing assessments are initiated and completed on each patient according to ICU and/or Step-Down guidelines.		40	36	32	22	0	
2. Data collection includes pertinent patient information regarding the health state/self-care activities.		30	27	24	17	0	
3. Alterations in the health state and self-care deficits are identified.		30	27	24	17	0	
4. Learning needs are identified, teaching goals established and where appropriate, return demonstration of new learning is evaluated.		30	27	24	17	0	
5. Status of self-care concerns/desired outcomes is noted.		30	27	24	17	0	
6. Nursing care is evaluated and revised.		65	58	48	33	0	
Subtotal		(225)	(202)	(176)	(123)	(0)	

Figure 4-1 *Qualifications, responsibilities, and performance standards for clinical nurses used to develop core curriculum. (Source: Georgetown University Hospital, Washington, DC. Reproduced with permission.)*

Georgetown University Hospital
Performance Evaluation Addendum
Knowledge and Skills

Performance Standards

Department of Nursing Staff
Staff Nurse–ICU
(N4410GI.S64) (page 2 of 4)

B. Planning Care

	PS	Outstanding	More than Satisfactory	Satisfactory	Less than Satisfactory	Unacceptable	Total Points
1. Initial/on-going nursing assessment, medical plan of care, and patient/significant other goals are in the nursing care plan.		40	36	32	22	0	
2. Input from other units/ disciplines is incorporated into the planning of nursing care (i.e., Transferring Unit, Social Services)		35	32	28	19	0	
3. Patients' care plans are written according to Department guidelines.		35	32	28	19	0	
4. Clinical assessment and knowledge of the physiological and psychological occurrences in the unstable and/or unpredictable patient with complex clinical problems is in the care plan.		55	49	44	30	0	
5. Transfer information is appropriate.		20	18	15	11	0	
Subtotal		**(185)**	**(167)**	**(147)**	**(101)**	**(0)**	

(continued)

Georgetown University Hospital
Performance Evaluation Addendum
Knowledge and Skills

Performance Standards

Department of Nursing Staff
Staff Nurse–ICU
(N4410GI.S64) (page 3 of 4)

C. Implementation of Care

PS	Outstanding	More than Satisfactory	Satisfactory	Less than Satisfactory	Unacceptable	Total Points
1. Nursing actions are appropriate, based on scientific knowledge, initiated and performed according to the patient's self-care requirements.	100	90	79	55	0	
2. Medications are administered correctly and safely and knowledge of the therapeutic and/or nontherapeutic effects is known.	80	72	63	44	0	
3. All treatments and patient related activities are performed accurately and knowledge of the therapeutic and/or nontherapeutic effects is known.	80	72	63	44	0	
4. Changes in the patient's condition are noted and appropriate action is initiated.	40	36	32	22	0	
5. Patient report reflects the status and the plan of nursing care and is given succinctly.	40	36	32	22	0	
Subtotal	(340)	(306)	(269)	(187)	(0)	

Figure 4-1 *(continued)*

Georgetown University Hospital
Performance Evaluation Addendum
Knowledge and Skills

Performance Standards

Department of Nursing Staff
Staff Nurse–ICU
(N4410GI.S64) (page 4 of 4)

	PS	Outstanding	More than Satisfactory	Satisfactory	Less than Satisfactory	Unacceptable	Total Points
D. Documentation							
1. Documentation/report reflects the patient's status, the plan of nursing care and follows unit/department procedures/guidelines.		40	36	32	22	0	
2. Physician's orders are transcribed correctly.		40	36	32	22	0	
3. Delegated activities in the Quality Assurance Program (e.g., audits) are completed and documented.		30	27	24	17	0	
4. Attention is given to detail and accuracy when utilizing computer systems.		30	27	24	17	0	
5. The narcotic system is utilized correctly.		30	27	24	17	0	
6. The patient classification system is accurately utilized.		20	18	15	11	0	
Subtotal		**(190)**	**(171)**	**(151)**	**(106)**	**(0)**	
E. Orientation of new personnel is provided as assigned		40	36	32	22	0	
Subtotal		**(1000)**	**(900)**	**(790)**	**(550)**	**(0)**	

Place the total in the boxes for knowledge and skills on pages 1 and 4

Grand Total _____
Divide by 10 _____
Total _____

employee has the *cognitive knowledge* required to meet the competency. If, for example, one of the expectations is that the employee in an oncology area demonstrates knowledge of the therapeutic and the nontherapeutic effects of chemotherapy, then one may use a written test to evaluate the employees basic knowledge of commonly administered chemotherapeutic agents. Failure to achieve a passing score on such a test may be used as the criteria for entry into a remedial course. Alternatively, successful completion of the chemotherapy test may also be a criteria for completion of probation. In a diabetic treatment unit one might have similar requirements regarding the use of insulin or therapeutic diets.

If, as in the above examples, the knowledge required to care for patients is specialized then the use of written testing to assess competencies may have limited application at the departmental level. Unit or clinical area specific testing is often more appropriate. If patient populations are mixed, then departmental or generic testing may be useful.

In addition to assessing the *cognitive* competencies, strategies have been developed to evaluate *psychomotor* or skill-based competencies. The two most commonly used strategies are simulation exercises and observation of direct patient care. The most common example of a simulation exercise is the mock-code. During a mock-code the participants' actions are observed and evaluated by an instructor, and feedback about their performance is provided at the end of the simulated code. Other examples of simulation exercises include

- Lifelike anatomical models for teaching the initiation of peripheral IV lines
- Computer simulations of dysrhythmias to teach ECG interpretation
- Capillary blood glucose monitoring instruction using both test solutions and peer testing

Simulation exercises, although a very effective teaching strategy, are both resource and labor intensive and are therefore an expensive assessment approach. The use of simulation exercises should, in most cases, be reserved for skills which, if performed incorrectly, place the patient at high risk of injury or unnecessary discomfort. Infrequent performance of a complex skill is an additional reason for using simulation exercises to assess competency.

Observation of actual performance is the most commonly used approach for assessing competencies. These observations may be performed by a variety of people: a preceptor, supervisor or head nurse, staff development specialist or clinical specialist. More important than who performs the assessment is that the characteristics of "competent performance" be defined, so that both the performer and observer are aware of the critical elements.

The competency assessment approach selected will depend on the type of knowledge (cognitive or psychomotor), the potential risks involved, and the resources available. Baseline competency assessment can be an invaluable tool in planning the learning opportunities for an employee. However, depending upon the approach selected it can be very resource intensive.

Standard Programming

The staff development program consists of programs that are commonly expected or standard to most organizations. These standard programs are designed and implemented in a variety of ways. Program objectives developed for each activity specify the anticipated outcomes. These may differ from one organization to another. More common is the similarity of these programs across organizations. Articles in the *Journal of Nursing Staff Development* frequently report innovative and ingenious approaches to these standard programs. Evaluations of these common programs occasionally yield data that indicate a change is needed. Consulting the literature and talking to colleagues is a good way to find out how other organizations manage problems commonly associated with standard programs.

Orientation

The orientation of new employees is a major focus of the staff development program. Orientation can be regarded as having three levels:

- Hospital
- Department
- Unit or clinical area

Within each of these levels the new employee needs to be made aware of the institution's philosophy or mission, and its organizational structure and operating patterns.

Philosophy/Mission

While all hospitals are clearly dedicated to the provision of high quality patient care, there are varying ways in which this commitment is actualized. Community hospitals and university teaching hospitals have complementary but distinct missions. The degree to which an institution is committed to the provision of primary, secondary, and tertiary care is usually articulated in its mission. The institutional commitment to the education of health care professionals and to basic and clinical research are also evident in the mission statement.

It is important for all employees to have an understanding of how their employers define the institution's mission. An employee who cannot support the institution's mission will be neither happy nor productive. Thus it is essential to review and clarify the philosophy and mission of the institution during orientation.

Organizational Structure

The organizational structure of an institution is in part depicted on its organizational chart. The chart diagrams the chain of command and the relationships among the various components of the organization. The are several major types of organizations:

- Centralized versus decentralized
- Functional versus service line or matrix

Centralization refers to where decision making and accountability are seated within the organization. A centralized organization will locate these features with a limited number of managers and administrators. A decentralized organization establishes decision making and accountability as close to where the decision impacts as possible. The organizational charts of these two types of institutions will be quite distinct. A centralized organization generally has a more multilayered, vertical chart where decisions are made at the top and carried out by the lower levels. A decentralized organization has a flatter, more horizontal chart where there are fewer layers between the decision maker and the action.

Functional versus service line refers to the degree of integration built into the structure of the organization. In a functional organization, departments are comprised of specialized services such as nursing, social work, and housekeeping. Each function has its own department. In a service line organization, the functions needed to provide service to a group of patients, such as cardiac patients or pediatric patients, are integrated into service line departments.

Organizations come in various combinations of these four types of structure. It is important that all employees have an awareness of the institutions structure. Knowledge of the institution's organizational structure will assist the employees in understanding their relationship to the other members of the organization.

Operating Patterns

Operating patterns refer to the processes which are used to carry out work within the organization. Hospitals are 24-hour-a-day operations, but not all areas are open 24 hours a day. How are services provided in off shifts is an example of the type of information learned in a discussion of operating patterns. All institutions have formal and informal rules or guides for getting things done. The sooner new employees learn these rules the more effectively they will be integrated into the system.

The degree of specificity and the length of time devoted to each level of orientation will depend on the degree to which the institution's organizational structure and operating patterns are centralized or decentralized. A centralized organization, one in which there are few policy and procedural differences among patient care units, tends to have more in-depth and longer departmental orientation programs. Departmental orientations in a centralized organization provide orientees from diverse areas with an in-depth orientation that is applicable in all of their clinical areas. Decentralized departments, those with many policy or procedural differences among patient care units, will have briefer, more general departmental orientations.

While remaining mindful of the impact of the institutional or departmental organizational structure, the goals of orientation remain the same, that is, to introduce the new employee to "how things are done here." At each level the orientation program will include information related to the

- Organizational structure of that level
- Personnel policies
- Clinical policies
- Administrative policies
- Relationships among the various units within the level

Hospital Orientation

Orientation to the hospital at-large is usually a one day overview of the institution. The mission of the institution and the major components of its organizational structure are described. Overarching policies and practices such as equal employment opportunity policies, universal precautions techniques, and fire and safety practices are also introduced. In addition, this time is usually used to review the benefits program and to complete processing paper work. In large institutions a hospital-wide orientation is conducted as often as weekly for all new employees. Employees are then sent to their departments for continued orientation to their respective duties and responsibilities.

Orientation to the Department of Nursing

While the goal of a department-based orientation is similar to that of the hospital orientation, the focus is much more specific. Orientation to the department introduces the new employee to how the department functions. It does this both formally, through the content, and informally, through the process by which orientation is conducted.

Orientation to the department provides the employee with both information about and insight into the department and its culture. Because the orientation process will form the basis of the employee's perception about the department, it is a critical component of the department's retention program. The employee will also be given a message of how he or she is valued by the department. The depth to which information is addressed, the timeliness of speakers, the physical setting, the clarity and quality of materials distributed all provide the orientee with clues as to how the department functions and how much it respects the members of the staff. First impressions last a long time. Thus the importance of a well-orchestrated orientation program can not be over emphasized.

The time and effort spent in mapping out a departmental orientation program that welcomes the new employee and demonstrates the importance of integrating the new employee into the department is not to be either underestimated or undervalued. Coordinating such an effort on a regular basis is an awesome task but one that is critical to the effectiveness of any recruitment and retention effort.

Who should participate in the departmental orientation will depend on the organizational structure of the department. Each layer of nursing administration should be represented to orient the new employee to the roles and relationships within the department. Departments with whom the orientee will be expected to interact should also have a role in orientation. Typical departments include the operating room, dietary, social work, and others.

Staff resources on whom the orientee may call should also be introduced. These may include infection control practitioners, legal affairs, educators, and other nurses with specialized skills such as enterostomal therapy or patient education. The involvement from management, ancillary and support departments, and staff resource areas teaches the orientees how to use the organization's resources to effectively do their job.

Orientation Content

The content of the departmental orientation will vary depending on the organization, however, a reasonable check list of information includes the following:

1. Mission and scope of the department
2. Philosophy and nursing practice model of the department
3. Organizational structure of the department
4. Standards of nursing practice
5. Quality assurance
6. Policies—both administrative and clinical
7. Physical facilities
8. Records
9. Educational opportunities
10. Legal and ethical responsibilities
11. Infection control practices
12. How to access resources
13. Emergency response procedures
14. Evaluation

When selecting and developing the orientation content it is important to keep in mind that, in order for the program to meet the orientees' needs, it must also meet the department's needs. Ongoing assessment of the departmental needs is essential to the success of the orientation program. An initial assessment should be conducted with the first line managers to develop the initial orientation plan. Follow-up evaluation should be conducted on a regular basis with the managers as well as orientees. Figure 4-2 exhibits an orientation program in a large university teaching hospital.

Establishing the Culture

The department's culture, its norms, its formal and informal systems and networks, its values, and how it communicates are consciously or unconsciously taught to new employees during orientation. How the orientation program is structured, the methods of instruction used, the degree to which the orientee is expected to actively participate, and the degree of involvement of other members of the organization tells the orientees a great deal about their new employer.

A passive lecture approach, loosely organized and presented solely by a member of the staff development group communicates something wholly different from a highly interactive, well-managed program which has active participation from nursing administration, nursing management, and non-nursing department heads. Program planning for the former is clearly easier. However, it is the rare institution that truly wants to tell their new employees that they have such low expectations. Not only is the effectiveness of the teaching-learning experience enhanced by varying the methods of instruction and the presenter, it also indicates to the orientees that their commitment to the organization is valued.

Inservice Education

Nursing practice and the technologies of care are changing at an ever-increasing pace. New technologies are introduced almost daily. Patient care providers must be assisted in keeping up with these new technologies, their safe use, and how to troubleshoot problems which inevitably arise.

In addition to new technologies and procedures, the biochemical explanations of many disease processes are changing. Prostaglandins, among other recent discoveries, are only beginning to be understood. It is imperative that patient care providers continue to develop their knowledge base.

Inservice education is one vehicle for maintaining the skill, knowledge, and awareness of members of the department of nursing. Inservice education is a term ordinarily used to refer to brief teaching-learning experiences that take place during the work day within the work setting. The providers range from product/technology representatives, to members of the nursing and medical staff, to representatives from other departments within the hospital.

The role of the staff development specialist ranges from planning and coordinating to presenting the inservice program. The role assumed will depend upon the content and the expertise of the individual. The teaching-learning strategy used to provide inservice programs can cover the full range of methods covered in Chapter 5.

Skills Training

The development and maintenance of clinical skills is essential to maintain the quality of care provided. Thus programs which either introduce or maintain technical skills are a critical component of a staff development program. Skill development programs are frequently provided in response to the proposed introduction of new technology. Often the product or technology representative is the primary instructor.

The program design used to teach manual or technical skills will depend on the nature of the skill and the target level of the employee. Teaching an employee to use a modified form of an existing technology will require a less intensive program than adding a new technology.

When designing skills training sessions to introduce a new technology it is useful to look closely at the current practices within the clinical area to find parallel or comparable skills that can be built upon. Additionally, these

Georgetown University Hospital Nursing Department Orientation/July 1990

For more information call Nursing Education and Research: Ext 42591

Wednesday July 18	Thursday July 19	Friday July 20	Monday July 23	Tuesday July 24	Wednesday July 25
Hospital Orientation	**Conference Room A**	**Gorman Conference Room**	**Conference Room A**	**Computer Training**	**Computer Training**
8 AM through **4 PM** Conference Room A	**8:00AM** Welcome Distribute Packets *Carol Scott*	**8:00AM** Support Systems Coordinator *Carol Hester*	**8:30AM** Medication Test	As Needed "S" Level CCC Bldg	As Needed
	8:30AM Coffee	**9:00AM** Nursing Division Directors Meeting	**10:00AM** Processing	**8:00–11:30** OR **12:30–4:00** Schedule to be Announced	**12:30–4:30PM** CPR, BCLS
	9:00AM Overview *Carol Scott*	•Medicine *Shelia Hamel* (6 BLES Conference Room)	**10:45AM** Discharge Planning, Social Work, Home Care Visiting Nurse Assn. *R. Raspet*		Recertification
	9:30AM Overview of Nursing Department *Carol Scott*	•Surgical *Joan Fargo* (BLES 6036)	**11:45AM** Lunch		
	10:15AM Break	•OB/GYN/ MHCU/PEDS *Elizabeth McPherson* (B 3035)	**12:30AM** OR/RR *Nancy Blasko*		
	10:30AM QA Patient Classification *Ginny Dodds*		**1:00PM** Infection Control *Cheryl Blane*		
	11:30AM Hospital Tour				

Lunch

1:15PM   Nursing Education
         Carol Scott
         Joan Kelly
         Ramone Rayle

Gorman Auditorium

2:30PM   Insurance

Conference Room A

10:15AM Nursing Department Administration
         Eunice Kautzman

10:45AM Retention and Recruitment
         Pam Feinstein

11:15AM Role of Staffing Coordinator
         Peg Mooney

12:00   Lunch

1:00PM   Care of Vascular Access Devices
         Helen Roach

2:00PM   Code Response
         Judy Curtis

2:30PM   Nursing at Georgetown University Hospital
         Carol Scott

3:00PM   Math Review
         Carol Scott

2:00PM   Break

2:15PM   Dietary
         Peggy McGovern

2:30PM   Enterostomal Therapy
         Teresa Yang

3:30PM   Legal Affairs
         Sheila Zimmet

4:30PM   Evaluation of Orientation

Figure 4-2 Nursing orientation program schedule. (*Source: Department of Nursing, Georgetown University Hospital, Washington, DC. Reproduced with permission.*)

programs should be designed to stage learning. That is the participant should be introduced to the critical elements—the "must know"—and allowed to assimilate that knowledge prior to being presented with all of the background or detailed knowledge that supports the use of the technology. Adults learn what they need to know. Thus, the greater the apparent relevance to safe practice, the more likely the learner will feel a need to know the information. Once the immediate challenge is mastered, employees may then be ready and interested in knowing the less immediately applicable information.

Continuing Education

Continuing education is frequently used to refer to programs that will assist the attendee in growing and developing in ways that are organizationally desirable but not required. The employee will be better prepared after having attended the program, but attendance may not have been essential for the employee to meet performance expectations. These programs are usually longer in length than inservice or skills training courses.

The term "continuing education" may be reserved for those programs that meet the documentation requirements of accrediting bodies such as the American Nurses' Credentialing Association (ANCN). Workshops of four or more hours in length are usually considered to be continuing education offerings. Workshop offerings will depend on the needs of the organization and the interests of the staff.

Differentiations Between Types of Program Offerings

The American Nurses' Association (ANA) has defined continuing education[2] as

Learning activities intended to build upon the educational and experience bases of the professional nurse for the enhancement of practice, education, administration, research or theory development to the end of improving the health of the public.

They defined inservice education as

Activities intended to assist the professional nurse to acquire, maintain, and/or increase competence in fulfilling the assigned responsibilities specific to the expectations of the employer.

The distinction seems to rest on the motivation to seek education and not the program itself. Nurses and their professional organizations have traditionally placed a higher value on continuing education. Given that the employers of nurses and the profession of nursing tend to have a common goal of providing high quality health care to the consumers of their services, the distinction made between the two forms of additional education seems less than real—a distinction without a difference.

When considering whether an offering falls into the inservice or continuing education category it is important to contemplate several key concepts:

- Recognition or valuing
- Transferability
- Sponsors
- Stakeholders
- Goals

Recognition Issues

Contact hours are awarded for a variety of on-going education. The ANA continuing education program approval process is one in which nonacademic nursing programs may be granted approval to award contact hours to program attendees. The contact hours awarded through this mechanism are often recognized by other credentialing bodies such as boards of nursing and certification groups like the Association of Operating Room Nurses (AORN) and others. The standard used by the ANA and most other approving bodies is that one contact hour is awarded for every hour of class. The ANA and other professional nursing organizations' certification programs require evidence of continuing education to maintain certification. Some states have mandatory contact hour requirements for relicensure. Most often these requirements can only be met by attending programs that fall into the continuing education category rather than the inservice category. Thus, in many instances, despite a lack of difference in the quality of the educational offering. Thus the pseudovaluing of continuing education programs over inservice education programs.

There are some instances, however, where inservice education programs are deemed to be of equal or higher value. These are mostly intrainstitutional applications. For example, clinical ladder programs often weight attendance at either type of program equally. Nurses may attend inservice education programs to prepare them for internal credentialing which is highly valued within the institution. Attendees at inservice education programs in many institutions are awarded organizational contact hours for attending these sessions.

Transferability

Historically, organizations or associations accepted any evidence of ongoing education as valid. Colleges of nursing and a variety of for-profit continuing education providers offered programs of widely varying quality. Because of the disparities of the education programs available, the ANA established an accreditation process so that consumers could predict whether or not a particular program met minimal standards. This has been helpful to both consumers—the nurses and the requirers (i.e., state boards of nursing and professional associations). However, as with all well-regulated approval processes there are a substantial number of requirements that a program must meet to be approved. These steps must all be performed in a sequential manner that necessitates substantial prior planning. Inservice programs are by nature more spontaneous and more driven by immediate need. They rarely meet the planning process requirement for awarding of ANA approved contact hours. Thus continuing education programs are more likely to be transferable to external organizations.

Sponsors

Inservice programs are primarily sponsored by employers or product manufacturers. They usually take place on or close to the patient care units. Continuing education may be sponsored by employers, professional associations, colleges of nursing, for-profit education vendors, and product manufacturers. They usually take place away from the immediate work site.

Stakeholders

A stakeholder is anyone with an interest in the outcome of an event. Inservice education stakeholders include the employers, the employees, and the patients. Continuing education's stakeholders include the sponsor, the attendees and less directly the patients cared for by the attendees. The difference in these two groups of stakeholders is primarily the intimacy of their interest in the outcome. The inservice stakeholders have a more personally vested interest in the outcome.

Goals

Similar to the differences seen in the issue of stakeholders the primary difference in goals between inservice and continuing education is one of immediacy. Inservice education has an immediate application in addition to supporting future growth objectives. Continuing education has a less immediate or defined application.

Leadership Development

Developing the leadership potential of prospective, neophyte, and experienced leaders is usually part of the staff development mission. A wide variety of programs fit under the umbrella of leadership development. Programs to teach attendees how to run a meeting, time management, or how to do a presentation may be helpful to the aspiring staff nurse. Programs on how to manage conflict or how to handle the difficult employee may be helpful to both new and experienced managers. When planning leadership development programs, it is important to identify programs to meet the needs of the three major target audiences: staff, newly appointed leaders, and experienced leaders.

While the staff nurse may avail herself of the more generic leadership or management offerings, programs intended for the new and experienced leader must, in addition to assisting these individuals to enhance their leadership skills, provide them with a basic knowledge of management policies and procedures. Supervisory training programs are a vehicle for providing new supervisory personnel with a basic understanding of the applications of equal employment opportunity requirements, disciplinary procedures, and strategies for motivating and evaluating employees. Advanced workshops can provide experienced supervisors with the opportunity to further develop their repertoire of techniques for motivating and managing employees.

There are two major types of leadership development programs—formal workshops and structured on-the-job training. The stability of the leadership within the department will dictate the frequency with which an organization offers the formal development programs. That is, a department with little turn over in leadership positions will have fewer workshops and will instead focus on the structured individual training approach. Departments with more frequent turn over are more likely to offer workshops which, because of the volume of new leaders, can be cost effective.

In either case leadership training programs usually include content related to

- Fiscal management: budget construction, monitoring and control
- Personnel management: interviewing, hiring, counseling, disciplinary action, employee development
- Systems management: communication networks, reporting relationships, team building

As with all other development programs, it is important to design leadership training programs which are reality based and provide the attendees with the chance to use the suggested leadership and management strategies during the training. Simulation exercises, role playing, and application scenarios are useful teaching strategies. It is often advisable to develop several levels of training so that skills can be assimilated over time.

Some objectives can be met fairly expeditiously. For example, a one-day, department-head orientation program provides newly appointed department heads and assistant department heads with the opportunity to meet with the leaders of the ancillary and support departments. This type of session will provide new leaders with contact persons to whom they can relate in each of these areas.

Charge nurse workshops are one of the more frequently offered leadership development programs targeted to staff nurses. These programs are designed for staff nurses who are assuming shift-based leadership responsibilities. They provide an opportunity for role clarification and the development of problem-solving skills, often through the use of case studies.

As previously mentioned, programs on how to run meetings, time management, and presentation skills are also useful leadership development programs. This type of programming provides staff nurses and unit leadership with assistance in developing emerging skills and talents and helps prevent the frustrations inherent in the trial-by-fire approach so commonly used.

New Graduate Programs

The difficult transition from student to practitioner can be significantly eased through the use of a specifically designed new graduate orientation program. In the 1960s internship programs were developed by hospitals for graduates from baccalaureate programs. It was believed that when compared with diploma graduates, BSN graduates required additional supervised clinical experience prior to assuming the responsibilities of a staff nurse. Internship programs ranged from six to twelve months and included rotations through several specialties prior to assignment to the area of employment.

Few institutions could afford elaborate internship programs. Based on the work of Kramer,[3] many hospitals initiated transition programs designed to support new graduates through the "reality shock" encountered on entry to the work place. These programs were primarily used to augment unit-based clinical orientations and used group meetings over the first six to twelve months of employment to identify and discuss common concerns of the new graduate.

Both internships and reality shock programs became victims of the cost-cutting efforts of the mid 1980s. The nursing shortage and concern for retention as well as the decline in nursing school enrollments and the increase in competition to hire new graduates has resulted in a resurgence of some interest in new graduate orientation programs. The investment in the development of the skills and confidence of the new graduate is predicted to increase loyalty to the organization as well as contribute to the more rapid development of the new graduate's abilities.

The type of new graduate program developed, again, depends on the organizational structure and operating patterns of the institution. In general these programs are consistent with the orientation programs offered to experienced nurses.

Generally, new graduate programs consist of a basic review of anatomy and physiology, pathophysiology and the nursing technologies commonly associated with the pathophysiology, medication administration, documentation systems, priority setting, and organizing daily activities. Programs frequently include or incorporate a review course to assist the new graduate nurse pass the NCLEX exam used to license registered nurses. Occasionally, programs are also designed to assist the new graduate practical nurse, but these are rare. One sample new graduate program includes

- NCLEX review course during the fourth week of June.
- Two new graduate skills days offered immediately following Core Orientation. These two days include medication administration, use of IV equipment, documentation exercises, priority setting, and organizing of daily activities.
- Systems and technologies review: a four-day series spread over four weeks. Content includes Code Response training, working with patients experiencing cardiac, pulmonary, renal, gastrointestinal, neurological, psychiatric, and surgical problems; care of the patient with

diabetes mellitus; skin and wound care; hyperalimentation; therapeutic nutrition; pain and analgesia; and care of the oncology patient.

Time is also set aside for the new graduates to discuss issues of concern, for example, role adjustment and handling stress.

This program is designed to give the new graduate and the nurse manager flexibility. Together they can identify the sessions most appropriate for the new graduate. New graduates who are working with adult medical or surgical patients are encouraged to attend all of the sessions. However, new graduates working in post-partum may attend only the NCLEX review and skills sessions. In a decentralized system flexibility is the key to program success.

Certification and Credentialing

New health care technologies are introduced every day. As these new technologies are integrated into the scope of nursing practice, new programs must be developed to teach and maintain the skills required to competently perform the technologies. For example, several years ago, nurses began doing capillary blood glucose testing in order to more effectively monitor and control the administration of insulin. The introduction of this technology necessitated the development of training programs to teach nurses how to accurately use the equipment and interpret the results. Also, because of the risks inherent in incorrect use of this technology, it is important to update and validate the nurses continued competence.

In addition to new technologies, the role of the nurse has expanded to providing primary interventions in high risk situations such as cardiac and/or pulmonary arrests, chemotherapy administration, dysrhythmia interpretations and others. This has led to the initiation of programs that update and evaluate the maintenance of the requisite knowledge and skills.

In response to the need for increasing technical skill and knowledge, many organizations have initiated targeted certification or training programs. The difference between certification and training warrants some discussion. While it is important not to put too much importance on a name, certification is usually used to describe a requirement. If certification is required, then all employees who use the technology must be certified. While this is a worthy goal, it can create a management nightmare. New employees would need to be given the certification classes during their orientation. Employees who were unable to master the certification training would be unable to continue their employment. There are some skills for which these implications are warranted. Skills that are very high risk and not regularly used are ones for which many organizations require certification. Examples include cardiopulmonary resuscitation and defibrillation.

Training programs that have been developed to meet and maintain the knowledge and skill needs of staff using technologies that do not meet the certification risk threshold are often referred to as credentialing programs.

Examples of these types of offerings include chemotherapy administration, skin care, dysrhythmia interpretation, and intravenous catheter insertion.

Cardiopulmonary Resuscitation

It must be acknowledged that there are external requirements that affect the types of repeat training programs that are offered. JCAHO and most state accrediting bodies require that direct care providers have either annual or biannual cardiopulmonary resuscitation training. This is often interpreted as a requirement for BLS certification offered by the American Heart Association or for CPR certification offered by the American Red Cross. The 1991 Nursing Care Standards Scoring Guidelines of the JCAHO[1] clearly indicate that this is not the case. Hospitals must assure that the nursing staff can

1. Summon assistance (for example, "call a code")
2. Maintain a patent airway, breathing, and circulation in the patient until such time as assistance arrives or a physician makes the decision to cease (p. 29).

The American Heart Association and the American Red Cross offer standardized curricula to teach basic life support. These curricula teach participants the Heimlich maneuver, responding to the unconscious patient, one and two person resuscitation for adults, and resuscitation of infants and children. Instructor certification is required to award a "certification" card to individuals who successfully meet the requirements of these courses.

Georgetown University Hospital offers Adult and Pediatric Code Response Classes as alternatives to BLS. This decision was based on a review of the "Code" evaluations which indicated that the staff nurses were uncomfortable with medications used in codes. It was determined that staff needed more than an occasional mock code activity to gain confidence in their skills. This was particularly true in clinical areas where sudden death of a patient or "code" rarely occurs. The Code Response class includes

- Completion of a code response Self-Learning Packet which reviews the code-related policies and procedures
- Lectures on the medications commonly used in a code
- Mock code in which the faculty assume the roles of the physician and code team nurse and the participates serve as either the "cart nurse" or recorder
- Skill stations for practice in each competency of CPR and the code cart

Chart 4-1 outlines this program.

Completion of the Code Response Class or BLS certification and completion of the Code Self Learning Package meet the annual training requirement for cardiopulmonary resuscitation. Many nurses elected to maintain their BLS certification as well as attend the Code Response Class. This choice speaks to the generalizability of the BLS certification and to the value of the content in the Code Response Class.

C hart 4-1
Code Response Workshop

I. Welcome	**Scenario I**
	With Assistance from Participants
II. Code Drugs	**Scenario 2**
III. Code Cart	**Stations**
IV. Recording	O_2 Therapy
	EKG/Defib
V. O_2 Therapy	Code Cart
	Compressions/Ambu
VI. Pediatrics	**Evaluation/Post-Test**

Chemotherapy

The qualifications of nurses who administer chemotherapy agents is not currently regulated by external accreditors. However, many hospitals have defined this as a skill requiring additional training. Programs to ensure minimal competence have been developed. Most programs include both a didactic and a clinical practice component. A sample proposal for a chemotherapy administration course with objectives is presented in the Appendix at the end of the chapter.

IV Insertion

The insertion of peripheral intravenous lines is another skill for which certification or training programs are commonly required. Again, these training programs include a didactic portion in which the practice issues like indications and complications are reviewed, policy and procedure are presented, and techniques are demonstrated. Practice on lifelike manikins is a critical component. The formal training session is usually followed by supervised intravenous insertions in the clinical setting. Class times range from two to four hours depending on class size.

Other Standard Programming

Each organization must respond to imperatives that are unique to that organization. The approach used to outline unusual performance expectations frequently includes learning activities offered through the staff development program. These activities should be supported through hospital policy.

Mandated Training. External regulators, such as federal agencies, state accreditors, and voluntary accreditors, all place training requirements on hospitals. These include fire and electrical safety, infection control, and use and disposal of hazardous materials. Staff development specialists are usually asked to assist the organization in meeting these training requirements. The design of these programs is best done in collaboration with the departments involved. For example, the infection control programs are usually the responsibility of the infection control practitioner. However, the design of the program should be done in consultation with the clinical services because the infection control issues vary significantly across specialties. Intensive care units require more frequent programs and, in some instances, different programs than do general units. The staff development specialist's role is one of coordinating the design and implementation of these programs.

A variety of training strategies can be used to meet the standard training requirements cost effectively. Video tapes, self-learning packets, games, or crossword puzzles are tools that can be used. Annual training days are also used by many organizations to assist staff in meeting the minimal requirements. These sessions are offered frequently enough to accommodate the demand. In large departments they are offered four to six time a year. In smaller departments they may be offered less frequently.

Preceptor Programs

Many institutions have come to rely on staff to assist in the training of new employees. New employees are assigned to work with one or several experienced staff members who assume the role of preceptor. The preceptor is a coach, an instructor, a guide, and mentor for the new employee. Historically, staff were simply assigned this role. Recently, however, more emphasis has been placed on assisting staff in developing the knowledge and skills necessary for successful preceptoring. Preceptor workshops are now a standard part of most staff development programs.

The content of the preceptor workshop varies according to the role expectations of the organization. One sample curriculum includes sessions on

- The roles and responsibilities of a preceptor
- The application of adult learning strategies
- The evaluation process: How to critique performance?
- Problem solving
- Negotiating with challengers

Teaching strategies used within a preceptor training program should role model those which the preceptors will be using on the units. Thus, it is important to design a highly interactive program which allows the preceptors to identify their learning needs and to discover the concepts.

Some organizations have found that it is beneficial to develop a two-tier design for preceptor workshops: one for new preceptors to introduce them to the role, and one for experienced preceptors to assist them in expanding their skills. Advanced preceptor workshops build on the initial curriculum. The intent is to draw on the preceptors experience and to assist them with learning from each other. A sample course includes sessions on

- Rights and responsibilities: preceptor and preceptee
- Roles: change over time
- Challenges: working with difficult, slow, aggressive learners

Workshops for preceptors offer the additional benefit of providing an educational vehicle for demonstrating to the preceptors that they are valued members of the department. Devoting the time and money to augmenting the skills and self worth of this critical group is time and money well spent.

Summary

There is a natural tendency in organizations to believe that programs simply happen, and that the success of a program is mostly happenstance. Nothing could be further from the truth. While designing staff development programs is time consuming and resource intensive, the benefits far outweigh the disadvantages. Well-designed programs meet an organization's needs, conserve the institutions resources, and have significant positive effects on the vitality of the organization.

Mapping the strategic plan for the department is a primary responsibility of administration and management. Once this has been accomplished, it is the responsibility of the staff development specialists to design learning situations that will assist employees in growing into their future.

References

1. Joint Commission on Accreditation of Healthcare Organizations (1991). *Accreditation Manual for Hospitals.* Chicago: Author.
2. American Nurses' Association (1984). *Standards for continuing education in nursing.* Kansas City: Author.
3. Kramer, M. (1974). *Reality shock.* St. Louis: Mosby.

APPENDIX: CHEMOTHERAPY COURSE PROPOSAL

The chemotherapy course will include both a didactic and clinical component. Successful completion of both components will be required for certification.

The didactic course content is designed to prepare the nurse to administer chemotherapy, and concentrates on the science of chemotherapy and the nursing management of the patient receiving chemotherapy. The content is taken from the Oncology Nursing Society Cancer Chemotherapy Guidelines (1988). Eighteen to twenty-four hours of classroom time will be required to cover this component. At the completion of the didactic component of the course, a written test will be administered. A passing score of 85% is required in order to proceed to the clinical component.

In the clinical component of this course, the focus is on the need for the nurse to apply the knowledge gained in the didactic component in direct patient care situations. Emphasis is placed in the clinical competencies the nurse must demonstrate prior to being considered qualified to administer chemotherapy. A competency-based skills checklist will be used. It will be necessary to demonstrate proper technique for administration of three chemotherapy drugs to successfully complete the clinical component.

Objectives

At the completion of this course, the nurse will be able to demonstrate the following behaviors:

1. Describe advances made in the field of oncology related to the utilization of chemotherapy as a major treatment modality.
2. Describe the basic cellular kinetics of tumor growth.
3. Define disease staging and tumor classification systems.
4. List the various classifications/categories of antineoplastic drugs and describe their mechanisms of action.
5. Explain the rationale for combination chemotherapy.
6. Explain the rationale for continuous versus intermittent infusions of chemotherapy.
7. Describe tumor response criteria and other methods by which response to treatment is measured.
8. List three reasons for treatment failure and tumor recurrence.
9. Define the phases of clinical trials for testing new anticancer drugs.
10. List the major principles to be followed in the preparation and administration of chemotherapy.
11. Describe safety precautions recommended to minimize exposure of health care personnel, the patient, the family, and the environment to the potentially harmful effects of chemotherapy.
12. Describe the nurse's role in ensuring informed consent.
13. State the various routes used to administer chemotherapy and describe the rationale for selecting a route.
14. List four methods of intravenous administration of chemotherapy and

describe the indications for each method.

15. List the specific nursing assessment parameters for the major side effects of chemotherapy.
16. Differentiate between expected and untoward side effects of chemotherapy and describe the basic pathophysiological mechanism for the major organ toxicities.
17. Develop a nursing management plan based on the specific treatment regimen and the expected side effects for the patient receiving chemotherapy.
18. Develop a teaching plan, which includes the patient's family, for patients receiving chemotherapy.
19. Identify the signs and symptoms of extravasation of a vesicant and outline the nursing measures to minimize tissue damage.
20. List the signs and symptoms of an anaphylactic reaction and outline appropriate nursing measures to manage this complication.
21. Describe the more common latent and long-term complications that can occur with chemotherapy.
22. Demonstrate knowledge of the legal issues involved in the administration of chemotherapy, the documentation of nursing interventions, and the role of institutionally approved policies and procedures.

Didactic Course Content

I. ADVANCES IN ONCOLOGY
 A. Overview and Advances in Oncology
 B. History of Cancer Chemotherapy
II. PHARMACOLOGY OF ANTINEOPLASTIC DRUGS
 A. Chemical Structure Classification
  1. antimetabolites
  2. antibiotics
  3. alkylating agents
  4. vinca alkaloids
  5. hormones
  6. miscellaneous agents
 B. CELL LIFE CYCLE CLASSIFICATION
  1. cell-cycle specific drugs
  2. cell-cycle nonspecific drugs
III. PRINCIPLES OF CANCER CHEMOTHERAPY
 A. Goals of Treatment
 B. Staging TNM and Histological Classification
 C. Tumor Cell Kinetics and the Cell Life Cycle
 D. Rationale for Drug Selection
 E. Limitations of Chemotherapy
 F. Reasons for Treatment Failure
 G. Therapeutic Strategies
 H. Rationale for Drug Dosing Schedules
 I. Response Criteria
IV. PREPARATION, STORAGE, AND TRANSPORT OF CHEMOTHERAPY
 A. Drug Preparation
 B. Institutional Policies and Procedures

V. HANDLING AND ADMINISTRATION OF CHEMOTHERAPY
   A. Determination of Drug Dose
   B. Drug Administration
   C. Venous Access: Special Considerations
   D. Drug Interactions
   E. Sequencing of Agents
   F. Duration of Drug Administration
   G. Institutional Policies and Procedures
VI. DISPOSAL, ACCIDENTAL EXPOSURE, SPILLS
   A. Disposal
   B. Accidental Exposure
   C. Spills
VII. NURSING ASSESSMENT AND MANAGEMENT
   A. Pretreatment Assessment Phase
   B. Patient/Significant Other Education
   C. Side Effects
      1. alopecia
      2. anemia
      3. anorexia
      4. cardiac toxicity
      5. constipation
      6. cystitis
      7. dermatitis
      8. diarrhea
      9. flulike syndrome
      10. gastrointestinal ulceration
      11. hepatic toxicity
      12. leukopenia
      13. metabolic alterations
         a. hypocalcemia/hypercalcemia
         b. hypoglycemia/hyperglycemia
         c. hyperuricemia
         d. hypokalemia/hyperkalemia
         e. hypomagnesemia
      14. mood alterations
      15. nausea and vomiting
      16. neurotoxicity
      17. ototoxicity
      18. pulmonary toxicity
      19. renal toxicity
      20. reproductive dysfunction
      21. sexual dysfunction
      22. stomatitis
      23. thrombocytopenia
      24. venous fibrosis/phlebitis
   D. Latent Effects of Chemotherapy
   E. Allergic/Anaphylactic Reactions
   F. Extravasation
   G. Handling of Patient Excreta
VIII. DOCUMENTATION OF CHEMOTHERAPY ADMINISTRATION

chapter 5

Needs Assessment: The Essence of Staff Development Programs

Belinda E. Puetz

*Learning needs assessment forms the basis of the nursing staff develop-
ment specialist's planning process. Without determination of employees'
and the organization's learning needs, the educator will not be providing programs that are targeted toward improved employee performance
and meeting organizational imperatives. Malcolm Knowles[1] defined a
learning need as the "gap between the learner's present level of competence and a higher level of performance which is defined by the learner,
the organization or society" (p. 85). The cultivated ability of the staff
development specialist to inquire into the actual and perceived needs of
the organization and its nursing personnel is crucial to success. This
chapter discusses how to appraise the necessity for a learning needs
assessment. The discussion begins with an exploration of planning and
implementation methods, and concludes with a review of strategies to
evaluate the learning needs assessment process.*

Keys to Successful Needs Assessment

Three key elements in learning needs assessment summarize the
framework for the process: investigation, validation, and communication.
Each of these three components must be present for learning needs assessment to be efficient and effective.

Investigation

Learning needs assessment is an investigative process: the nursing staff
development specialist searches for learning needs that must be met in order

for nursing staff to perform to an expected and defined standard, and to meet the organization's mission and goals. Knowles'[2] definition takes into account the need for staff development specialists to develop skill in "helping adults discover and become interested in meeting their real needs, rather than just their interests" (p. 82). It is these "real needs" that the staff development specialist assesses during the needs assessment process. Since many adults are not commonly able to identify their own learning needs, the nursing staff development specialist starts by assisting employees and managers in defining what they need to know in order to do their work. The manager is involved in this process since it is the manager who is held accountable for performance. Knowles[1] further described the impression of institutional management of training needs: those changes that *should* be made in employees' skills, by educational techniques, to further operation efficiency and mission accomplishment. The staff development specialist has the added challenge of helping managers understand the limits and potential of educational interventions to change behaviors. The specialist initiates the investigation, rather than waiting to be asked to conduct an assessment, or worse, told by someone in the organization that a learning needs assessment is necessary.

In conducting a learning needs assessment, the staff development specialist makes an effort to link the process with the organization's mission, goals, objectives, and future directions. Finding out about these aspects of the organization may require a significant amount of persistent investigation. Some within the organization may need the assistance of the specialist in understanding why this data is essential to the staff development program. These individuals may not make the connection between successful implementation of new programs and services and the competence of the staff involved in these services. Others may not know how staff development specialists help with transitions and competency development. These individuals may also be clients who have simply never used or been offered staff development services. In general, these individuals must be helped to understand the key role they play in defining the staff development needs of nursing personnel.

The outcomes of the learning needs assessment may also have to be altered as additional information becomes available or as the organization changes plans for the future. A well-developed network of individuals who can provide needs assessment data is crucial to the success of this activity. This dynamic and ongoing activity may cause the staff development specialist to change educational programs already planned. However, this training will be more relevant if it is responsive and in keeping with the future directions of the organization. In addition, the specialist who maintains a futuristic orientation in learning needs assessment and program planning will be perceived as being on the cutting edge.

In the investigation, the staff development specialist assesses not only individual but also organizational learning needs to find out what the current problems are and what difficulties amenable to educational investigation are anticipated for the future. The investigation is ongoing, not just an annual affair. Staff development specialists concerned about developing programs that are viewed as valuable by their organization, as well as their learners, must complete a thorough needs assessment before embarking on program development.

Needs assessment data then is used as a baseline for evaluation activities. The investigation in the evaluation component involves data collection to help measure the overall impact of the staff development program on the organizational and individual needs.

Validation

The nursing staff development specialist uses a variety of techniques in order to be certain that the needs identified actually are learning needs. The specialist asks the question, Do the problems stem from a lack of skills or knowledge among employees or are they due to a lack of an administrative system that sets clear performance expectations? If the answer is affirmative related to the lack of knowledge or skill, then the need is one that can be met through a staff development intervention. If the answer to the question yields data that indicate a lack of an administrative or management system, then the staff development specialist should identify it as such. The intervention is different for administrative problems and may or may not involve the staff development department. For example, if a needs assessment activity consistently yields information that indicates misunderstanding about a standard of performance related to a common skill, the staff development specialist may refer the problem to the Policy and Procedure Committee requesting that a standard be set. Another example is when the lack of knowledge and skill is due to a lack of adequate supervision and feedback about performance. The learning need may be identified as one in which the manager needs to learn coaching, counseling and feedback skills. To differentiate between the two areas, Mager and Pipe[3] suggested a performance analysis approach that begins with asking the question, Could they do it if their life depended on it? If the answer is yes, it is probably not a learning need, rather it is a system or administrative problem.

Many needs assessment data collection and validation efforts uncover complex issues that require both administrative and staff development interventions. These complicated issues usually require the collaborative effort of both staff development and management to resolve. However, it is often through staff development needs assessment activities that these problems are identified.

In the validation process of learning needs assessment, the focus is primarily on the needs of the organization, rather than just the needs of individual employees. The nursing staff development specialist uses triangulation strategies to synthesize the two sets of data.[4] The staff development specialist checks the results of learning needs assessments with relevant individuals in the institution, asking, Does this finding truly reflect a learning priority in the organization? Because everyone may not agree on educational priorities, the process of synthesis and validation is essential to obtain valid and reliable learning needs. If differences in perception between organization and individual occur, generally that points to another learning need.

Communication

In conducting a learning needs assessment, the staff development specialist informs everyone in the institution who is involved in the process about the purpose of the needs assessment. The goal of this communication is to help all involved view the activity as an institutional project, rather than a staff development effort. In addition, it will help focus the assessment on the needs being investigated. For example, perhaps an assessment is needed on the skill level of nurses related to physical assessment. The needs assessment will be conducted differently, as discussed later in this chapter, than if the needs assessment were designed to collect all learning needs.

People are informed about what the needs assessment is for as well as what it is *not* for,[5] that is, the learning needs assessment will not solve all of the organization's problems. Communication about the needs assessment also serves to let the organization know that its purpose is *not* to provide "nice to know" programs, when the organization is committed to providing only "need to know" information.

In communicating the results of the learning needs assessment, the nursing staff development educator summarizes the needs assessment in written and verbal forms. The final report does not contain any unpleasant surprises, such as learning needs based on a lack of appropriate orientation, in which one particular unit or department is identified.

The final report of a comprehensive needs assessment is in written form and should include purpose, dates, objectives, methods, sources of data, analysis, results, actions to be taken, and recommendations. If the report is lengthy, an "executive summary" of one to two pages should be included. The summary condenses the study methodology, emphasizes findings and defines actions to be taken as a result of the needs assessment. The executive summary is placed at the beginning of the report. Copies of resources used are added as appendices.

The written report of the learning needs assessment is distributed widely throughout the institution. The staff development specialist further communicates these findings by writing letters or memos of thanks to those who participated in the plan.

Other means of communication about a learning needs assessment include writing an article for the organization's newsletter, a one-page summary of results for distribution with employees' paychecks or a brief note for posting on bulletin boards throughout the institution. The staff development specialist also reports verbally at every possible meeting: results are reported at all inservice, staff development, and continuing education programs in order to disseminate the findings of the learning needs assessment as widely as possible. Announcements are made at the beginning of those educational offerings planned as a result of the needs assessment so that participants know the program was designed to meet their identified learning needs. Staff development specialists can also use these opportunities to assist management with clearly delineating performance expectations by linking those programs to the competency expected as an outcome of the classroom experience.

These methods of communication serve to inform the institution's administration and nursing staff about the learning needs assessment process and outcomes. These strategies also sensitize people to learning needs, and a serendipitous benefit may be enhancement of the reputation of the staff development specialist for contributing to the achievement of the organization's goals and objectives.

Planning Learning Needs Assessment

In planning a learning needs assessment, the nursing staff development specialist first decides what the purposes of the study are, as these will determine the depth and scope of the learning needs assessment. Jazwiec[6] stated that the most frequently given reasons for a learning needs assessment are

- Identification of previously unknown learning needs
- Validation of those needs
- Program marketing/promotion

Bell[7] identified three typical purposes of learning needs assessment as

- Identifying organizational problems
- Assessing educational deficits
- Meeting organizational requirements

The staff development specialist should consider carefully the purpose of the needs assessment as each will cause the specialist to select somewhat different strategies for the implementation of the process. For example, assessment's sole purpose is to assess learning needs. An additional purpose may be to market and promote staff development services. In the latter case, the staff development specialist may use an interview process to obtain information about learning needs as well as to promote selected services. During the interviews, the staff development specialist gathers data about how to tailor the selected services to best meet the perceived needs of the identified group of employees or specific units within the organization.

The choice of needs assessment strategies also depends on several other considerations. Questions that should be answered during the planning phase of the needs assessment process include the following:

- What specifically will the department do with the needs assessment data?
- What resources can be allocated for this function?
- How will staff development services continue during this process?

The learning needs assessment should be planned for the purpose of answering questions that need to be answered in order for a complete staff development action plan to be developed. The needs assessment results should contribute to ongoing decision making about programmatic as well as administrative aspects of staff development in the institution. Through careful planning of the needs assessment, the staff development specialist will find that the time and energy expended will yield useful data that become essential and integral to ongoing staff development efforts.

Implementing the Learning Needs Assessment

The process of conducting a learning needs assessment involves the use of a variety of data collection methods, selecting those that will provide the most reliable and valid data on which to base program planning decisions. The method selection process also considers the learning styles and preferences and the demographics of the potential respondents.

Methods are selected based on ease of use as well as the advantages they offer in comparison with other methods.[8] Jazwiec[6] identified formal, semiformal, and informal methods of needs assessment. Formal methods are written assessments, group methods such as nominal group process, and individual interviews. Semiformal types of assessment include asking staff and managers in the organization on a random, but ongoing basis for their identified learning needs: random observation also can be used as part of this semiformal process. Jazwiec further described informal methods of assessment as pursuing comments such as "we need...." from managers and staff and then exploring in more depth what the real needs may be. While there may be higher use of the formal approaches by a staff development department on an episodic basis, the staff development specialist will rely on the semiformal and informal methods of gathering needs assessment on a day-to-day basis. Among the most commonly used learning needs assessment methods are questionnaires, interviews, observation, and group discussion.

Questionnaires

Questionnaires have the advantage of being relatively simple to construct and use. Data also can be collected from a large group at a single time. The major disadvantage of questionnaires is that they do not permit much interpretation of the responses: someone who marks "no" to an item, for example, often does not provide the rationale for doing so. The content of a learning needs assessment questionnaire should avoid eliciting information about interests rather than learning needs, the "nice to know" rather than the "need to know." The focus of the items should be on assessing the difference between actual and optimal employee performance.

All of the questionnaire items should be job-related and should attempt to determine what behaviors are being performed on the job. The next step in the learning needs assessment is to assess not only the proficiency, but the criticality and frequency of the behavior specified. Rosetti[9] suggests it is important to

- Find out how well an employee can perform a specific behavior.
- Determine how important it is that the employee perform that particular behavior.
- Determine how often the employee is called on to perform the behavior.

Staff development activities then are targeted toward those behaviors that are essential for the employee to perform often and that they currently are not proficient in performing.

A learning needs assessment should include items on demographics only if they will be used in targeting educational programming to a specific audience: for example, if educational activities will differ for the night shift, then such a question is appropriate. If level of education will not make a difference in the type of programs planned for various educational levels, then an item on basic or highest level of education should not be included.

Where behaviors are specified that relate to future organization plans, the consciousness of staff can be raised about these future plans and, consequently, the learning needs that derive from them. To accomplish this, the staff development specialist can include in the beginning of the item a statement such as, "Management has forecast the introduction of bedside computers on all units by 1994. Indicate your learning needs to become competent about the following aspects of computer technology."

Because the emphasis of a learning needs assessment is on work-related learning needs, all items on the questionnaire should describe on-the-job performance. Chart 5-1 illustrates a variety of typical examples and suggests improved items that will accomplish this goal. Similarly, items on an educational program evaluation form that ask about "other content of interest" should be rephrased to ask, What else is needed to do your job? so that the focus on learning for performance is consistent.

A panel of experts can be used to design the learning needs assessment questionnaire. Other nursing staff development specialists can provide useful information gained from experience with their own learning needs assessment tools. Pre- or pilot testing is recommended to be certain the items are clear, concise, and comprehensive. Groups of learners can be asked to complete and critique the form. Suggestions should be incorporated and the questionnaire retested until the staff development specialist is satisfied that the responses obtained truly represent learning needs.

Interviews

Interviews are a method that is useful, particularly for individuals in management positions, who may consider themselves too busy to complete a questionnaire. The interview can cover the same items as a questionnaire, but have the advantage of allowing the interviewer the opportunity to provide as well as receive information. Interviews also are useful in validating the needs identified through questionnaires.

Interviews should be brief, no more than thirty minutes long. A schedule of interview questions should be prepared and used in each exchange. If several staff development specialists will be conducting interviews in their respective areas, the use of a schedule of questions is essential. Interrater reliability between and among specialists may be of some concern if the interview data will be aggregated. A discussion about how to avoid bias and a clear understanding of the purpose of the assessment will help increase the reliability of the recorded responses to the interview questions.

Informal interviews also occur between staff development specialists, managers, and learners on a day-to-day basis. Information from these experiences is helpful when used to modify planned programs, and makes them more meaningful to learners and relevant to managers.

Chart 5-1
Sample Needs Assessment Items

Typical

Which of the following workshops are you interested in? Rank in order of priority from most interested (5) to least interested (1).

Alternative

What I most need to learn about in order to do my job better is:

In order to improve their practice, my colleagues need to learn more about...

Typical

What other topic would you like to see in 199_ ?

Alternative

What is your most critical job-related problem?

What part of your professional knowledge should be improved?

What do your nursing colleagues most need to learn improve their practice?

Typical

What do you like best about (name of offering)?

Alternative

In (name of offering), what is of value to you in your practice?

What information in (name of offering) is most useful to you?

Typical

What do you like least about (name of course)?

Alternative

In (name of course), what are you least able to apply in your practice?

What information in (name of course) is least useful to you in your practice?

Typical
Were your personal objectives for attending this course met?

Alternative
Please rate your agreement with each of the following statements:

Statements	Never	Sometimes	Often
In my practice, I am expected to (behavioral objective)	☐	☐	☐
I can perform (behavioral objective)	☐	☐	☐
My supervisor would say I perform (behavioral objective)	☐	☐	☐
My colleagues would say I can perform (behavioral objective)	☐	☐	☐
As a result of attending this course, I can (behavioral objective)	☐	☐	☐
In order to perform (behavioral objective), I need to…	☐	☐	☐

Nominal Group Technique

This learning needs assessment technique permits input from individuals as well as groups. It can be used at the end of an educational activity, though time would have to be allocated for this purpose. The process also can be used as a scheduled part of an ongoing needs assessment plan.

In nominal group technique, people are placed into small groups of six to eight. A leader is chosen by the group members. Individuals, working alone, then write down three learning needs based on what they need to know to perform their job proficiently.

After five to ten minutes, each person presents one item. The leader writes them verbatim on newsprint. Items should be presented in round robin sequence until all items have been presented and recorded. No discussion, censorship, or evaluation of the items as they are being listed is permitted.

Then, the leader displays the newsprint and duplicate items are eliminated. Each of the remaining items on the list is thoroughly discussed. During this step, the groups should clarify each item and indicate their support or lack of support for the inclusion of that learning need.

When the list of items has been discussed, group members individually rank the remaining items in order of priority as learning needs. During this step, the participants are voting for items that are considered more important. The members should be instructed to use a 1 for the lowest learning need and higher numbers for the learning needs perceived as higher priority. The leader combines the individual rankings or votes to arrive at a group total or score for each item. The item with the highest score then is ranked with the priority number of 1. The second highest score is ranked with a 2, and so on. The new list is written on newsprint and represents the group's perceived learning needs. The final step in this process is to validate the learning needs list developed by each group with the entire group. The final step in the process can use a consensus approach. All small group members become part of the large group and again have the opportunity to vote/rank priority items after similar items are deleted.

Group Discussion

As with the nominal group technique, group discussion can be conducted as a planned activity after a meeting or program, or it can be conducted when time is unexpectedly available. The discussion should be limited to fifteen or twenty minutes. Questions to be discussed should be provided to each group on an index card or posted on newsprint. Again, results should be displayed and validated as part of the process.

Individual Appraisal

Testing is one method of learning needs assessment using individual appraisal. However, many adults are uncomfortable with testing. Testing should be used only in situations where required by program design, or where alternative methods of learning needs assessment are not available or feasible.

When testing is used, a map or blueprint of the proposed test will assist the nursing staff development specialist to prepare the test in such a way as to capitalize on the test's ability to tell the difference between good and poor learners. The test map is constructed by identifying content to be tested; only critical content is included. Trivial matter is omitted.

Next, learner outcomes, or the educational process, are identified. The outcomes should be stated in behavioral and measurable terms (much like course objectives).

A content/process matrix is the next step in the process. In this step, the relationship between the subject matter, observable behaviors and the number of test items is defined. For example, definition of terms may comprise five items, while searching for alternatives may be a critical component of the course, thus, twenty test items are devoted to the process of searching for alternatives in the content area.

In the final step, test items are selected for their ability to measure the achievement of the outcome process in the specific content area. Specific test items best measure particular types of learning. Chart 5-2 illustrates some principles of test construction.

Test items should be subjected to an item analysis to assure that they do assess the desired learning. Items that do not meet the established criteria should be eliminated.

Other individual appraisal methods include computer assisted instruction (CAI), competency models, performance checklists, and preceptor ratings. These can be used to discover existing learning needs. As with other learning needs assessment methods, these instruments should be designed to focus on work performance and should include the aspects of criticality and frequency as well.

Delphi Technique

The Delphi technique in a learning needs assessment uses "rounds" of questionnaires to achieve consensus on learning needs.[10] The method is fast, inexpensive, convenient and avoids the problems of "group think" or dominance that may occur in group rather than individual approaches to learning needs assessment.

The content of a Delphi survey is generated from the target audience either from previous responses to evaluations, interviews, or other data collection methods. The content should be validated for clarity with others before the instrument is sent to the respondents.

The steps of a Delphi survey involve sending three consecutive rounds of a learning needs assessment questionnaire to the participants. In the first round, the questionnaire content consists of learning needs items suggested by the subjects, but arrayed on the form by the nursing staff development specialist. The questionnaire is completed by the respondents and returned to the staff development specialist.

The questionnaire for the second round is formulated from the responses to round one. The items may be reorganized, duplicates eliminated, and other items added if necessary. The staff development specialist uses some discretion in this process, as changing the questionnaire substan-

Chart 5-2
Principles of Test Construction

Alternate Response Items (true/false; agree/disagree)

Confine the statement to one simple idea. Avoid specific words such as always, never, usually. Directions must be exact. There should be approximately equal numbers of false as true items.

For example:
1. The purpose of a needs assessment study is to assess the probability of attendance at specific programs.
True _____ False _____

Multiple Recognition

All alternatives (possible responses) should agree grammatically with the stem. Do not use "a" or "an" with the alternatives. Use at least four alternatives with each item. Avoid alternatives that may give clues to the correct response.

For example:
1. Multiple approaches to needs assessment are used to:
   (a) obtain additional information from the same population
   (b) validate the accuracy of the needs assessment data
   (c) discover which method results in the most information
   (d) experiment with various methods to find the best one

Completion Items

Blanks should be placed at the end of the sentence. Avoid using too many blanks in each sentence. Key words should be the ones omitted from the sentence. Only one answer should be possible for each blank.

For example:
1. Learning needs are best identified by _____ .

Matching Items

More choices should be offered than can be matched. Terms should not give clues to the expected response. The matches should be unambiguous but not obvious.

Essay Questions

The nature of the task should be clearly stated ("discuss…" is not sufficient). The exact limits should be defined. The desired outcomes should be the basis for grading.

Situation Analysis

The situation should be geared toward the learner's knowledge and experience. Sufficient information should be included to assure clarity. The description should be of reasonable length. A variety of test items can be used to assess the analysis of the situation.

Critical Incident

The critical incident should be sharply focused. No extraneous information should be included. Questions should relate only to the information provided.

Decision Making

Criteria for judging the adequacy of decisions made should be specified in advance. A variety of test items can be used to assess competency in critical thinking.

Source: Puetz and Associates, Inc. © 1988. Reproduced with permission.

tially defeats the purpose of the Delphi technique in achieving consensus.

In this second round, respondents rate the importance of the topic items on a scale of 1 to 5, where 1 is "of little importance or need," and 5 is "of significant importance or need." The second round questionnaires are distributed and collected.

In the third round of the Delphi needs assessment, the staff development specialist calculates means and modes for topic responses. Any comments that respondents made are added to the items and the questionnaire then becomes the one distributed in round three.

In this round, participants not only review their own learning needs, but the addition of the mean and mode to each item allows the respondents to assess the item's significance to their colleagues. In this way, consensus on the importance of various learning needs is achieved.

When questionnaires are collected in round three, the nursing staff development specialist again calculates means and modes and summarizes comments. The report of the results of the Delphi technique learning needs assessment should be provided to the participants, but additional rounds generally are not advisable; if consensus has not been reached by round three, further attempts to achieve it will probably not be productive.

Focus Groups

Focus groups involve a small number of individuals who meet to discuss a prearranged topic or set of questions. Focus groups involving consumers, for example, are used in business or industry to obtain information on new products or services.

Focus groups as a learning needs assessment method are most useful when setting future directions; individuals involved in planning or research and development for the institution should be invited to participate. The group usually is comprised of from four to twenty people; ten to twelve generally is recommended. It is customary to invite more than needed to the session since some individuals will not be able to attend.

A moderator who knows how to conduct a focus group session is essential; the moderator should be someone who has no investment in the discussion or its outcome. The moderator must maintain control of the group, but be flexible enough to flow with the group if the value of the information in process warrants a departure from the prearranged topic. In addition, the moderator has to insure that every person contributes on every item, knows what is needed and at what level of detail, and what will be done with the information obtained as well as how confidential it is.

Participants in the focus group should sit in a circle; the moderator should be part of the circle, not seated apart. Two hours is the maximum time for a focus group.

If the individuals invited to participate are not homogenous, it may be necessary to convene more than one focus group, since members in a heterogenous group may focus more on each other's contributions (discussion, disagreements, arguments) rather than on the topic at hand. An agenda or script is needed to keep the discussion on track and to assure that all the topics are covered adequately.

The nursing staff development specialist may choose to send a questionnaire before convening the focus group to stimulate thought before discussion. To determine whether a focus group is the appropriate strategy to use, responses to the following questions are needed:

- What does the staff development specialist want to know?
- Who has the information?
- What resources are available to obtain the data?
- What is the best way to get potential respondents to provide the data?
- How can respondents give the needed information?

Focus groups should only be used to address major issues, since the cost and time involved are likely to be considerable. The value of the information obtained from a focus group, in some cases, however, makes the expenditure of resources worthwhile.

Resources

Resources already available to the staff development specialist are also a foundation of needs assessment data. These resources include

- Meeting minutes
- Accident/incident reports
- Exit interviews
- Satisfaction measurements and indices
- Preceptors' perceptions
- Chart audits

One of the most serviceable sources of needs assessment data is that collected through the organization's quality assurance program and monitors. These data—when generated using an approach of monitoring important aspects of care or service that are high risk, high volume, or problem-prone[11]—will provide staff development specialists with data on areas of high need. These data then can be used to provide programs that are directly linked to improving the competency of the nursing staff.

Media

The media also can provide another source of needs assessment data. This method often identifies current state-of-the-art practices that may support the need for staff development programs. Current buzz words in the literature often will become tomorrow's staff development program. Some caution should be exercised by the staff development specialist as information in the print media (in professional books and journals, for example) may already be outdated. The challenge for the staff development specialist is to take the information found in these sources and then design a program that is relevant to the staff's particular learning needs.

Other Sources of Needs

Bille[12] described several additional approaches to needs assessment, including group problem analysis, job analysis, performance appraisals and behavioral evidence. Group problem analysis is a technique in which a group is asked to discuss a specific problem and identify solutions. For example, an increase in medication errors or patient falls can be presented to a unit-based group and the group guided to analyze the modifications needed to effect change. The staff development specialist then may facilitate the implementation of these changes and coordinate any educational intervention associated with these problems. In many cases, these problems are related to administrative or system issues that must be addressed in order to resolve the problem. This method is frequently used as part of monitors completed during quality assessment action plans.

Job analysis and performance appraisals also may be a useful source of needs assessment data. Nurse managers can be helped to channel learning needs discovered as part of the performance appraisal process to the staff development specialist. The staff development specialist may be able to help the employee change behaviors through a learning contract or other individualized learning plan to achieve satisfactory performance.

Through direct observation in the clinical area during routine unit visits, the staff development specialist may collect a rich variety of information that will help identify the gaps between actual and desired behaviors. Although behavioral evidence is frequently used by the staff development specialist, this information may not always clearly indicate a learning need.

A final needs assessment strategy described by O'Connor[13] is the telephone survey. The telephone survey is similar to standard interviews, but the interaction is not face-to-face. Surveys of ten to fifteen people in the target population may yield a representative picture of learning needs. The interviewer must orient the respondent quickly to the process and, using a prepared set of questions, complete the survey in five minutes or less. Telephone surveys have the advantage of brevity over interviews. The disadvantage is that rapport generally is not established with the interviewee, and, thus, the quality of information collected may be adversely affected.

Knowles[1] also reminds providers of staff development services of the fact that "in every organization, situations occur repeatedly which produce obvious training needs" (p. 97). These include

- New employees
- New job assignments
- New procedures and products
- New equipment
- Changes in the mission or structure

While there are a variety of learning needs assessment methods from which to choose, no needs assessment strategy is perfect. Each technique has advantages and limitations. Using a variety of strategies will help the specialist become proficient in learning needs assessment and obtain valid and reliable data on which staff development programming can be based. Proficiency in learning needs assessment is achieved with practice; trial and error efforts will lead to competency. Another result of working at obtaining expertise in learning needs assessment efforts occurs when others are oriented to the fact that needs assessment is a standard component of nursing staff development practice.

Problems in Needs Assessment

Common problems that occur in learning needs assessment involve

- Lack of knowledge
- Excessive cost
- Methodological concerns
- Political considerations

Generally, these problems can be addressed through judicious use of existing resources, making certain that the effort expended is justified by the outcome of the study. Specific gaps in knowledge can be remediated through self-study or in consultation with peers.

Mager[14] provides a sound framework to assist the staff development specialist with a resolution of some of the problems associated with needs assessment activities. In his discussion of human performance, Mager differentiates between instructional technology, performance technology and management. He describes performance technology as the procedures used to change performance capability, such as demonstration, presentation modeling and reinforcement. These are the techniques and procedures in which staff development specialists influence what learners *can do.*

Instructional technology, however, is a subset of performance technology. That is, the techniques and strategies used are intended to facilitate the performance that people *already know,* but are not performing as desired. Strategies such as job and performance analysis, policies, feedback, job/performance aids, and task redesign are used within this domain. Mager also describes the instructional and performance technologies as a subset of management. Management includes the allocation and control of available resources toward the accomplishment of goals and objectives. Examples include people, money, materials, facilities and others.

This framework can be used to help staff development specialists and managers understand and explore which learning needs may be amenable to staff development intervention. It also will help differentiate those needs which will require a collaborative effort between management and staff development.

Prioritizing Learning Needs

Collecting and analyzing learning needs assessment data leads the staff development specialist to setting priorities for programs to meet the identified learning needs. Several ways have been identified to set these priorities.[15] The staff development specialist may plan programs based on the number of requests for education on a specific topic, or the decision can be made on the basis of the available resources. For example, programs may be planned on the basis of whether faculty are available within the institution to teach on a particular topic. Advisory committees and other groups external to the staff development department may provide useful input on setting priorities.

Nursing managers can be used to help set priorities for staff development programs. In a method described by Straka,[16] a ranking and valuing mechanism is employed by selected managers to assist in priority setting for staff development efforts. Participating managers are asked to rank items from a list of possible programs and/or projects provided by the staff development specialist. The items can be written in terms of objectives reflecting the outcome of the program or project. The group of managers is asked to rank order each of the items from most to least important.

In the next step, managers are asked to establish a value for each of the items. Participants are asked to place a value of at least 10 next to the least important item. Then the participants are asked to place any value higher than 10 by the next least important item. For example, if a manager selects a value of 10 for the least important item, and the next least important item is compared and deemed not much more important, a value of 15 might be assigned. Participants may use any value that will communicate the importance of the item to the staff development specialist; no upper limit is placed on the value of a particular item. The only restriction in the valuing is that the least important item be assigned no less nor more than 10 points. This procedure continues until all items have a "value" number next to them (see Chart 5-3).

In the final step, the staff development specialist "normalizes" the rank and value of each item. Normalizing is accomplished by averaging all ranks and values to come up with a single value. Using this process allows the staff development specialist to confirm the importance of the information collected from participants in the learning needs assessment, and involves managers in setting priorities for staff development services. This technique of setting priorities helps assure that the educational programming provided will meet organizational goals and objectives, and focus on performance of nursing staff.

Using Needs Assessments

Upon completion of the process of setting priorities for the learning needs assessed, the work of using the data begins. The needs assessment data can be used as a basis for educational programming, to demonstrate accountability to the organization, and to solve organizational problems. The most common use of learning needs assessment information is to plan staff development educational programs. Learning needs assessment also is a requirement for accreditation of the institution's continuing education program as a provider by the American Nurses' Association accreditation mechanism. The results of a learning needs assessment can be used by decision

Chart 5-3
Priority Rating Form (Example)
Allegheny General Hospital

Name: ....
(person completing)

Directions

Four goals for Nursing Staff Development are listed below in the Worksheet.

1. In the left column, place the rank you think each goal should have (1 = most important to 4 = least important)
2. In the right hand column, assign a value to each goal.
   a. Give the least important (#4) goal a value of 10.
   b. Look at the goal you have ranked number 3. Decide how much more important this goal is compared with number 4 and write the appropriate value at the right. (For example, if you think #3 is only slightly more important than #4 you might assign a value of 14. If you think it's fifty times more important, you would assign a value of 500.) There is no upper limit on the number of value points you can assign to the objectives. Your only restriction is to assign 10 value points to the least important one.
   c. In the same manner, assign a value to each remaining goal, moving from the least important to the most important goal.

Worksheet

Rank	Goals	Value
....	Examine models of Clinical Nurse Specialists utilization to increase cost-effectiveness and provide advanced clinical practice.	....
....	Improve the quality and cost effectiveness of nursing orientation programs.	....
....	Identify and implement activities to enhance nursing staff's professional growth and role satisfaction.	....
....	Expand research to support educational and administrative information analysis as well as clinical research.	....

Source: Department of Nursing, Allegheny General Hospital, Pittsburgh, PA. Reproduced with permission.

makers at various levels in the institution. At a minimum, learning needs assessment data is the crucial link between the learners and the providers of educational services.

Evaluating the Needs Assessment

The results of the planning and implementation process for the learning needs assessment should result in affirmative responses to the following questions:

1. Will the method measure learning needs?
2. Is the method easy to administer?
3. Is the cost reasonable?
4. Are others involved in the process?
5. Are the instruments comprehensive, reliable, and valid?
6. Have the data analysis methods been identified?
7. Have actions in response to the results been determined?

Affirmative responses to each of these questions will assure the staff development specialist that the learning needs assessment is efficient and effective. The evaluation criterion of significance for a learning needs assessment is whether the assessment resulted in information that will be functional in program planning to address the identified learning needs.

Summary

A learning needs assessment is an integral part of the nursing staff development program. Without a learning needs assessment to set directions for the staff development program, the specialist basically is without direction. The assessment is a road map, providing direction for successful implementation of the overall staff development effort.

References

1. Knowles, M. S. (1970). *The modern practice of adult education: Andragogy versus pedagogy*. New York: Association Press.
2. Knowles, M. S. (1980). *The modern practice of adult education: From pedagogy to andragogy*. Chicago: Association Press.
3. Mager, R. F., & Pipe, P. (1984). *Analyzing performance problems*. Belmont, CA: Lake Publishers.
4. Puetz, B. E. (1987). *Contemporary strategies for continuing education in nursing*. Rockville, MD: Aspen.
5. Bowman, B. (1987). Assessing your needs assessment. *Training, 24*(1), 30–34.

6. Jazwiec, R. M. (1985). Learning needs assessment: A complex process. *Journal of Nursing Staff Development, 1,* 91–96.
7. Bell, E. A. (1986). Needs assessment in continuing education: Designing a system that works. *The Journal of Continuing Education in Nursing, 17*(4), 112–114.
8. Bell, D. F. (1978). Assessing educational needs: Advantages and disadvantages of eighteen techniques. *Nurse Educator, 3*(5), 15–21.
9. Rossett, A. (1989). Assess for success. *Training, 26*(4), 55–59.
10. Chaney, H. S. (1987). Needs assessment: A Delphi approach. *Journal of Nursing Staff Development, 3*(2), 48–53.
11. Berman, S., & Wilkinson R. (Eds.). (1988). Step by step through the monitoring process. In *Examples of monitoring and evaluation in special care units*. Chicago: Joint Commission on the Accreditation of Healthcare Organizations.
12. Bille, D. A. (1982). *Staff development: A systems approach*. Thorofare, NJ: Slack.
13. O'Connor, A. B. (1986). *Nursing staff development and continuing education*. Boston: Little, Brown.
14. Mager, R. F. (1988). *Making instruction or skill bloomers*. Belmont, CA: Lake Publishers.
15. Puetz, B. E., & Peters, F. L. (1981). *Continuing education for nurses: A complete guide to effective programs*. Rockville, MD: Aspen.
16. Straka, D. (Speaker). (1989). *Integrating management values into total program planning: A quantitative approach*. (Cassette Recording No. 7). Philadelphia, PA: Medical College of Pennsylvania.

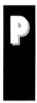

chapter **6**

Planning Programs: Strategies for Success

Phyllis J. Miller

The planning of educational activities consumes a large portion of the staff development specialist's time. Meticulous planning is essential for the ultimate success of any staff development activity. The planning process begins with an assessment of learning needs, followed by a deliberate planning procedure that ensures that the design of an educational activity will promote optimal learning. This chapter will explore a variety of teaching–learning designs commonly used by staff development specialists. In addition, conference planning activities will be discussed. Finally, issues related to marketing staff development programs will also be described.

Balancing the Program

As discussed in the previous chapter, needs assessment data will yield the requirement for many different types of programs. Balancing the staff development program to meet the myriad needs of the nursing staff and the organization is one of the most pivotal challenges for the staff development specialist. The demands of many individuals must be balanced with the needs assessment data. Staff development programs will differ from organization to organization depending on these needs and demands. A skillfully balanced program will take all available data from many sources and meet the needs of a broad assortment of customers using limited resources efficiently and effectively. A balanced program will also use a collection of teaching and learning strategies that will challenge the nursing staff to participate in a process of life-long learning and development.

The Basis of the Program Plan

Data derived from needs assessment data provide the basis of any sound program plan. Information gathered from individuals, the organization, professional literature, and the nursing community is essential in program planning. Based on these data, a learning activity appropriate to the expected outcomes, level, and experience of the learner can be designed. Discussed in the previous chapter, the integration of these data is essential to the success of any staff development activity. Savvy staff development specialists will use the needs assessment process as an opportunity to build commitment to the educational process and help managers and staff understand staff development services.

Domains of Learning

The design of educational activities will vary depending on the material to be learned. Staff development specialists will also need to plan educational activities in diverse ways to match the subject matter to be learned. An education plan begins with a description of what the learner is expected to know, do, or feel at the end of the educational experience. This usually takes the form of learner objectives developed from the perspective of what the participant will be able to do as a result of participating in the learning activity. A common first step in the development of the objectives is to write a statement like, "At the completion of this program, it is expected that the participant will...."

The use of a taxonomy of educational objectives[1] has been the time-honored approach of staff development specialists in the development of objectives for learning activities. This classification, often referred to as Bloom's Taxonomy, divides learning into three domains. The first domain is described as cognitive and deals with discrete information and knowledge. The second is the psychomotor domain, which has to do with learning motor skills. The final domain, the affective, deals with feelings, attitudes, and values. Most learning can be primarily categorized into one of these domains. Though learning may fall into several of the domains, it is up to the staff development specialist to decide which domain is the dominant one.

This classification helps staff development specialists structure learning activities in different ways. Using the dominant domain, the specialist selects a teaching and learning strategy that is compatible with the identified domain. For example, if the needs assessment yields data which indicate a knowledge deficit, the objectives would be derived primarily from the cognitive domain. The design of this activity would include an assortment of strategies such as lecture, discussions, drills, and case studies.

If the needs assessment indicates the staff are unable to perform a skill, the objectives would be drawn primarily from the psychomotor domain and include strategies such as demonstration, practice, and return demonstration. A common limitation of programs designed in the psychomotor domain of learning is the lack of adequate time to practice to a predetermined skill level. Staff development specialists can avoid this design problem through careful planning that allows time for each participant to practice the skill and using additional faculty to assist with groups larger than five.

Planning for learning in the affective domain is most challenging. Needs assessment data will usually indicate the need for staff to be willing and motivated to do what is expected to meet organizational goals. The data will also support the fact the staff *know how* to perform but are not performing as expected. Learning activities planned to achieve objectives in the affective domain must include a high level of participation by the learners. For example, a frequent approach to program design in this area is the use of small groups assigned to answer a question such as, "Describe what happens to patients' sense of dignity when they enter the hospital." In learning designed to change behaviors in the affective domain, participants must be able to discuss the issues that may be causing them to exhibit observed behaviors. These behaviors are the result of long-held values, beliefs, and feelings. These feelings can be explored through learning activities. Other strategies used to accomplish objectives in the affective domain include, but are not limited to simulations, games, role playing and other group activities.

The identification of objectives to be achieved in the learning experience is usually a major step in designing it.[2] The development of objectives is a challenging task, yet it is the hallmark of a well thought-out educational plan. Objectives declare the actual intended result of learning. Within the staff development program, they are the justification for existence.

Teaching and Learning Strategies

The stated objectives will help the staff development specialist determine which teaching learning strategy to select. While objectives from several domains may exist, the strategies selected should contribute to the overall design of the experience. Several of the most familiar strategies used in nursing staff development are

- Lecture
- Group discussion
- Skills training
- Case studies
- Self-learning packages
- Study guides

Each of these approaches can be used in a variety of ways to meet learning objectives. Some basic principles should be used to add the probability of success to the learning experience.

Lecture

In her article on preparing lecture presentations, Alspach[3] refers to the lecture as the "most widely used, misused and abused method of instruction." Despite this comment, it is a time-honored approach to present factual information in a logical and coherent manner. O'Connor[4] defines the lecture as a carefully organized oral presentation of subject content by a qualified expert. The criticism often levied against the lecture is usually the result of the learners' experience in lectures which are not carefully organized. The staff development specialist can master the use of the lecture as a teaching strategy through careful planning and practice. At the end of each lecture presentation, the specialist should systematically and thoughtfully review the experience and determine what should be done differently the next time a lecture is planned. In other words, the staff development specialist also learns from the lecture experience!

When the lecture is used as the only teaching strategy, it may be ineffective. There are a number of reasons for this; one of which is the presentation is auditory, not visual. The availability of high tech entertainment media also causes learners to bring different expectations to the experience, particularly if they watch a great deal of television. Another reason the lecture alone may not be effective is the limited involvement of the learner. The learners function in a passive mode rather than engaging in the learning and participating in the exchange of information. Most nurse learners bring myriad experiences to learning activities and are usually able to judge the usefulness of the information presented. If not given the opportunity to do so, the learner may discount the knowledge as erroneous since it does not match the experiences of the nurse.

The lecture can be used to convey cognitive information and to emphasize and reinforce knowledge previously learned. It is helpful and efficient for imparting information and can add details not commonly available to learners. A lecture can also provide the basis for the application of cognitive and psychomotor skills.

When planning a lecture, it is important to identify the key objectives of the learning activity. The staff development specialist should ensure that the scope of the objective and subsequent lecture is not too broad. Present only the essential content to meet the objectives. Avoid the tendency to overload a lecture with trivial material. The specialist should develop an introduction along with a summary that is presented with the main content of the lecture. The age-old adage to "tell them what you're going to tell them, tell them, and then tell them what you told them," still works.

Other stylistic features the staff development specialist can employ to enhance a lecture include the following:

- Use dialogue, rather than the straight lecture format, to engage the group in discussion of major points.
- Use groups of two, three, or more learners to discuss the content. Instruct them to be prepared to report relevant learning and questions for clarification to the large group after ten minutes of discussion.
- Break up lecture time with group participation activities, such as a case study or clinical judgment example.
- Reinforce learning by stopping every few minutes to ask the group a question related to the information just presented.

- Provide a note-taking outline with the main points of the lecture listed, and encourage the participants to use the space provided to fill in the outline as the lecture proceeds.

Any enhancement that will encourage participation and create an environment that is conducive to learning should be tried and improved with each lecture given. Movement around the room and the use of audio-visuals to reinforce learning are helpful to enhance the lecture. Use of varying voice pitches and patterns have also been reported by learners as aiding their acquisition of knowledge in a lecture. In addition, the lecture should be prepared to cover information in twenty minute blocks of time, unless other learning activities are incorporated into the planned experience.

The determining factor to the success of any lecture is preparation. Staff development specialists who take the time to plan their lecture presentation carefully and completely, review their notes before the presentation, modify it as new information becomes available and respond to needs for changes within the lecture will have achieved mastery with this teaching strategy.

Group Discussion

The use of group discussion as a teaching strategy is firmly rooted in adult education theory and recognizes learners' previous experience and learning. The most important element in using group discussion is to design them with a clear focus and goals. Otherwise, the discussion will quickly diverge due to misunderstanding of the task at hand. Subsequently, the opportunity for maximal learning may be lost.

Cooper[5] emphasizes that attention should be given to climate-setting for optimal function of the small group. The staff development specialist lets the group know at the outset, the time available for the activity. Introductions should be facilitated if the group does not know each other. The staff development specialist may also use an instruction sheet that outlines the tasks for each group. This will provide a ready reference for the groups' tasks to be completed.

It may be appropriate in some learning designs, particularly those with objectives in the affective domain, to have each small group report back to the larger group with information developed in their group. Care should be exercised to avoid extending group discussions for long periods of time. In general, a ten to twenty minute discussion period should be enough to accomplish most tasks assigned using this method.

The effective use of questioning techniques is another factor in the successful use of discussion as a teaching strategy. Questioning learners will encourage the exchange of ideas. It assists the specialist with determining what the learners may already know from previous learning. It can also teach critical thinking and will enhance class participation.

Questions should be framed carefully to accomplish the intended result. Three main categories of questioning have been developed by Verduin, Miller, and Green.[6] The first, recall questioning, is thought of as a lower-level question and is the most frequently used. The questions are used to help learners retain, recognize, and memorize information, and can also be used to reinforce materials already learned. Words such as

- State
- Name
- Identify
- Describe

will assist with recall questions. An example of this level of questioning might be "describe the flow of blood through the heart."

The next level of questioning involves a higher level of thinking. This level is called evaluative thinking and the learners are asked to analyze information and make a judgement. This level of questioning fosters critical thinking and decision making. Words used for the method of questioning include

- Compare
- Contrast
- Differentiate

For example, "compare and contrast the nutritional and pharmacological treatment plans for this disease."

The final level of questioning is the highest order and is referred to as creative questioning. It involves helping nurses create or invent something different and new to them and think beyond the subject matter being studied. Words used to convey this level of questions include

- Create
- Design
- Invent
- Predict
- Develop

An example for this category would be to "develop a plan for your unit to respond to the nursing shortage."

Effective staff development specialists will evaluate their learning objectives in light of these three levels of questioning and then formulate discussion questions that will contribute to the accomplishment of those objectives.

Skills Training

When designing a program in which a psychomotor skill is the expected outcome, the staff development specialist should focus on the what, why, and how of the skill. The first step is to help the learners focus on the skill to be learned and then tell the learners why it is necessary to learn the skill. It is much easier for nurses and others to learn skills if they are able to articulate reasons for knowing the skill. The next step is the "how to" step. This is often referred to as demonstration. Skills training differs in that the steps include the following:

- Focus on the task at hand and why it is to be learned.
- Demonstrate the task from start to finish without interruption.
- Demonstrate each step in the skill again with an explanation and pause for questions and clarification.
- Repeat the demonstration as a "master" or "model."
- Immediately assign learners to a practice period with simulation models if available.
- Supervise and assist learners through the practice session.
- Allow each learner to perform a return demonstration.

Expect learners to vary in their skill acquisition ability. Some nursing staff will pick up manual skills very quickly, while others may need more time to practice with the model. It is advisable to have reading material and other activities available for those learners who master the skill quickly; alternatively, these quick learners can be conscripted to assist the slower learners as long as the specialist judges that the quick learners will be helpful.

Performance checklists are also a part of skills training sessions. These checklists can be derived from a variety of sources such as

- The specialist's knowledge
- Journal articles
- Other performance checklists of related skills
- Procedure manuals

The checklists serve as a guide for the learner and a performance test for the return demonstration.

The key to a well-planned skills training session is adequate space, facilities, simulation aids, equipment, and supplies. In addition, adequate numbers of faculty to supervise and check off learners as they acquire the skill is essential to a quality skills training session.

Case Studies

The use of case studies as an educational strategy was instituted in the 1950s at the Harvard Business School. This strategy has enjoyed wide use within nursing staff development activities. Armistead[7] has identified several case study categories. Those that are most applicable to nursing are the following:

- **Exercise case study:** The learner is assisted in practicing the application of specific procedures.
- **Situation case study:** The learner reads the case study and is asked to analyze selected information.
- **Decision case study:** The learner goes a step beyond the analysis of the situation case study and presents plans for solving the problem presented.
- **Critical incident case study:** The learner is provided with parts of the situation for analysis and determination of the action to be taken. As each step is correctly concluded, additional information is provided for further analysis and problem solving.

Some computer-assisted learning programs use these formats. Some are programmed with high levels of sophistication and the learners' choices for problem resolution, right and wrong, are advanced through pathways until the learner arrives at a final "right" and "wrong" situation.

To assist learners through some case studies, decision trees and algorithms may be provided. While these are useful adjuncts, care must be exercised to help the learner understand that these decision tree "cookbooks" are guides to help learn judgment but should not replace the thinking process that must occur with any problem-solving skill development.

When developing the case study, the staff development specialist must again evaluate the objectives of the learning activity, and structure the case study to meet those objectives. Elements from real-life situations should be incorporated to any case study written by the staff development specialist; the more realistic the case study, the more relevant the learning.

A final caution with this strategy is in order. Use the case study as an application of content (often taught with a lecture), not a substitute for that content. An exception may be one in which a group of experienced nurses must review familiar cases and the case study combined with group discussion is used to explore and reinforce strategies to improve care of the patients selected for the case study. Competency *assessment* activities frequently use case studies to measure nurses' management of patient care.

Self-Learning Packages

Another effective and efficient teaching strategy used often in nursing staff development is the self-learning package (SLP). Described by del Bueno in the mid-seventies and expanded by Miller[8] later, SLPs are a self-contained unit of instruction that focus on a single concept or topic and contain a few well-defined objectives. An SLP utilizes the concepts of adult education theory and competency development.

One advantage of SLPs is their efficiency for subjects that need to be taught over and over to many groups of nurses. This method also acknowledges the different paces at which learners acquire information. The SLP also provide specific, consistent information over time because there is no variation in instructors.

Disadvantages of the SLP as a teaching strategy include differences in preferences of learning style in which some staff may need a more prescriptive or traditional approach to the acquisition of new knowledge. Other members of the nursing staff may be unsure of their ability to learn on their own, lacking confidence in their skill with this method. Others, in some nursing positions, may not have a high enough literacy ability to read the SLP and may need an alternative. Some learners may feel a sense of depersonalization, since the face-to-face interaction that occurs in the classroom is not present. The staff development specialist may also need to adjust to less classroom time for topics selected for SLPs and may also experience a sense of depersonalization.

The staff development specialist must plan for more than the usual amount of up-front development time with an SLP, as the package is designed to be a stand-alone unit and no content can be left open to question. In general, the specialist may need as much as ten to fifteen hours to develop the first SLP that takes a learner one hour to complete. Though this time is reduced with skill development in this area, it is one of greatest disadvantages to the staff development specialist who has an already full schedule. Despite this, the SLP is a cost-effective alternative to classroom teaching, and with nursing staff socialization toward the concept, can be a successful adjunct to the staff development program.

There are *three components* to a self-learning package. The first component is the evaluation method, which in its purest form is both a pretest and a posttest. The second component is the actual learning content in the SLP. This content must be presented in small, sequential steps with much repetition. The final component of the SLP is feedback. This helps the learner bridge the gap of an absent instructor. The feedback activities in the SLP give immediate reinforcement to the learner on how well they have acquired presented knowledge through short questions throughout the SLP. Answers are also provided.

SLP development begins with topic selection. Usually, SLPs can best be used for teaching cognitive information. If the staff development specialist wants to use an SLP for psychomotor skill development, it can only relate the concepts needed to perform the skill. The specialist will need to plan follow-up skills training activities such as demonstration, practice and return demonstration to evaluate learning. SLPs are generally not used for learning in the affective domain.

Once the topic is selected, the staff development specialist develops learning objectives. This will give focus to the SLP content and help identify the areas of the package that must be reinforced through feedback. Because of the finite nature of the SLP, staff development specialists must focus very narrowly and specifically on what the learner needs to know about the subject.

An overview of the package and how to use it must always be included. This will help orient the first-time user. The experienced learner may skip this page if it is known information, or review it quickly—a hallmark of this method of learning, that is, it is not necessary to spend time on learning already acquired knowledge.

The writing style of the SLP is informal and conversational in tone. A warm, sincere, and sometimes humorous approach will appeal to most learners. This will also settle some of the feelings of depersonalization discussed earlier. Other techniques that will help make the package more attractive to the learner is the use of diagrams, sketches, characters that "talk" to the learner, clip-art, or comical illustrations. Staff development specialists who integrate their own "style" into the package will find this communicated to the learner.

As the content of the SLP is being developed, a general suggestion is to hone the content so the SLP will not extend beyond thirty or forty pages. In addition, each page should not have more than thirty to forty words. This allows the learner to think about each bit of information as it is presented.

Feedback activities should be incorporated about every five to ten pages and after each essential point. These feedback activities are usually in the form of questions, informally asked (perhaps by the comical character used as the "voice" of the package). Two to five relevant questions are asked and the answers, with references to the SLP and suggestions for reviewing the section, are included on the next page.

Once the content of the SLP has been developed along with the feedback sections, the evaluation instrument is developed. This instrument, usually in the form of a test, is specifically oriented to the objectives and tests only the content related to the objectives. The staff development specialist establishes criteria for satisfactory completion of the package by judging the criticality of the information.

Once the package is complete, it should be pilot-tested before it is released to learners. It is helpful to pilot test the package with people with content expertise, people with SLP process expertise, and target audience members. Generally, about six to ten individuals are needed to conduct a good test of the package. These individuals should be instructed to judge the clarity, accuracy, and flow of the package. The staff development specialist elicits feedback from the test pilot group and makes revisions as needed. Following these revisions, the package is released to the target audience. Additional announcements and flyers about the availability of the SLP are necessary due to its unusual nature.

Like other staff development programs, the SLP must be managed. The staff development specialist is also responsible for grading and returning post tests, posting credit if awarded and reviewing and updating the SLP annually.

The staff development specialist can make a significant contribution to the organization in the form of "returned patient care hours." For each learning hour using an SLP, rather than a classroom hour, about one patient care hour is returned.

Study Guides

A study guide, as a teaching strategy, is also an efficient method to transmit information. Frequently used to disseminate information related to policy and procedure revisions, the study guide can also be completed at the learner's convenience. The body of information that needs to be transmitted is organized into a document by the staff development specialist or the actual policy and procedure is used. A series of specific questions to guide the acquisition of the information is written. The nature of these questions is different than the usual test question, in that the learner is expected to "find" the answers in given material, therefore the questions may be trivial by design. It is expected that learners will read the policy and be exposed to the information as they "search" for answers to questions.

The study guide is also an efficient strategy that can return patient care hours to the organization.

Other Teaching–Learning Strategies

Many other teaching–learning strategies exist and are available to the staff development specialist in other educational sources. Two other available methods are

- **Poster displays:** A new or revised procedure or form can be readily displayed on posters stationed within nursing units. These displays may or may not have an evaluation tool, usually to award credit, in which nursing staff complete a series of questions related to the information displayed.
- **Nursing rounds:** A group of patients, a specific situation, or a challenging case can be identified on a nursing unit, and the staff development specialist leads a discussion in which nursing care options and alternatives are identified and discussed.

The proficient staff development specialist will learn a variety of teaching–learning methods. Each presents challenges, advantages, and limitations. As a method is used and refined, the specialist builds a repertoire of available methods that may be accessed as the situation demands.

Planning the Staff Development Activity

The staff development specialist engages in a logical step by step planning process. Using needs assessment data, the specialist decides, in collaboration with others, how the event will take shape. With knowledge of outcome expectations in the form of learning objectives, the specialist designs and plans the staff development activity.

Documentation for this process can take a variety of forms, but should include as a minimum:

- Topic
- Date(s), time(s), and place
- Faculty
- Coordinator
- Source of need
- Learning objectives
- Target audience
- Evaluation method
- Contact hours
- Outline

Chart 6-1 illustrates a sample documentation form that meets these criteria and can be used for brief learning activities of a half to one hour in duration. Chart 6-2 shows a format that may be used to document activities that are longer, such as a one-day conference or a four-day course. Additional documentation may be necessary to meet regulatory and accrediting body requirements and should be incorporated into the staff development documentation system.

Each of these items may be viewed as questions the staff development specialist can ask during the planning process. For example, what is the *topic* about and how should it be worded to best communicate to the nursing staff.

Chart 6-1
Sample Documentation Form for Brief Learning Activity
Center for Nursing Education

CNE use only
Code _____

Learning Activity Record
_____

Program Title:

Coordinator:

Date/Time/Place:

Faculty:

Source of Need:

Learner Objectives:

Teaching Strategy:

Target Audience:

Aids or Equipment:

Contact Hours:

Evaluation Method:

Evaluation:
(Completed after activity)

Please attach course outline to this form

Source: Greater Southeast Community Hospital, Washington, D.C. Reproduced with permission.

Chart 6-2
Sample Documentation Form for Lengthy Learning Activity

Syllabus

Title:

Date/Time/Place:

Coordinator(s):

Faculty:

Program Description:

Source of Need:

Planning Process:

Objectives:

Target Audience:

Evaluation Method:

Contact Hours:

Add DCNA Offering Approval Form
to this documentation

Source: Greater Southeast Community Hospital, Washington, D.C. Reproduced with permission.

The next question to ask is the *source of need*. How did this learning need come to the attention of the staff development specialist? Was it during annual needs assessment activities or as a result of a quality of care monitor? Did a nurse manager observe poor performance related to this topic or was the knowledge deficit identified as a result of a specific incident? What are the staff behaviors that indicate this learning activity is necessary and how did these behaviors come to my attention? The answer to the source of need question is documented and serves as a follow-up source as well. In addition, accrediting agencies look for the relevance of the staff development activity and how it relates to improving patient care and staff competency. Answers to the source of need question will show that relationship. Any educational activities conducted as a result of quality monitoring should be noted as such.

Learning objectives are developed as discussed earlier and should answer the question, What is the learner expected to be able to do at the completion of this staff development activity? Written in behavioral terms, the objectives are the framework of the activity.

The staff development specialist then proceeds to ask the question about the *target audience*. Who is this information prepared for? Whose behaviors need to change? Information targeted to all members of the nursing staff is prepared and presented differently than to a homogenous group of only RNs. While it may be common practice to include all levels of nursing personnel in staff development activities, the staff development specialist designs the program for a target audience, the group that is expected to change as a result of the activity.

The next to last step is the identification of a *planned evaluation method*. Depending on the criticality of the information and skills taught, evaluation methods may range from a reactionnaire to a written test. Many evaluation methods are available to the staff development specialist and are discussed in Chapter 8. The careful selection of an appropriate method during the planning process is essential. Without this step, the learners will not be informed about expectations and the measurement of their learning.

The final step is the determination about how long the learning activity will take. Usually recorded in clock or contact hour form, the staff development specialist should again ask questions as the program is planned. How long is it anticipated that this learning will take? How many people are expected? At a single session or multiple sessions? How much time can be spared from patient care?

The evaluation of the activity is completed after the program and documented in the record. Chapter 8 addresses evaluation strategies in detail.

While each of these steps in the planning process seem to flow in a logical fashion, in reality they do not. The answer to each question causes the staff development specialist to think of the learning activity as a whole and to consider how each element will affect the whole. For example, if the topic is related to a new, but somewhat simple skill expected of all nurses throughout the organization, such as a new way to discard hazardous biological waste, the specialist must consider how to best reach a critical mass of nurses with skill demonstrations and arrange practice and return demonstrations. However, if the skill is more complex, for example, the administration of chemotherapy, then the staff development specialist will design a program for the target audience that will give adequate detail, opportunity for questions, policy support explorations, and ample knowledge and skill acquisition opportunities.

The time spent in the actual planning of the program details will vary depending on the complexity of the educational design. It is important to begin this process far enough in advance so that adequate planning is possible. Individual organizations may differ as to the lead time necessary, but most will have a general guideline based on experience. For shorter learning activities that are one to two hours in length, three to five weeks is usually sufficient. For a longer activity that will be conducted over one or two days, more lead time is needed. In general, fourteen to sixteen weeks is needed. Conference room space must also be reserved and a budget for the activity developed within the guidelines of the organization. Chart 6-3 provides a sample budget planning form.

Despite all effort to allow adequate time for planning, most experienced staff development specialists have so many demands and such limited time for other activities that planning time gets delayed. It is up to the specialist to protect planning time and give it equal importance to other staff development activities.

Many detailed activities are factors of a well-planned staff development activity. In addition to the elements identified above that begin the planning process, the staff development specialist must also accomplish the following:

- Negotiate agreements with nurse managers and others for mutually acceptable dates and times for the activity.
- Identify and secure faculty for the activity—agreements about services should be communicated. Charts 6-4 and 6-5 provide samples of letters and an agreement in which no honoraria is included. If the agreement includes honoraria and any other financial stipulations, this should also be communicated. Charts 6-6 and 6-7 show a format that will help accomplish this task. All negotiations for honoraria and other financial agreements are the responsibility of the staff development specialist who, in turn, is held accountable for the program budget.
- Ensure that adequate information about the learning needs of the target audience is identified and shared with the faculty. If the faculty do not know the audience, begin communications with a description of who the anticipated learners are and follow with their needs. A description of the patient population for clinical topics is also helpful for faculty unfamiliar with the organization. Finally, share any desires for information the learners themselves have expressed.
- Market the program as soon as possible and let all involved parties know how the program plan is progressing.
- Contact and confirm all support services needed well in advance of the program. These may include environmental services, food services, the security department, and the audio-visual department, depending on the organizational structure. Systems to request services within each organization are often defined; if not, simple memos will suffice that alert the department of the event and request their help.

Chart 6-3
Sample Budget Planning Form

Budget Planning Worksheet

Program Title _____ Code _____

Scheduled for _____

Program Coordinator _____

Co-Sponsored by _____

Expenses

Anticipated Side A	Item	Actual Side B
_____	Faculty Honorarium/Fee	_____
_____	Faculty Travel	_____
_____	Faculty Lodging, Meals and Other	_____
_____	Brochures/Printing	_____
_____	Postage	_____
_____	Purchase Materials/Handouts (cost per unit x no. participants)	_____
_____	AV Rental/Purchase	_____
_____	Conference Materials (cost of folder/name tags x no. participants)	_____
_____	Catering (cost of A.M. break + P.M. break x no. participants)	_____

Source: Greater Southeast Community Hospital, Washington, D.C. Reproduced with permission.

Anticipated Side A	Item	Actual Side B
_____	Special Catering (*ex:* speaker luncheon – cost per lunch x no. guests)	_____
_____	Other (specify)	_____
_____	_____	_____
_____	_____	_____
_____	**Total Expenses**	_____

Income

_____	Non-(hospital name) participants x fee	_____
_____	Other (specify)	_____
_____	_____	_____
_____	_____	_____
_____	**Total**	_____

Signatures

_____	Program Coordinator	_____
_____	Director	_____

▐ hart 6-4
▐ Sample Faculty Confirmation Letter with No Honoraria

199_

Dear _____:

I am delighted that you will be able to participate as a faculty member for our conference, "_____ ," to be held on , _____ 199_ , in the Health Education Center Auditorium here at Greater Southeast Community Hospital.

Your audience will be primarily Greater Southeast nurses. We will be marketing this conference to metro-area nurses also. Other interested health care professionals may attend.

Your session is entitled "_____ " and is scheduled from _____ .

As we discussed, I would like you to focus on the following:

I have enclosed a *faculty agreement* for you to sign as well as to indicate your *audio-visual equipment* needs, and a *biographical data form* from DCNA for you to complete. Because of changing accreditation guidelines from the ANA, we can unfortunately no longer accept a C/V or resume instead of this form. Also enclosed is the *Offering Approval Documentation Form* for you to record your outline as well as teaching strategies. I would encourage you to develop *handouts* for the participant packet. Our participants have indicated that they especially like note-taking outlines. I would be happy to duplicate the handouts if you can provide me with one clear copy. I will need all of the above materials returned to me by _____ .

If you have any questions, please feel free to contact me at (202) 574-6762. I am enclosing some of the program brochures for your use. I look forward to working with you on this program!

Sincerely,

Phyllis J. Miller, RN, MS, FHE
Education Specialist
Center for Nursing Education

Attachments

C hart 6-5
Sample Faculty Agreement Form with No Honoraria

Greater Southeast Community Hospital
Department of Nursing Education and Research

Faculty Agreement

Greater Southeast Community Hospital is pleased that you have agreed to serve as faculty for our program. We will reproduce all support materials, as provided, within reasonable limits, and provide audiovisual equipment necessary to the effective implementation of your program. We reserve the right of approval on all materials.

Your acceptance of this invitation includes your agreement to effectively organize a professional learning experience for the conference registrants within the guidelines described in the accompanying letter. Your cooperation in meeting established deadlines for submitting data to Greater Southeast Community Hospital is also appreciated.

I accept your invitation to speak at the (title of conference) which is scheduled for (date).

Topic: (topic l)

_____

Date   *Signature (speaker's name)*

AV Needs: _____

_____ 35-mm Slide Projector
_____ Overhead Projector
_____ Flipchart
_____ VCR—3/4-inch tape
_____ Electric Pointer
_____ Other

Please return no later than (return date) to: _____

Your name
Center for Nursing Education
Greater Southeast Community Hospital
1310 Southern Avenue, S.E.
Washington, D.C. 20032

_____

Received   *Associate Director, Nursing Education and Research*

Source: Greater Southeast Community Hospital, Washington, D.C. Reproduced with permission.

hart 6-6
Sample Faculty Confirmation Letter with Honoraria

199_

Dear _____:

I am delighted that you will be able to participate as a faculty member for our conference, "_____ ," to be held on _____ 199_ , in the Health Education Center Auditorium here at Greater Southeast Community Hospital.

Your audience will be primarily Greater Southeast nurses. We will be marketing this conference to metro-area nurses also. Other interested health care professionals may attend.

Your session is entitled "_____" and is scheduled from _____.

As we discussed, I would like you to focus on the following:

Please accept our honorarium of $ __ for this work. I have enclosed a *faculty agreement* for you to sign as well as to indicate your *audio-visual equipment* needs, and a *biographical data* form from DCNA for you to complete. Because of changing accreditation guidelines from the ANA, we can unfortunately no longer accept a C/V or resume instead of this form. Also enclosed is the *Offering Approval Documentation Form* for you to record your outline as well as teaching strategies. I would encourage you to develop *handouts* for the participant packet. Our participants have indicated that they especially like note-taking outlines. I would be happy to duplicate the handouts if you can provide me with one clear copy. I will need all of the above materials returned to me by _____ .

If you have any questions, please feel free to contact me at (202) 574-6762. I am enclosing some of the program brochures for your use. I look forward to working with you on this program!

Sincerely,

Phyllis J. Miller, RN, MS, FHE
Education Specialist
Center for Nursing Education

Attachments

Source: Greater Southeast Community Hospital, Washington, D.C. Reproduced with permission.

hart 6-7
Sample Faculty Agreement Form with Honoraria

Greater Southeast Community Hospital
Department of Nursing Education and Research

Faculty Agreement

Greater Southeast Community Hospital will pay an honorarium of
$ _____ for your presentation. Greater Southeast Community Hospital
will also produce all support materials and provide audio-visual equipment within reasonable limits necessary to the effective implementation
of your program. We reserve the right of approval on all materials.

Your acceptance of this invitation includes your agreement to effectively organize a professional learning experience for the conference
registrants within the guidelines described in the accompanying letter.
Your cooperation in meeting established deadlines for submitting data
to Greater Southeast Community Hospital is also appreciated.

I accept your invitation to speak at the (title of conference) which is
scheduled for (date).

Topic: (topic l)

_____

Date   Signature (speaker's name)   Social Security Number

AV Needs: _____

_____ 35-mm Slide Projector
_____ Overhead Projector
_____ Flipchart
_____ VCR—3/4-inch tape
_____ Electric Pointer
_____ Other

Please return no later than (return date) to: _____

    Your name
    Center for Nursing Education
    Greater Southeast Community Hospital
    1310 Southern Avenue, S.E.
    Washington, D.C. 20032

_____

Received   Associate Director, Nursing Education and Research

---

Source: Greater Southeast Community Hospital, Washington, D.C. Reproduced with permission.

Chart 6-8
Sample List of "Things to Do" Before Workshop Conference

Before Workshop Conference

		Completed
*1	Reserve conference room space	☐
*2	Develop course syllabus and evaluation tool for ANA file	☐
*3	Develop budget sheet and submit to Associate Director with syllabus for review	☐
*4	Letter of confirmation to speaker—confirm fee, how they will be paid, and request faculty agreement, DCNA bio & outline forms, A/V requests, handouts, and other needed material	☐
*5	Design brochure or flyer; select paper and ink; send to print shop..	☐
6	Design signs and send to print shop (4 weeks)..........	☐
7	Send printing for packets to print shop (2 weeks).....	☐
8	Order catering for breaks and/or meals (1–2 weeks)	☐
9	Order meal tickets and parking passes for faculty. (1–2 weeks)...	☐
10	Notify Environmental Services of room design. (5–7 days)...	☐
11	Assemble packets (3–5 days)	☐
12	Compile roster sheet of registrants, type name tags, and obtain program code number (1–3 days)	☐
13	Make arrangements for help with registration and provide with necessary materials (1–3 days)..............	☐
14	Inform Security and Dietary about number of conference attendees (1–3 days)................................	☐
15	Confirm catering (1–3 days)	☐

*14–16 weeks in advance of program

Source: Greater Southeast Community Hospital, Washington, D.C. Reproduced with permission.

The aspects of program planning are abundant. Checklists to help remember these components are helpful; several samples are provided in Charts 6-8, 6-9, and 6-10. The attention to detail paid by the staff development specialist during the program planning and design process will yield many benefits. In particular, the care and comfort of the learner, to the degree possible within organizational resources, is an essential component of any well-planned staff development activity.

Chart 6-9
Sample List of "Things to Do"
on Day of Workshop/Conference

Day of Workshop Conference

		Completed
1	Put up directional signs	☐
2	Verify room set-up and catering	☐
3	Assist with registration	☐
4	Announcement at beginning of workshop	☐
5	—location of restrooms	☐
6	—arrangements for meal	☐
7	—ANA credit/program code no./In-house and out-of-house attendance verification	☐
8	—announce "no recording" if applicable	☐
9	—upcoming program	☐
10	—evaluation sheet	☐
11	Call pulse editor for coverage of seminar	☐
12	Sign verification slips and/or certificates	☐
13		☐
14		☐
15		☐

Source: Greater Southeast Community Hospital, Washington, D.C. Reproduced with permission.

Promoting the Program

Before marketing staff development programs, the department will need to consider some issues. The answers to the issues will dictate a consistent approach to marketing that will use resources efficiently. Since thousands of dollars can potentially be spent on marketing plans, the staff development specialist must determine what resources are available and how

Chart 6-10
Sample List of "Things to Do"
Following Workshop/Conference

Following Workshop Conference

Completed

1   Compile and summarize evaluations. .... ☐

2   Submit check request for speaker(s). .... ☐

3   Thank-you letter to speaker(s). .... ☐

4   Turn in completed program file to registrar. .... ☐

5   Submit names of nonattendees to registrar for payroll deduction. .... ☐

6   Send out certificates to participants if not given out the day of the conference. .... ☐

7   .... ☐

8   .... ☐

9   .... ☐

10   .... ☐

11   .... ☐

12   .... ☐

13   .... ☐

14   .... ☐

15   .... ☐

Source: Greater Southeast Community Hospital, Washington, D.C. Reproduced with permission.

those resources will be spent in order to gain the most benefit. Following are several questions/issues that will help the staff development specialist make sound marketing decisions.

- What is the department's mission in providing staff development services?
- What staff development programs and services are available?
- Are programs considered a benefit of employment? Or will the employees pay part or all of the costs—for all programs or for selected programs?
- Who is the intended market or customer for these services? Is the market the nurse manager, the staff nurse, or nurses in the community?
- Is there a desire or need to tap new markets for staff development services? What are the benefits to the organization if new markets are tapped?
- How much resource is available (and from whom) to dedicate to marketing efforts?
- If programs are marketed to an audience other than members of the organization, then what would be the revenue expectations? How would that revenue be used?

The answers to these questions will significantly affect the marketing plan of most staff development programs.

Resources within the organization are often available to the staff development specialist to help with these decisions. For example, most health care agencies have an individual who is responsible for communications, marketing, media, and/or public relations. This individual can bring insight into many marketing issues and their advantages and disadvantages. Once the questions have been answered, specific marketing strategies can be selected to accomplish the overall marketing plan.

Most staff development departments use a blended approach to marketing programs. Approaches to internal and external marketing have commonalities and differences. While these approaches can be used creatively in a variety of ways, in general, marketing to an external customer requires some additional strategies that may not be required for the internal audience.

Once the staff development specialist defines the target audience during the planning process, the audience is questioned about whether nurses from other organizations may also benefit from the program. Programs that include information that can be applied in a variety of settings will appeal to nurses from the community; however, programs designed to help nurses learn a procedure very specific to one organization, use of forms for documentation, for example, will not appeal to other nurses.

Once the market has been determined, a marketing plan specific to the individual program is developed by the staff development specialist. Kelly[9] advocates the use of a familiar nursing model for thinking about this plan— the nursing process. This plan may be part of a larger plan or may be a prototype for an emerging plan. The marketing plan may be written and available for a reference or it may simply exist as an idea, concept or image that the department is attempting to project.

The marketing plan should begin with an assessment of the organization's needs or the internal environment. If the target audience include nurses from the community, it may be appropriate to determine the needs of that group (which serves as the external environment). This can be done simply through informal surveys and questions of participants or quite elaborately with formal marketing surveys. This assessment also includes an estimation of how much money and resource are available for marketing. If funds are limited, the marketing effort must also be limited. Greater funds will allow the marketing plan to include professional assistance with image projection, brochure development, direct mail services, and analysis of each strategy. Fewer resources may mean that the staff development specialist will develop brochures and flyers internally, on available equipment, and manually address and send the promotional piece to the target market. The range of marketing options is primarily driven by the available resources and occasionally by the creativity of the staff development specialist. Data gathered during the assessment will determine the type of marketing plan possible.

The planning process of the marketing plan will specify how all available resources will be used. If new markets are to be penetrated, the marketing products will have to be developed. If a design for marketing products is already in place, the planning process may only include using the organization's system to develop the marketing piece. If the decision is to limit a program to the internal audience only, a simple flyer may be all that is needed to effectively market a program. The department may also have a standard format in design, color, typeface, and type of information that is included in all promotional pieces. In these cases, the planning step merely selects the appropriate vehicle. The planning phase also includes a timeline for release of materials and products related to the program or programs in the marketing plan.

Once the plan is developed, implementation begins with the development of the actual materials for distribution. Using the timeline developed in the planning phase, the staff development specialist coordinates the development and distribution of promotional materials. These are often in the form of calendars, brochures, and catalogs. They may take other forms such as letters and invitations. Receptions, special events, and meetings are occasionally used to promote new services and programs.

The most important issue during the implementation stage is timing. Using the planned timeline, marketing materials must be received by potential participants within a timeframe that allows them to make a decision. Most participants will need to arrange schedules to participate. This takes time, particularly when the individual is part of a staffing system. Generally, the timeline should include an eight- to twelve-week notice for participants. This means program information and brochures, particularly those sent in the mail, should be developed sixteen weeks before the planned program and be ready to mail twelve to fourteen weeks in advance of the program. Internally marketed programs may require less time; however, less then eight weeks notice may have an effect on participation, unless the program is required and administrative plans are made for participation.

External Marketing

Direct mail is the most common form of external marketing used by staff development specialists. Direct mail pieces send many messages and the staff development specialist should consider carefully what message will be sent with any promotional piece sent from the organization. Does the piece *promote* the organization and the staff development program? What message does the piece communicate? Marketing professionals may be able to help answer these questions with several examples. However, staff development specialists can also use their own experience as recipients of direct mail pieces used to promote programs. To do this, asked to be placed on mailing lists of colleagues and other providers of programs. Watch the mail for other promotional materials. Look for style and design differences and similarities that are attractive. As the department begins to develop a feel for what is attractive, these feelings will need to be verbalized and put into graphic form. Graphic artists are often used to help conceptualize images into a tangible form such as a brochure or flyer.

The promotional pieces must be geared to the department's identified customer. The image of the department's institution is also reflected in the materials. For example, a very conservative institution will use a more staid approach to the marketing brochure and other direct-mail pieces. Many health care organizations have some sort of identifying logo. It is not uncommon for this logo to be required on all materials released from the organization.

Once a design is developed for direct mail and other promotional pieces, it should be used consistently on all pieces. This approach will enhance the staff development program in the market. If all brochures, flyers, and catalogs look similar, name recognition will follow. The design can also be incorporated into conference folders, name tags, and other conference materials. Thus, the department's image is further represented.

Brochure copy, the most important component of the promotional piece, should focus on the benefits to the customer. Everything in the brochure should be written in terms of the gains the nurse will experience as a result of participation. Copy should also be written in the second person and familiar language used. For example, "If you attend this program, you will increase your knowledge and ability to care for...." or "Tired of not getting it all done? If you attend this program, you will learn thirty ways to perform your patient care more efficiently!"

The cover of the brochure is also an essential element in catching the potential participant's interest. The title should provide enough information to draw attention. The phrases used in the titles of programs should be consistent with the image, and care must be exercised to clearly state titles to the potential respondents. The cover of the brochure should also include the sponsoring organization in a prominent position.

The brochure or promotional piece should include at least the following information:

- Title
- Date, time, and place
- Program description
- Objectives
- Target audience
- Program schedule
- Faculty biography
- Registration information

- Contact hour information
- Cancellation/refund policy
- Phone number for additional information

It is better to err on the side of giving too much information than not enough. Research has shown that nurses are more likely to attend a program if the above information is provided as a minimum.[10]

To begin writing brochure copy, the staff development specialist should think about the person for whom the program is planned, and then write copy directed to that person. How will the program enhance the participant's professional development? The copy should match the person to whom it is being sent in terms of personalization, sophistication, and tone. Sample statements can include items like "our faculty will help you recognize key elements of interpretation of common dysrhythmias," or "we will assist you in developing your skills with...," or "you will leave the conference with a nursing management plan for...."

Another way to feature program benefits is to use a bulletin board to highlight benefits for attending the program. Alternatively, several questions might be presented, followed by a statement such as, "Attend this program and get answers to these and other questions!" Testimonials from participants of previous offerings may also be used to sell the benefits of attending the department's programs; however, permission from the participant is necessary if the individual is identified.

Some of these same principles can be used by the staff development specialist for internal marketing. Informational flyers are more commonly used and the amount of detail may be limited by space. However, the principle of appealing with language to the potential participant prevails.

Internal Marketing

Internal marketing of the staff development program to the organization's own nurses cannot be overlooked or minimized. These nurses represent the core of customers for any staff development program based within an organization.

Successful staff development programs do not just happen. They are the result of careful planning and deliberate intervention. Successful programs are tightly linked to the organization's goals and objectives. They look at the genuine needs of the organization and focus on its mission and goals. This immediately builds internal credibility for the program, as staff know that this program can help them meet organizational goals. It is clear how these efforts market the program internally.

The savvy staff development specialist knows where the organization is going and assists with the journey. They know what new programs and services are planned for the future and forecast the anticipated learning needs. The staff development specialist knows what services are being phased out and begins to temper energies devoted to development in those areas. On a day-to-day basis, the specialist is in tune with the areas the organization is concerned about and is planning and/or providing programs that address those needs.

Successful staff development specialists are often considered the eyes and ears of the organization. They have contact with many people and can listen for common themes among the nursing staff, and essentially "take the pulse" of the organization. The specialist also has the ability and perspective to step back and look to where the organization is headed and determine answers to questions. These questions might include, What are the values? What is the corporate culture?" and What are the norms? Successful staff development specialists then work to have an impact on that culture through building coalitions among appropriate players to make the necessary changes. One of the most common formats for assisting the change process is education. Thus, the importance of using information gleaned from internal sources to design the internal marketing effort is recognized.

The work accomplished by the staff development specialist with the program participants and their managers is the most important aspect of the internal marketing effort. Gaining commitment from these individuals is crucial to the achievement of the staff development intervention. From the first contact in which needs are identified to the last evaluation report, elements of marketing are used. These elements include the following:

- Work with the manager to meet perceived and actual needs.
- Obtain frequent feedback to ensure that needs are adequately addressed.
- Involve learners early in program development.
- Remain enthusiastic about the potential effects of the program.
- Continue to talk about the benefits to the unit and staff as a result of participation.
- Ask for the order, that is, gain commitment about how many participants will attend the program.

Involving learners at the outset of the program planning process is another essential component of internal marketing. This should occur during the needs assessment phase when the potential participants are asked to identify their own needs related to the topic planned. The staff development specialist can ask the learners for their ideas about program content, program focus, and data for case studies. These learners are clinical experts and can provide the clinical reality and credibility needed to resolve patient care problems and issues on a day-to-day basis. They will have unmatched, first-hand, experience-based knowledge to contribute. This acknowledgement of their experience also positions the learners and the staff development specialist as partners engaged in a mutual effort to improve practice, each with something to offer the other.

Another way to continue the staff development process, achieve commitment, and help nurses fully recognize the need for life-long learning is to use selected staff nurses as faculty members for portions of programs. This approach provides positive feedback for their recognized abilities and is an excellent developmental opportunity. It provides a chance for the nurses to enhance their teaching skills and gain new knowledge. Through coaching and supportive exchanges, the staff development specialist can assist the nurse as the requisite teaching skills are developed. Using similar processes used by the specialists themselves, the nurse can be helped to learn about and use the teaching–learning strategies necessary to impart knowledge and skill.

The first and final comprehensive aspect of internal marketing is the continual involvement of the customer in all elements of the planning process. This involvement will directly affect the success of the program as it becomes "owned" by the consumer, and as all become committed to the success of the staff development program.

Projecting Costs and Benefits

Accountability for the effectiveness of the staff development program is an economical organizational expectation. The staff development specialist is in a unique position to demonstrate how the development of personnel can benefit the organization. Through the use of selected formulas and reports, the effectiveness and benefits of staff development can be measured and explained.

Though the financial analysis of staff development is an evolving one, specialists can modify and use formulas and approaches used in other fields to suit their purpose. The difficult issue is the effort to quantify the quality-of-life questions that arise in any financial analysis strategy in health care. Regardless, staff development specialists are expected to use measures and demonstrate productivity and effectiveness to the organization. In organizations where this does not occur, the staff development program may be an early victim of cost-cutting measures during times of scarce resources.

Cost Analysis of Staff Development Programs

The analysis of staff development activities takes many approaches. The specific approach used is grounded in the decision the staff development specialist needs to make. Several common approaches are as follows:

- Project selected direct costs, such as the speaker fees, materials, and food costs
- Project selected indirect costs, such as electricity and space costs
- Project staff development specialist time for program planning, implementation, and evaluation
- Project learner costs
- A combination of the above

Kelly[11] has enumerated other costs that may be included in a cost analysis:

- Planning costs—including the salary and benefit costs of the planning committee and specialist
- Cost of curriculum development—usually the specialist's salary, though it may include resources such as books and library search costs

- Faculty fees—including travel, lodging, and occasionally the development of materials and audio-visuals
- In-house instructor salary and benefits
- Coordinator salary and benefits
- Secretary and clerical support and benefits
- Program material expenses—such as folders, work materials, and name tags
- Cost of software and hardware—prorated over the life of materials such as films, videos and equipment
- Marketing costs—including brochure development, printing, postage, and mail handling
- Telephone expenses
- Program administration costs
- Cost of overhead—rental space for the staff development department
- Cost of miscellaneous supplies
- Learner salaries
- Replacement costs for learners in the clinical areas if overtime is necessary to replace learners

Learner Salary

The most significant cost to any organization for staff development is the loss in patient care hours while staff are acquiring new knowledge and skills.[11] Identified as "learner salary" in most approaches, it remains the single most costly feature of staff development. Therefore, staff development specialists must be very judicious in their design of programs and use staff time spent away from patient care very efficiently. These costs represent an investment by the organization in its staff, and the outcome of staff development should be viewed as a return on that investment.

A quick way to calculate the learner salary is to calculate (or ask personnel to calculate) an average salary of various learners and multiply that salary by the number of anticipated learners and the number of hours spent in the staff development program. For example, if the RN average salary is $20/hour and 25 nurses are expected for an eight-hour program, the learner salary is calculated by multiplying $20/hourly salary x 25 learners x 8 hours in class = $4000. This figure should be used by the staff development specialist to raise the consciousness of managers and learners about the investment of the organization related to the staff's knowledge development.

Reporting Results of Cost Analyses

In general, reports of costs without an indication of outcomes, effectiveness, or benefit are incomplete. Most specialists use an approach in which the costs are reported in ratio to the effectiveness or benefits of the program. Cost-effectiveness and cost-benefit analysis formulas are commonly used. Cost-effectiveness analysis compares the dollars spent in a program with educational outcomes (effectiveness). Cost-benefit analysis compares the dollars spent on the staff development program with the dollar benefits expected of the program.

Decisions regarding which of these tools to use for financial analysis must be made by the staff development specialist based on how the information will be used. The best use of these data is for improvement of the efficiency and effectiveness of the program. If the staff development specialist can demonstrate the efficient use of resources and analyses in which efforts to improve efficiency and effectiveness are enacted with results, the specialist will experience success with this area. However, if the specialist is not able to show cost analysis and resource allocation decisions based on these analyses, then the staff development program may not be viewed as a contribution to the achievement of goals within the organization.

The decision regarding which costs to collect is also an element of how the results will be used. For example, for overall budget planning purposes, it may be necessary to collect only direct costs related to faculty fees and honoraria, materials, and supplies. In other cases of a more comprehensive analysis, additional costs may be analyzed.

Cost-Benefit Analysis

Cost-benefit analysis examines the costs incurred by a staff development program compared with the dollar value of the benefits achieved by the program. Programs are used as strategies for changing the behavior of staff. Many benefits can be realized through an educational program:[12]

- Improved patient care
- Decreased length of stay
- More efficient care delivery
- Decreased errors and incidents
- Reduction in turnover
- Decreased absenteeism
- Less medical supply use
- Fewer workman's compensation claims
- Decreased litigation costs
- Fewer grievances
- Increased productivity
- Less turnover
- Higher employee job satisfaction

The calculation of these costs may provide a challenge to the staff development specialist. With persistent questions of key members of selected departments of the organization, for example, personnel and legal affairs, the staff development specialist's investigation will yield cost data that can be used for analysis. Explanations about how the information will be used will be necessary in most cases. Assistance should be sought to understand how to best use the data as they become available. If approached diplomatically, with an explanation of the cost-benefit analysis project, most employees of other departments will assist with cost data collection.

Many benefits will be calculated with an estimation of what could be saved. For example, reduced litigation expenses can be calculated by using the average cost of each litigation currently facing the organization and estimating which if any can be reduced as they relate to the program under analysis. The calculation of reduced turnover may be estimated based on the cost of recruiting new staff members and projecting a percentage of this cost that may be reduced as a result of the staff development program under analysis.

Most of these items and others can be compared with the costs of conducting the staff development program. Using these figures, decisions can be made about resource allocation. These figures are expressed as a benefit to cost ratio as follows:

$$\frac{\text{Benefit}}{\text{Costs}} = \text{Benefit:Cost Ratio}$$

To interpret the figures, the staff development specialist should think, "for every dollar (cost) invested in this program, a potential benefit of X dollars may be realized." An example of this analysis applied to a body mechanics program is provided in Table 6-1.

Cost-Effectiveness Analysis

Another method for analyzing the financial costs of a program is to use a cost-effectiveness formula advocated by del Bueno and Kelly.[13] This method requires a calculation of total program costs and computes a value based on the "cost per participant hour." This cost per participant hour value is then compared with an outcome value. If the two values are in ratio—that is, equal—then the program is considered to be cost-effective. If, however, the cost value is higher than the effectiveness value, then the program is inefficient and should be revised to achieve better outcomes or use less resource.

This formula is useful in comparing different instructional modalities, in making decisions about investing human and financial resources in a new program, and in making decisions about continuing a program.

Cost Comparisons

Elements of these financial analyses can also be used to compare the costs of one teaching strategy with another. Table 6-2 provides a comparison of the costs of a traditional lecture format in a classroom setting with those of a self-learning package. Decisions about strategies and their cost to the organization can be made on the basis of these comparisons.

Generating Revenue

Some staff development departments are expected to generate revenue. Others may be asked if revenue generation is possible. And yet others may choose to generate revenue to make a contribution to the organization. The decision to generate revenue is a serious one and should be made cautiously. The following questions must be considered:

- How much revenue will be generated?
- How much resource is available to begin the process of revenue generation?

Table 6-1
Cost-Benefit Analysis for a Hypothetical
Body Mechanics Program

Costs

Planning/Development	
Based on no. of hours of instructor time =	
3 x Salary of $15/hr	$45.00
Implementation	
Instructor salary	
Salary at $15/hr x 1-hr class	$15.00
Learner salary	
Salary at $10/hr for 35 learners	$350.00
Total Cost of Program	**$410.00**

Benefits

Reduced worker's compensation claims	
6 cases less per year @ $600 per claim	$3600.00
Reduce cost of processing claims	
Hospital representative @ $25/hr x	
2 hrs each claim x 6 claims	$300.00
Reduced absenteeism	
6 employees x 2.5 weeks =	
600 hours x $10/hr employee salary	$6000.00
Total Projected Benefits	**$9900.00**

Total benefits: $9900.00
Total costs: $410.00

Benefit:Cost ratio = 9900/410 = $24.15 Return on investment

Statement: For every dollar invested in this program, a potential return of $24.15 is projected.

Note: The staff development specialist would calculate the actual benefit during a follow-up evaluation of this program to measure actual benefit.

Table 6-2
Cost Comparison of Traditional Inservice Program and SLP

Cost Comparison
Program Title: Infection Control
Estimated number of participants: 500 per year per program

Traditional Inservice		SLP	
Planning/Development	$30.00	**Planning/Development**	$150.00
Based on no. hrs instructor time (3) x salary ($10/hr)		No. hrs spent developing (15) x salary ($10/hr)	
Implementation		**Implementation**	
Instructor Salary	$250.00	*Covers*	$25.00
Salary ($10/hr) x no. actual hrs taught (25)		Cost of covers ($0.50) x 50	
Learner Salary	$4000.00	*Copying*	$25.00
Salary ($8/hr) x no. hrs in class (1) x no. participants (500)		Cost ($0.50) x 50	
Materials	—	*System*	$10.00
		Instructor salary ($10/hr) x 1 hr to maintain system	
Total	**$4280.00**	**Total**	**$60.00**
Evaluation		**Evaluation**	$50.00
		Instructor salary x no. hrs to grade post-test	
Total cost	$4280.00	Total cost	$260.00
Total no. participant hrs	500.00	Total no. participant hrs	500.00
Cost per Participant Hour	$8.56	**Cost per Participant Hour**	$0.52

151

- How will the revenue be used?
- How will the accounting system be set up,
- Who will participate in the process?
- What happens if projected revenue is not generated?
- What are the benefits and costs of such an effort?

Each organization's staff development department approaches revenue generation differently. Some must provide a certain level of programs that will generate a predicted amount of revenue and an individual is often dedicated for that sole purpose. Subsequently, if the programs fail to generate the projected revenue, that individual is at risk. Other staff development departments market selected programs to the community of nurses, charge a fee, and generate revenue from these fees. These fees may offset some of the costs of the program. However, it is the rare case in which the costs of the entire staff development effort can be offset with this approach. In fact, the organization should not expect it to generate enough revenue to cover all costs.

The staff development program is a service to the organization and exists to assist the organization in reaching its goals. Therefore, it also has inherent costs to the organization, as any investment would. The staff development department usually represents less than 1% of the total operating budget of the organization, and the contribution made by most departments far outweighs the cost of the program.

A decision to generate revenue can be made using the following steps:

1. Review the department's mission statement. If the mission statement is totally focused on internal services, yet the organization is focused on new revenue-generating initiatives, the mission statement may need to be revised or at least questioned.
2. If revenue will be generated, decide what products the department will sell. Some products will require a significant effort and others will require less. For example, selling self-learning packages and other work manuals requires a strategic plan to generate revenue that will exceed the costs of the effort. Marketing selected programs to the local market may require less effort and resource, particularly if it is done on a trial basis using internal resources.
3. Set reasonable limits on the amount of resource and effort used for the purpose of revenue generation. In some organization, so much energy is dedicated to revenue generation that normal, expected, and required staff development activities suffer. The department may lose credibility within the organization if it is unable to meet its primary mission. Decide where the revenue will go—a staff development department's image may be enhanced if revenue is contributed to the general fund, rather than maintained within the department, since the revenue was generated using resources from the general fund.
4. Recognize all benefits to a revenue generation project. For example, if a program is marketed to the community of nurses and they subsequently decide to work within the organization, a spillover benefit of recruitment is experienced. If employed nursing staff see nurses

from other organizations participating in their education programs, it may be a source of pride and increased job satisfaction and thus contribute to retention.

5. Report all results to key individuals in administration, including actual costs and actual revenue generated after a specified period of time. Make recommendations about continuing, expanding, or terminating the effort. Include costs of each recommended option.

Other benefits of marketing staff development programs to the community include an increased visibility and image projection opportunity. For example, if the nursing department has a desire to position itself as a progressive one, the marketing plan to generate revenue should include specific strategies to project a progressive image. This includes the careful development of copy and materials to accomplish this goal, in addition to revenue generation. If no particular image projection project is identified, the organization can be positioned as supporting staff development within an active, growing environment that is interested in the continuing development and education of their nurses.

Summary

This chapter has presented elements of the program planning process essential for the staff development specialist. Included in this process is the use of needs assessment data, the selection of appropriate teaching and learning strategies, and the design of those strategies to accomplish learning objectives. Strategies for internal and external marketing were outlined along with financial analysis methods such as cost-benefit, cost-effectiveness analysis and cost comparison. The staff development specialist will find this chapter a valuable resource for planning comprehensive staff development programs.

References

1. Krathwol, D. R., Bloom, B. S., & Masia, B. (1964). *Taxonomy of educational objectives, Handbook II*. New York: David McKay.
2. Houle, C. O. (1978). *The design of education*. San Francisco: Jossey-Bass.
3. Alspach, J. (1982). How to prepare a lecture presentation. *Focus on Critical Care, 9*, 27–32.
4. O'Connor, A. B. (1986). *Nursing staff development and continuing education*. Boston: Little, Brown.
5. Cooper, S. S. (1983). *The practice of continuing education in nursing*. Rockville, MD: Aspen.
6. Verduin, J. R., Miller, H. G., & Green, C. E. (1978). *Adults teaching adults*. Austin, TX: Learning Concepts.
7. Armistead, C. (1984). *How useful are case studies? Training and Development Journal, 38*, 75–77.

8. Miller, P. J. (1989). Developing self-learning packages. *Journal of Nursing Staff Development. 5,* 73–77.

9. Kelly, K. J. (1987). Marketing. In Puetz, B. E., *Contemporary strategies for continuing education in nursing.* Rockville, MD: Aspen.

10. Kelly, K. J. (1983). *Marketing continuing education programs: Study preferences of Washington Metropolitan area nurses.* Master's thesis. Virginia Polytechnic Institute and State University, Blacksburg, VA.

11. Kelly, K. J. (1985). Cost-benefit and cost-effectiveness analysis: Tools for the staff development manager. *Journal of Nursing Staff Development, 1,* 9–15.

12. Maryland Chapter of the American Society for Healthcare Education and Training (MASHET) (1985). *Measuring accountability in healthcare education.* Unpublished manuscript. Chicago: American Hospital Association.

13. del Bueno, D., & Kelly, K. J. (1980). How cost effective is your staff development program? *Journal of Nursing Administration, 4,* 31–36.

Chapter 7

Implementing the Staff Development Program: Organizing to Meet the Institution's Needs

Judith F. Warmuth

Staff development departments are responsible for providing a total program that uses resources efficiently to assess, maintain, and develop the competencies of nursing personnel. To accomplish this task, a typical week of staff development activities may include

- *Manager workshops on quality assurance*
- *Unit support for computer changes in the order entry system*
- *New nursing employee orientation*
- *Basic dysrhythmia interpretation classes*
- *Unit-based inservices on new intravenous therapy pumps*

   How do these things happen? Who organizes them? What does it take to implement them? The schedule above is an actual one. It reflects the activity of a department in a 400-bed community hospital. The activities reflect only basic programming—that which is required for the organization to successfully achieve its mission. This chapter discusses the operation of a staff development department; how to get it organized, how to schedule programs, how to use resources efficiently and effectively, and how to decide if the need has been met. Based on the combination of knowledge and experience, this pragmatic chapter also includes good questions to raise as program decisions are being made. Answers to these questions will differ in each organization. However, the questions will provide the staff development specialist with a framework from which good program decisions can be made.

Purpose

Staff development departments can serve many purposes and provide many services. Unfortunately, departments usually cannot provide all the services frequently expected, due to limited human and financial resources. For example, a department may develop an annual orientation schedule, including reserving rooms and assigning staff only to be requested to provide orientation for new nurses on a demand basis. Another example of this issue of expected versus available service is the response of a nurse manager to a carefully planned major program with the feeling that the program is not specific enough to meet unit needs. A departmental goal of increasing efficiency by increasing class size may conflict with an institutional goal to decrease dollars paid for classroom time.

Developing and communicating a purpose statement may help resolve some of these issues. It is a requisite component of department design and program decisions. It is also a key to guide the appropriate response to requests and expectations from consumers of staff development services. A clear statement of the purpose and mission of the staff development department and program lays the groundwork for resource allocation and program requests. Routine appraisal and monitoring of the effectiveness of the program is also based on this purpose, answering the question, Are we doing what we set out to do?

There are many ways to develop a mission or purpose statement. Most strategies could also be used to evaluate or revise an existing statement. A strategy that surveys the users and consumers of staff development services is an effective one. Managers and staff can be asked about what functions are the most valuable in their view, and what services are valuable but need improving. These same groups can also be asked what needs are essential to meet. Interviewees can also be asked to rank and value identified needs and goals in order to build a staff development program that is responsive to client needs. Forced choice questions can also be asked to focus the program. For example, a series of questions in which the client is forced to select the more important one from two such as "orientation on demand *or* regularly scheduled using preceptor support." Other interview strategies could include an analysis of answers provided to a question such as What constitutes the ideal staff development department? or When is the staff development department most helpful to you? Least helpful? Developing a consumer focus is not a new idea, but a structured assessment of the customer's perspective will strengthen the department's purpose.

Another method for developing a mission or purpose statement would be to use the members of the department to create a description of what exists. A document that communicates the current scope and function of a department communicates to the institution a description of the current situation and sets a framework for expectations. It could include services provided, individuals providing the service, limitations, and methods used. Charts 7-1 and 7-2 illustrate an example of this approach.

If your institution has a strategic planning process in place, a written statement which indicates the contribution that staff development makes to achievement of strategic goals may become the department's mission.

The mission statement can be worded in many ways. For example:

- Providing the resources needed by staff nurses in the giving of care is the purpose of....
- Staff development at (name of) hospital provides structured educational experiences....
- Orientation of new employees and limited consultation to units developing their own programs are provided by....
- Efficient use of limited resources requires the following priorities....

Chart 7-3 illustrates one mission statement, another can be found in Chapter 2. A purpose statement could also be a simple listing of services provided by the department or program.

In addition to describing the "what is" of staff development, development of the mission statement provides the opportunity to examine what could be. Staff development departments and programs can be structured in many ways, deliver many kinds of services, and provide very different resources. Listed below are nine questions which may be used to review the department's mission and purpose.

1. Who are the customers you seek to satisfy? (the organization, nurse managers, or staff nurses, all or some of those listed, others, are some more important than others?)
2. Do your learners come to you or do you go to them?
3. Are your services provided mainly in classrooms or in the clinical areas or both? If both, what is the ratio of class to clinical?
4. Do staff development specialists teach, coordinate, consult, or collaborate? Some of each or all? If all, in what ratio?
5. Do nursing staff teach, coordinate, consult, and collaborate with staff development?
6. Are staff development specialists also expected to be clinical specialists?
7. Is nursing leadership and management development part of the expected staff development program or not? If yes, how much programming is expected? And what resources will be used to provide the service?
8. Does the design of the staff development program use other than the classroom lecture method? If yes, are there interactive and learner-driven methods also available? If so, what are expectations about the use of these methods by nursing staff?
9. What goals are primary and fundamental? Are departmental goals more important that meeting changing needs? What dictates how the department will respond to requests for service?

Other questions may also be added to the list to help develop or refine the staff development mission and purpose statements. As institutions change and as health care changes, staff development programs and departments must also change and adapt to meet institutional needs. Three questions should always be asked during any review of a mission and purpose statement. The

Chart 7-1
Sample Scope of Services Document

Scope of Service

Center for Nursing Education

In this hospital, the Center for Nursing Education provides comprehensive staff development services for approximately 875 Patient Care Services personnel. Personnel in the Patient Care Services division include primarily:

- Registered Nurses
- Licensed Practical Nurses
- Medical Surgical Technicians
- Specialty Technicians (i.e., Operating Room Technicians, Emergency Room Technicians, Delivery Room Technicians)
- Unit Secretaries and Managers

Considered a management tool for achieving behavior change in employees, these services are based on identified organizational needs and priorities and include:

- Orientation
- Inservice Education
- Continuing Education
- Skills Training
- Leadership Development
- Group/Unit/Team Development
- Credentialing/Assessment Centers

Definitions of these services can be found in CNE 116 Nursing Education Program Definitions.

The following services are delivered through a variety of mechanisms and include:

---

first is "What are we?" The second is "What do we want to be?" and the third is "What could we be?" These questions help guide the many decisions made every day related to who gets what service, when, and in what way. In addition, the statements help the staff development specialist select strategies and goals for program implementation. Finally, the mission and purpose statements guide the use of limited resources and help the specialist decide what can and cannot be offered as a service of the staff development program.

- Direct Provision of Education
- Collaboration
- Support
- Coordination
- Counseling
- Consultation

Definitions of these service delivery mechanisms can be found in CNE-121.0 Service Delivery Mechanisms.

In addition, the staff of CNE serve on a variety of task forces and committees that help further the work of this department and the organization.

The services described above are provided by the following CNE staff:

- Education Specialists
  (4.0 FTE)
- Diabetes Educator (1.0 FTE)
- Enterostomal Therapist
  (1.0 FTE)
- Nutrition Support Nurse
  (1.0 FTE)

The department is administered by the Associate Director of Nursing for Education and Research. In addition, a CNE systems manager oversees the development and maintenance of automated and manual systems to enhance work flow and program management. Additional information about each of these roles is delineated in CNE 122 through CNE 130 Position Descriptions, CNE 118 CNE Structure, CNE 114 Education Communication Chart

The department hours are Monday through Friday from 8:30 A.M. to 5:00 P.M. However, services are provided on a routine and regular basis to all three shifts of personnel as dictated by program and development needs.

Resources

It is the people in a staff development department that make a program work efficiently and effectively. Instructional staff is usually made up of registered nurses with additional preparation in adult learning theory, teaching theory, curriculum and program planning, and design and program evaluation. Current recommendations for the staff development specialist role

hart 7-2
Sample List of Individuals Responsible
for Providing Staff Development Services

The Center for Nursing Education is composed of the following members:

Associate Director of Nursing for Education and Research   (l)

A nurse with demonstrated expert clinical practice and expertise in the teaching learning process and administration. Accountable to the Vice President for Patient Care Services, this individual is responsible for designing, implementing, and evaluating an educational program that supports the established philosophy and framework of the PCS department and the NER department. This individual is also responsible for budget preparation and control, education policy development, and supervision and development of CNE staff. In addition, this individual is responsible for facilitating the research process within the philosophy and guidelines of the PCS department.

Nursing Education Specialists   (4)

Nurses with demonstrated expert clinical practice and expertise in the entire teaching learning process. Accountable to the Associate Director, NER, these individuals are responsible for designing, implementing, and evaluating assigned educational programs *and* instruction in those programs. In addition, these individuals are responsible for participating in education policy development and other PCS committee activities that support the goals and objectives of the PCS department.

Nutrition Support Nurse   (l)

This individual is responsible for assessing and monitoring patients receiving enteral and parenteral nutrition support. A member of the Nutrition Support Team, this nurse is responsible for assuring that patients receiving nutrition support are receiving appropriate and relevant nursing care.

include a BSN and graduate preparation in the areas listed above. Licensed practical nurses and unit clerks, managers, or coordinators may also be part of the instructional staff if the department is also responsible for the preparation and orientation of assistive nursing personnel and unit assistants.

Staff Development Specialists

The job description for the staff development specialist is usually quite broad and includes the following:

Enterostomal Therapists (2)

Nurses certified by the International Association of Enterostomal Therapists, and who also demonstrate expert clinical practice in the areas of
ostomy care and wound and tissue trauma management. Familiar with
the teaching learning process, these nurses also demonstrate excellent
teaching qualities. Accountable to the Associate Director, NER, these
individuals are responsible for the delivery of enterostomal therapy services to patients and clinical consultation to nurses, physicians, and
other health care professionals. In addition, these nurses are also
responsible for participating in committees and other activities that support the goals and objectives of the PCS department. (2 ETs filling 1
FTE)

Health Educator (1)

A nurse prepared to conduct specific education programs including diabetes and community hypertension screening programs. Familiar with
the teaching–learning process, this nurse also demonstrates expert
teaching qualities. Accountable to the Associate Director, NER, this individual is responsible for organizing, implementing, and evaluating specific patient education programs.

Systems Manager (1)

Accountable to the Associate Director, NER, this individual designs,
implements, evaluates, and maintains automated and nonautomated
office systems that enhance the efficiency and effectiveness of the
department. Responsible for providing some secretarial support for
nursing education programs, this individual is also responsible for educational record keeping and maintenance. In addition, this individual is
responsible for participating in policy development for areas related to
records maintenance and program documentation.

Source: Greater Southeast Community Hospital, Washington, D.C. Reproduced with permission.

- Assessing learner and institutional needs
- Designing, implementing, and evaluating learning experiences
- Clinical instruction
- Problem solving and group leadership skills
- Well-developed communication skills
- Ability to motivate and stimulate
- Enthusiasm, flexibility, tolerance for ambiguity, and endurance

The description of the work of the staff development specialist may
seem exceptional but also may be congruent with organizational expecta-

Chart 7-3
Sample Mission Statement

The Division of Nursing Education, Practice and Research provides services to nursing personnel, patients, and families.

We provide educational services which include inservices, continuing education programming, orientation, and clinical teaching.

We promote quality care for patients and families by direct involvement and through consultation with nursing staff and other disciplines.

We assist nursing staff to integrate research finding into nursing practice and participate in research studies.

We provide leadership through involvement on committees, setting nursing standards, and promoting the professional image of nursing within Meriter and the community.

The Division is comprised of Nurse Educators, Clinical Nurse Specialists, a Patient Education Coordinator, a Nursing Information Systems Coordinator, a Nursing Quality Assurance Coordinator, an Administrative Assistant, and secretarial staff.

Source: Meriter Hospital, Madison, Wisconsin. Reproduced with permission.

tions. Staff development specialists need a well-developed capacity for self direction. In return, specialists have the opportunity to influence nursing practice through staff development interventions on an ongoing basis.

Staff development specialists have often been competent and successful clinical nurses. They have also demonstrated a willingness to be learners and have a flexible attitude toward job conditions. The specialist position is often a promotion for a staff nurse and a lateral transfer for a nurse manager. Staff development specialists generally enter the role without formal preparation and require development within the role. Support, education, and structured experiences for new staff development specialists are essential for successful orientation to this evolving role. Historically, staff development specialists learned the role through trial and error and on-the-job training. Today, much more is known about what works within staff development. Therefore, new staff development specialists should benefit from this history and be helped to learn the role in the same way clinical nurses are helped to learn their new roles.

A department with several instructors may have the luxury of a preceptorlike relationship between a new educator and a more experienced one. This relationship can have all the benefits of staff nurse preceptor roles including role modeling, immediate feedback, and incrementally complex assignments.

Clerical Staff

Clerical staff are critical to the efficient, day-to-day operation of a staff development department. Many department functions can be accomplished without the use of instructor time. Clerical staff may be responsible for the registration process and system, including creating rosters, name tags, and evaluation tallies. In addition, they can prepare learner packets and accumulate, copy, and distribute handout materials. They may also be assigned to prepare transparencies and slides for use during programs. Another common area of assignment for the clerical staff is the reservation of space for staff development programs. Routine class schedules, records, and reports are also within the scope of the staff development clerical personnel. Additional functions may include inventory control of regularly used handouts and packets, management of audio-visual and software previews, and purchases. The generation of regular reports to nurse managers regarding staff attendance at selected programs, such as CPR, fire safety, infection control, and other required programs, may also be assigned to a staff development support person. Chart 7-4 illustrates the role and responsibility of a staff development support person, titled Systems Manager, in a large community hospital.

Exceptional organizational skill, ability to deal with multiple issues, and a helpful, service-oriented approach are critical prerequisites for support staff. In an efficient department, instructional staff are often in the clinical area or classroom and support staff are the primary contact. If a staff development program or department is to be well-utilized by hospital staff, help must be available when needed or requested. For example, a knowledgeable, helpful response by a secretary to a nurse about scheduled programs will have a more positive effect on the nurse's willingness to participate in an activity than an unanswered phone.

Learner Time

Learner time may seem like an odd category of resource. It is essential that staff development specialists recognize that every moment spent in a staff development activity is a lost patient care moment. Learner time spent in learning activities can be justified as contributing to improved quality of care, and it is up to the staff development specialist to assure that the time is necessary and well spent—that there will be a return on the investment for the patient and the organization.

Discussions with nurse managers during the planning of staff development programs will yield greater cooperation and collaboration. As a result of these discussions, nurse managers will be able to plan and budget for classroom hours, as they are assured that classroom time will help the unit reach care delivery goals through the staff development activity. In addition, the staff development specialist will be able to plan and schedule programs to accomplish the greatest good. Negotiation and compromises about realistic goals for attendance and program format may need to be made between nurse managers and staff development specialists. However, mutual goal set-

hart 7-4
Roles and Responsibilities of Staff Development
Support Person

Position Title: CNE Systems Manager

Reports to: Associate Director, NER

General Responsibilities

The incumbent will design, implement, evaluate, and maintain office systems that will enhance the efficiency and effectiveness of the Center for Nursing Education (CNE) and related programs. The CNE produces over 500 educational offerings each year. The staff of CNE also administer several special programs including the Clinical Ladder Program, the Nursing Research Program, CPR, Self-Learning Packages, Diabetes Education, Dermal Ulcer Management, and Nutrition Support. In addition, selected programs are accredited by the American Nurses' Association, the American Heart Association, and the American Diabetes Association. These programs require a highly skilled and creative individual to develop and manage automated systems for documenting all related activities. The individual will supervise assigned clerical help to assist in the implementation of these programs. All activities are directed toward enhancing the efficiency and effectiveness of all services and programs offered through CNE.

Tasks Performed

Design, implement, evaluate, and maintain office systems, both automated and nonautomated.

Change or recommend change in office systems for greater productivity and effectiveness.

Supervise five users of NBI word processing system and all users of office PC.

Administer employee transcript system:
- Maintain data base.
- Post classes.
- Generate transcripts.
- Generate activity reports.
- Evaluate software used and enhance as needed for increased efficiency and effectiveness.

Maintain education program records system:
- Evaluate record for completeness.
- Maintain over 500 offerings into a retrieval system.

Manage the accredited CE program records:
- Generate faculty agreements and contracts.
- Maintain compliance to accreditation body requirements.

Administer CPR program:
- Schedule classes.
- Schedule employees for class.
- Retest selected employees.
- Comply with American Heart Association requirements.
- Pay faculty.
- Maintain CPR tracking system:
     Maintain data base.
     Post classes.
     Generate reports.

Design, implement and evaluate an automated departmental budget tracking system.

Design, implement, and evaluate a tracking system for all nurses in the Clinical Ladder Program to include:
- Application
- Six-month review
- Credentialing
- Bonuses

Maintain relationships and open communication with over fifty educational services and supply vendors and perform support activities as needed.

Supervise all personnel assigned to CNE through work-study programs, SYEP, volunteer office, temporary staff, and light-duty personnel.

Complete payroll for department.

Provide other support services as needed for the smooth operation of the Center for Nursing Education.

Source: Greater Southeast Community Hospital, Washington, D.C. Reproduced with permission.

ting and collaboration between these professionals will contribute to mutual success. For example, if the organization decides some program content is essential for all staff, or it is required by some regulatory body, the cost of learner time will vary greatly if the content is offered as a self-study or a centralized classroom session. The staff development specialist should consider the several designs to accomplish the goal and make the recommendations that include the cost of learner time. Chapters 6 and 12 can be consulted for cost determination strategies. However, budget implications for learner time in programs are significant. Other learner time questions that should be considered by the staff development specialist during the design phase include the following:

- Will the program be offered over a short period, that is, one month, or should it be offered over a year-long basis, or perhaps should it be integrated into the regular ongoing staff development program?
- Should the program be offered during evening and night shifts or can those personnel attend the program during the day? What will be the cost of evening and night shift attendance? Will it be overtime or educational leave time?
- Can the program be offered in a variety of formats? Is it efficient for the staff development specialist to design a variety of formats or not?

The issues of staffing and scheduling within health care organizations are important. Staff development specialists must develop a healthy appreciation for the cost of learner time and make efforts to predict this time and use it efficiently.

Supplies

Staff development specialists are also responsible for selecting support materials for programs. Items such as texts, videos, films and filmstrip/cassette programs, audio cassettes, and packaged programs are available to enhance education programs. In addition, many simulation aids, such as CPR manikins, intravenous arms, and ostomy care torsos, are available for learners to practice skills. Depending on the available budget and other resources, the staff development specialist may make purchase decisions about these items. Since many versions and models are often available, it is helpful to assess several before the final purchase decision is made. Specialists in other organizations can also be contacted to gather data about their experiences with various texts and simulation aids.

Planning

Staff development departments operate on a planning continuum. At one end of the continuum is the process used to schedule the routine activities such as orientation, CPR, and other ongoing programs. At the other end of the continuum are the unexpected activities that must be planned and coordinated to meet some urgent goal. Staff development departments should develop a plan and calendar that incorporates all planned programs that are anticipated on at least an annual basis. This plan can be updated quarterly, new urgent programs added, and others deferred.

Most staff development departments attempt to achieve a balance in the program plan that incorporates predictability and flexibility. The predictability of the program plan communicates those activities that will need to occur regardless of any organizational imperative such as orientation. A clear direction of planned staff development is communicated through the predictable activities. Flexibility is merged with the plan in such a manner that allows response to unexpected needs and organizational change. While this may seem an impossible task, the planning process begins with evaluation data from previous planning activities and review of currently accessible evaluation data. The following series of questions may help guide this process:

What to offer? Have programs offered in the past been appropriate? What should be added? Deleted? Are quality assurance monitors indicating a need for any significant new programming? Is the orientation program efficient and effective? Does the stable preceptor population require an advanced program to continue their development? Do new internal policies suggest some programs, such as Advanced Cardiac Life Support, be added as a regular program? Do changing systems require new programs? Is there any plan to update the patient classification or hospital information system used by nursing personnel? Are there any plans to change the nursing care delivery system? Are any new service or product lines planned that require competency development of the nursing staff? Has manager turnover been reduced to the point where regularly scheduled manager orientation is no longer necessary? Should the manager orientation program be converted to guided inquiry rather than a classroom experience? Are there other programs that need evaluation and/or conversion? Do new state or federal laws regarding nursing assistant (NA) certification make the current program obsolete? What new clinical information is needed? Institution and nursing service goals, strategic plans, and/or program changes may also be used as a guide. Attendance patterns, requests, complaints, and quality assurance monitors should also be assessed. Key customers must be involved. Nurse managers can be asked to identify their challenges to explore new programming ideas. Nursing staff may also be a source of information about desired competencies and information updates.

When and how often to offer? Actual data will help guide these decisions. For example, to make a decision about how often to offer a critical care course, data about turnover in the critical care area will help. To make a decision about how often to offer CPR recertification classes, data about how many staff are required to maintain current certification are essential. Scheduling classes too frequently will result in small class size, cancelled classes, and department inefficiencies. If classes are not offered frequently enough, customer dissatisfaction, lost learners, and classes added to meet the need will result. Logistical issues such as limited classroom availability and instructor availability may limit or even control the answers to when and how often. However, it is important to think about these questions as program plans and calendars are being developed. Otherwise a stagnant, repetitive, and unresponsive program plan may be the outcome. Examples of program plans that require such thoughtful reflection are those which the institution expects all staff to attend—perhaps a safety review, an update on AIDS, or a new policy or procedure. These could be scheduled in a variety of ways, such as (a) intensively, over a week or ten days, for all shifts and including weekends, (b) routinely, over a year, every Monday, or (c) for one quarter, as a three-month effort only.

What time to offer? Institutional patterns will help establish the best time for programs. Some staff scheduling patterns may be analyzed for days in the cycle when staffing is more conducive for attendance at educational activities. Units with shifts that overlap may be more able to participate in programs during the overlap. Classes at the end or beginning of the shift may facilitate or inhibit attendance. Managers may find that extended programs (e.g., 4–8 hours in length) are easier to schedule for staff participation than briefer sessions. Scheduling programs back to back, that is 7:30 A.M. to 11:30 A.M., and repeating the session from 11:30 A.M. to 3:30 P.M. may allow split shifts and sharing of patient assignments.

The timing question is a complex one, often with no best answer. Regular polling of consumers may yield preferences which can be met, but it is not uncommon for a time to be preferred by some and not by others. Staff development specialists use different strategies to accommodate various needs and preferences. Routine predictable time is helpful for routine programs, as all consumers will eventually learn and adapt to the routine. This is a successful strategy for part of the total staff development program. However, variable schedules will always be an integral part of the program, due to the service nature and work of the consumers of staff development.

When planning questions have been addressed, a master schedule is to be prepared. Blocking in the planned program for a defined period of time, usually a year, will help staff and consumers plan their workload. Staff development specialists and support staff prepare their work and planning schedule. Likewise, managers can use the plan to meet staff development and scheduling needs. Nursing administration can also use the plan for other projects and initiatives. All program titles need not be completely refined. For example, if the plan includes a blueprint to design a Medical-Surgical Nursing Skills Update, the calendar can simply list the idea as a potential topic with or without a brief description of the plan. The calendar may also be used in this way as marketing tool to generate questions and interest in a particular topic. Once developed, the plan must be communicated, usually in the form of a calendar. Information that should be included in this calendar includes

- Topic
- Date
- Times (if known)
- Place
- Target audience
- Contact hours planned
- Staff development person to contact for additional information

The calendar may also include additional information such as a brief description, purpose, and goals and objectives.

The staff development plan in the form of a calendar can be organized in a variety of formats. Some agencies distribute it as a packet of pages stapled together. Others organize the information into a large poster that can be put on a bulletin board, and still others develop a catalog of offerings that is updated and distributed periodically.

Regardless of the format, information about the plan should be disseminated in a variety of ways. For example:

- Schedules published in a newsletter
- Large whiteboard of activities scheduled for one or more quarters posted in area where staff receive paychecks
- A personal calendar provided for each staff member as a holiday gift
- Concise schedules posted in all rooms used for report and other unit-based meetings
- Breakfast meeting for nurse managers with brief overviews of each program on the schedule with purpose, presenter, and expected result or outcome

There are many strategies to communicate the staff development plan. The important issue is that the calendar is communicated in a variety of ways.

It is essential that the fixed or predictable schedule account for only a portion of available staff development time and resources. Planned programs meet many institutional needs; however, short-term, urgent, and unplanned needs will emerge. It is also imperative that the staff development department retain enough flexibility in any program plan that they are able to respond to these unplanned, yet crucial needs of the organization in a timely way. To commit all or most of staff development time to a fixed and predictable program may result in an inability to carry out the program when higher priority needs are identified.

Implementing the Plan for Required Courses

Most staff development departments must deal with classes that have been labeled "mandatory" or "voluntary." Mandatory classes are often required by accrediting agencies and are very specific in content. Organizations may also decide that some specific content or information is so important that a majority of the employees must be exposed to the information through a staff development activity. Employees who must attend these sessions are compensated in some way according to the organization's policy. Common examples include fire safety, infection control, CPR, and others. Other examples may include a change in charting policies or medication administration procedures, or a significant change in performance expectations.

Voluntary classes may or may not be paid time for employees. Organizational policies that define these practices are often developed based on available resources and philosophical beliefs about the responsibility of employees for continued learning. A wide range of topics is usually offered to assist nursing staff in maintaining and developing competence and related knowledge as they continue to improve their nursing practice.

Learners arriving for a mandatory class may not be interested in the content or appreciate the need for obtaining the information. Nevertheless, their attendance is usually predictable. Voluntary learners usually attend programs with a need or desire to learn and arrive as more interested learners. However, due to the voluntary nature of the learning, their attendance is less predictable. Indeed, they may fail to show up if another area of interest or need captures their attention. There are no easy answers to this common planning dilemma within staff development. One core strategy may help. A clear focus on the content and its value to their work is conducive to reducing the negative component of mandatory classes. A second strategy is the use of various and creative approaches to transferring the required information in order to give learners options and choices for meeting expectations.

To plan an adequate level of access to required programs, the staff development specialist should determine the number of staff required to have the information, and plan a strategy (classes, self-learning packages, study guides, or other methods) that will help all learners meet the organization's expectation.

Learners who are required to learn by an external source, such as an organization, present a significant challenge to the staff development specialist. Special efforts may be required for unique and careful design and scheduling of educational experiences for these mandatory topics. Enthusiasm for learning can be transmitted by an enthusiastic specialist. Meticulous, thoughtful planning by the staff development specialist may yield an exciting, worthwhile experience for participants and the organization.

Balancing the Program

Staff development departments must focus their efforts on the areas of need and content that are requirements for organizational success. Programs should focus on what learners need to know. Basic programs such as orientation must address the acquisition of basic competencies. *However,* a department that attends exclusively to currently needed skills and knowledge runs the risk of becoming mechanized and repetitive. Annual program development activities should explore the possibilities of new areas of development and new strategies to help staff maintain and develop new competencies that respond to the continually changing health care needs of patients. The staff development program planning process should include considerations that will expand knowledge beyond the status quo and assist learners in exploring new areas of knowledge. These program ideas may come under the heading of special programs or continuing education.

Outside funding may be necessary to support some of these unique programs, or learners may be charged a fee that offsets some or all of the costs. The programs may focus on health issues of the staff, rather than the patients, or it may focus on new trends and issues in the profession. Community health problems or controversies are also potential topics. Even if these topics are offered on a limited basis, they may offer learners a unique experience which may generate new interest and enthusiasm for their work. The staff development personnel may also benefit as they work on new and uncommon program themes and topics.

One way to address the potential interest of staff development specialists is to ask each one to contribute an idea that they would like to implement but have never considered a possibility. This process should take place during the routine program planning process. The incorporation of these ideas and the support to implement them may energize the staff development department and enhance an annual program plan.

Organizing Your Program

To deliver an effective and efficient staff development program, a framework must be used to help consumers of these services understand how they are delivered, who delivers them, and who is responsible and accountable for the variety of services offered. In earlier chapters, several service delivery models were discussed. The most common approaches used by staff development specialists can be categorized as centralized, decentralized, or a combination of both. Most departments are hybrids that have evolved over time to meet the varying and changing needs of the parent organization. While most share commonalities, many departments retain unique qualities that help them carry out their missions.

Generally, a centralized staff development department is organized to support all of nursing services, and designs a program that serves that nursing division as a whole. A centralized staff development department often attempts to meet the needs common to all nursing personnel and primarily provides classroom instruction on a regularly scheduled basis. This type of organizational model for nursing staff development is often very efficient because it serves a large population of learners and provides these services in a predictable manner. The centralized model also supports the concept of staff development content experts. For example, a centralized department may have an BLS/ACLS expert, an orientation specialist, a management development specialist, and an audio-visual technician. These specialized individuals provide their services to all of the nursing units.

A decentralized staff development program is often based within smaller organizational units, such as a defined clinical area like obstetrics. Staff development positions may also exist within midlevel divisions such as maternal-child health or critical care. These staff development specialists usually focus on the specific needs of their assigned area. Such specialists, while often clinically specialized, need to develop skills in instructional technology and program planning and design. Education evaluation skills are also a necessary component to the success of the specialist within this framework. Staff development personnel within the decentralized model often support all of the educational needs of staff within their assigned areas. These needs may include, but not be limited to, orientation, inservice education, new skills training, new product introduction, safety and infection control updates, and specialized clinical instruction. Staff development specialists within a decentralized model are often perceived as more responsive to staff and nurse managers and tend to have a stronger clinical focus. These specialists are often accountable to a mid- or upper level nurse manager, rather than a staff development director. Some redundancy and repetition across programs is an inherent limitation of the decentralized model as each specialist provides the same services to smaller groups. In addition, a lack of expertise in program planning, design, and evaluation may be evident. Opportunities to develop the specific staff development competencies related to these areas may also be unavailable on a regular basis. Specialists may not have the chance to engage in their own professional role development.

Many staff development departments design an organizational structure that provides the efficiency of the centralized model and the clinical relevancy of the decentralized model. Most staff development specialists have responsibility for both centralized and decentralized services. Some programming is designed for all nursing personnel, for example, CPR and basic orientation. Others programs provided by the same specialist may be designed very specifically for the staff of one clinical unit. For example, patients requiring continuous ambulatory peritoneal dialysis are centralized on one unit; only the nursing staff of that unit require the specialty training to care for these patients.

Management of a staff development department with a combined model is more complex. However, added credibility is generally enjoyed and specialists are often more satisfied with the many challenges this model presents. A staff development specialist who teaches in the clinical area can draw on those observations during more formal classroom instruction. In addition, comparisons between "what is" and "what is supposed to be" may also be made, leading to the development of rational approaches to continued professional development.

Staff development specialists who function primarily in a clinical role need routine opportunities to maintain their clinical expertise. The opportunity should be scheduled and maintained. Ideally, this practice is of a significant time, full shift for example, and involves a regular patient assignment. Staff development personnel become credible with the nursing staff by demonstrating a willingness to help and an interest in patient care activities. Specialists also can use this experience to provide the opportunity to assess learning needs, observe current practice, and talk with learners about issues that are difficult for them to manage. In this way, the staff development specialist role is expanded and may include opportunities to counsel nurses about stress management and organizing work. It may also yield other consultation opportunities to assist several staff members in dealing with a current problem. One common criticism of staff development specialists is an apparent lack of relevancy and realism. Routine visibility in the clinical areas may add to the credibility of this role.

Most combination models also include a staff development specialist who serves as a liaison to the clinical units. This assignment may vary from one to as many as twenty. Responsibilities are similar to the specialist in the pure centralized model but can be carried out in a more efficient way, as several units may have the same needs. Specialists within this model are usually not expected to provide ongoing clinical support and consultation. However, these individuals can attend staff meetings, meet regularly with nurse managers and preceptors, follow up with new employees regarding their orientation, and help with the transition to new services and requisite skill development. In addition, these specialists can encourage participation in planned, centralized programs, gather evaluation data to incorporate into future program plans, and provide consultation to individuals and groups. Liaison roles are beneficial to the staff development effort, as they provide the routine link to the consumers of services. These concepts are also discussed and contrasted in Chapter 3.

Organizing Classroom Programs

Classroom teaching responsibilities must also be organized to meet the institution's needs. In some organizations, individuals may be hired for their content expertise and be expected to design and implement all classes within their area of expertise. In other organizations, staff development specialists may be hired based upon their breadth of knowledge and experience and be expected to implement all programs for their departments. These two models are the most common approaches to providing instructional resources. However, while they are logical responses to needs and efficient use of scarce resources, they share a common pitfall. No back-up system is available. In the case of illness, emergency, or termination, staff development resources may need to be reorganized to meet a heavy schedule of essential programs. To assist in this reorganization and limit frustration among specialists, a secondary system that will support the program is necessary.

A common secondary system that will contribute to the ongoing availability of programs, despite specialist unavailability, is one in which lesson plans are an integral component. Essential programs offered on a routine and predictable basis should be supported with fully developed lesson plans. Most educational record keeping systems use lesson plans as a central element. These lesson plans can salvage a program when the specialist resource is unexpectedly unavailable. A lesson plan is a classic approach to classroom instruction and includes all information necessary to teach a course. A typical lesson plan will include session objectives, outlines, time frames, needed instructional materials, including audio-visual hardware and software, as well as the teaching strategy and evaluation method. The form varies from organization to organization and may include all or some of the elements listed above. Chart 7-5 illustrates a common approach to a lesson plan form.

Lesson plans serve several purposes:

- Frequently taught classes are taught the same way each time.
- Structure is provided for infrequently taught classes.
- The planning process is demonstrated through the illustrated relationship of objectives, content, method, and evaluation.
- Common delivery is assured for programs taught by several instructors.

Chart 7-5
Sample Lesson Plan Format

Lesson/Session Title: _____

Approximate Time Required: Lecture _____ Discussion _____ Practice _____

Objective	Content	A-Vs/Graphics/Examples

Source: Meriter Hospital, Madison, WI. Reproduced with permission.

Through the use of lesson plans, the staff development program provides consistency and well-developed and secure instructional delivery system, even in the event of unforseen transitions within staff development.

A second method for specialist backup is to assign secondary specialists for all, or at least major, courses within the staff development program. Departmental guidelines can be developed to define the role of the secondary specialist. For example, some organizations may expect the secondary specialist to assume teaching responsibilities, but not classroom arrangements. Others may require the secondary instructor to take full responsibility for the program, and still others may divide the tasks among all available resources. This effort may seem costly and even unnecessary, but some cancelled classes may be even more costly to the organization and the staff development program. In particular, if many nurses have been scheduled for a particular event, cancellation may result in anger, confusion, and staffing difficulties, and, perhaps, lost income. Courses that should be considered for a back-up system include any that take a significant block of time, for example, a full- or half-day session.

Another mechanism for ensuring that the staff development program will continue as planned with limited cancellation and rescheduling includes the use of instructor teams. With teams, a group of two or more people are involved in designing the program and developing lesson plans. This team is also responsible for program evaluation. Using a team approach to planning ensures that more than one person is familiar with the entire course and could, at least in an emergency, provide the classroom instruction. Teams do not necessarily need to be made up exclusively of instructional staff. Using staff nurses, nurse managers, or even directors will strengthen the planning process, the base of support for the offering, and the available resources. Staff can also be involved in multiple teams. In turn, this activity will also contribute to the various team members continuing professional development.

If content experts are used to provide instruction within the staff development program, consideration of a back-up system should be part of the contract negotiations. Cancellation of a program provided totally by an outside contractor may have the same negative effects, though staff seem to be more forgiving of faculty from outside the organization.

Instruction that can occur outside the classroom is increasing in importance for staff development departments. Learner time is usually the most expensive component of the education program. Alternative methods for conveying content have the possibility of reducing organizational costs without reducing programming. Staff development specialists should develop a wide range of design strategies that go beyond the classroom, including

- Video-taped demonstrations
- Audio-taped presentations
- Guided study
- Self-learning packages
- Other strategies that do not require classroom attendance

Another example of this diversification of skills for the staff development specialist include the incorporation of basic audio-visual and media development knowledge into the repertoire of skills. Traditionally, staff development departments have used media extensively to support classroom instruction. Staff shortages and program costs may cause a shift to the use of the media as the instructor. Further examples of nonclassroom methods that may replace all or part of routine programming include the following:

1. *Demonstration of all new products on video.* Many suppliers have professionally made tapes which are available at no cost. Institution-specific procedures may be added to the video or provided as supporting printed material. A monthly update of all new products could even be considered as an ongoing component of the staff development program.
2. *Pre-class learning in a variety of formats.* Intensive care classes may involve a librarylike system of materials that may be checked out, such as articles, readings in texts, video and audio tapes. Proficiency tests and case studies can also be used to strengthen entry skills in the areas of clinical decision making.
3. *Self-study specialty orientation.* Procedures very specific to a limited specialty area or those procedures used infrequently may be provided as on unit self-study materials.
4. *Electronic programs and media used to meet ongoing requirements.* CPR certification may be provided using selected electronic media, either the written or performance tests or both without the need for an instructor. Other required activities, such as infection control and fire safety, may be available through a guided video format.
5. *Computer-assisted instruction for selected programs.* Selected programs may be available in a computer-assisted instruction format. While many do not go beyond the electronic page-turning approach, the novelty may be appealing to some learners, particularly those with personal computers at home. Libraries may also be used to provide these services; however, available resources must be considered before this method can be used in a significant way.

All of these methods provide the benefits of flexibility for the learner schedule, reduction of direct instructor time and broad availability to users. Nurse learners often state a preference for classroom experiences, but may become enthusiastic consumers of other methodologies with time and positive experiences. Staff development specialists may also need encouragement to explore alternatives which are not familiar and may not reflect their personal preferences.

Consultation

Consultation is another activity in which staff development specialists may spend their time. For a variety of reasons, instructors may be sought out to consult individuals and groups about personal and professional development. Nurse managers may seek out the staff development specialist for help with resolving practice, procedural, discipline, or counseling issues. Discussed in detail in other chapters, it is essential for specialists to understand that consulting is not advice giving. Rather, it is another component of the professional relationship established with consumers of services, which uses a problem-solving process.

Judgment in Staff Development

Decisions are made daily in staff development. Which programs to offer, which needs to address, are resources being used on the right things? To answer these and the myriad questions that are routinely raised, the staff development department needs to collect data on a routine basis. These data are then used to make judgments about future improvements of the staff development program.

1. Request log: Most departments receive requests on a daily basis. Some are part of informal telephone calls, some are part of hallway conversations, some are in writing, and others come as part of committee functions or management requests. Some, perhaps most requests can be addressed. Others cannot. The extent to which the department responded and the reasons other requests were not fulfilled or denied is an important data source for future planning. A request log, maintained by all members of the department, is a tool that can be useful in several ways. It may help in developing priorities for the next budget period. Reasons for denials may cause a reexamination of mission and purpose statements. Sharing the requests log may help others understand the nature of a staff development department, which is part planned systematic programming and part response to requests.

2. Time studies: A second type of data which is useful to staff development departments are time studies. A time study provides a systematic mechanism for attributing staff development costs to programs. For example, routine time studies allow nursing management to know what percentage of instructor time is spent with RN orientation. In turn, this allows an institution to understand the actual cost of each new nurse employee. Many other questions can also be addressed with a time study. These include (a) the preparation time required for classroom teaching, (b) amount of staff development resource currently used to support committee work, and (c) amount of time specialists are spending in clinical areas. Any number of areas lend themselves to the collection of data related to time spent in various activities. These studies should be approached as helpful tools that will assist with decision making, rather than a personnel surveillance system. Time studies should also be carried out to collect data in a systematic way that will assure representation of the sample. If the decision is made to engage in a time study of all departmental activities, a commitment should also be made to analyze the data and demonstrate the myriad activities that are all components of the staff development process. A common approach to this type of total study involves two phases. During the first phase, the staff write down on a log the activities as they occur over prespecified time increments of 15 to 30 minutes, using narrative descriptions. Following the first phase, the group develops common definitions, categories of time, and a system for coding each category. The second data collection phase involves all staff using a similar time grid, similar definitions and coding, and a similar time frame to capture the use of staff time. Summarized data should be reviewed and discussed by the group as a whole. Full participation of the staff is essential to view findings as credible and accurate. The findings can be used to demonstrate services commonly provided and budget planning and preparation. If this type of data is collected routinely, they will provide trend data which may indicate changes in resource utilization. Subsequent reassignments may then be made based on the data. This approach to resource utilization has increasing value within the changing and more businesslike health care system.

   3. Cost-effectiveness analyses: The comparison of the cost of all or part of the staff development effort to the outcomes achieved is another source of information about a department. The most frequent use of this methodology is in program planning or at the proposal stage when a new approach or program is designed. The predicted costs and benefits of a program are outlined and presented with the proposal, or data are collected about past program experiences. As competition for resources increases, this methodology becomes more important for routine use. At budget planning time, programs that have clearly articulated costs and outcomes will be more positively viewed than those with unknown or ambiguous costs and outcomes. When resources become so constrained as to require program reductions, an analysis of alternatives using a cost- effectiveness framework for decision making is more desirable than across-the-board cuts which diminish all programs.

   4. Quality assurance: Quality assurance (QA) programs began as a mechanism for assuring accreditation and reimbursement agencies that the clinical care was of sufficient quality. In most hospitals and health care agencies, the scope of QA programs has expanded to all departments including staff development. Discussed in detail in Chapter 11, quality assurance within staff development is an emerging, essential characteristic of sound programming for nursing personnel. Standards of practice have been established by the American Nurses' Association and provide a framework for quality. Monitoring and evaluation activities are beginning to yield useful data needed to continually improve the staff development effort. Staff development is one quality assurance mechanism for patients, and the recognition of this feature is evident in most QA models. QA monitors completed by other nursing departments, as well as those conducted within staff development about internal processes, all provide a rich data source to assist in making judgments about services and programs needed by the organization.

   The above listed sources of data provide information to help the staff development specialist make decisions and judgments that will contribute to a well-developed program which, in turn, will contribute to the nursing divisions goals and objectives.

Issues to Ponder

Staff development services, programs, and departments are arranged in a variety of ways. Each has strengths and limitations. The key to the success of any effort is the organization of resources to accomplish the most good in assisting the organization in meeting its priorities and imperatives. Following are several additional characteristics of staff development departments. Each can be considered and reviewed during routine strategic planning endeavors. Each may contribute to the overall success of the staff development effort, but each must be considered within the overall utilization of scarce resources. Each consumes a significant amount of resource and must be compared with the benefits perceived by the entire organization.

To have an advisory committee? There are a variety of reasons to have an advisory committee including, (a) to assist with needs assessments, (b) to assist with program evaluation, (c) to provide the learners perspective, (d) to provide consultation to the staff development effort regarding its mission, purpose, philosophy, and (e) to market the department and program to its consumer groups. All of these are valid reasons and there may be others. Advisory committees can be particularly helpful in obtaining the consumers perspective about issues and problems facing the department. An advisory committee should be organized according to a written plan similar to that used for other organizational committees. Membership, terms of offices, meeting times, purpose, and leadership should be clearly identified. Agendas should be distributed prior to meetings, and expectations about members participation in meetings and agenda item discussions should also be communicated. A committee without this level of structure is unlikely to be productive. Frustration will result for the staff development department and the advisory committee members.

To seek approval from an SNA or accreditation from ANA? If the staff development program includes continuing education, it may be worthwhile to seek accreditation from approval bodies for these activities. The ANA has a mechanism or review and approval for continuing education. At the present time, no other mechanism exists for review and approval of the entire staff development program. The recent release of staff development standards, makes this is a logical next step. Asking the question and discussing the possibility of applying can be a constructive activity even if it does not result in an application. The first step in this process is to obtain a copy of the standards and carefully compare them with the department's standards. Does the department meet the standards? All of them? Some of them? Could you meet those standards not currently in place? What are the costs and benefits to the department and the organization? Will it help meet mission, goals, and objectives statements? If the answers to these questions are positive, and the decision is made to explore this option further, several more questions must be addressed. Acquiring a copy of the accreditation manual or SNA approval process will help with some of the basic questions. For example, are there policies related to eligibility which may be a problem? What are the hidden costs involved, such as those needed to maintain accreditation and record keeping requirements? How much time and effort will be needed for the application and self-study? Have other organizations attempted or completed this process?

What was their experience? Will help be available from the approving organization? Would it benefit the learner, who must meet requirements for relicensure or recertification? Would it meet the organization's requirement for external review? Would it enhance the organization's and department's credibility? The process of review which accompanies an application can be a positive, though time-consuming experience. It may also provide a mechanism to highlight the best activities of the staff development department and provide a stimulus to improve other areas using the same process.

Should staff development generate revenue? Two factors are increasing the frequency with which this question is asked. Increasing pressure to reduce costs in health care institutions is threatening the staff development department's ability to maintain staff and programs. Revenue generation is sometimes seen as a mechanism to offset decreasing institutional support, but maintain programs and staff. A second factor is the increasing entrepreneurship of health care. As institutions seek alternative sources of revenue and new strategies for maintenance and growth, creative and enthusiastic staff development specialists seek out similar alternatives. For departments that have long dealt with reductions, the idea of taking control of the future is appealing. The decision to commit to a revenue generation should be made after review of several questions, such as (a) Is this constant with the mission? (b) Would any internal customers receive less service? (c) What are the risks if revenue expectations are not met? (d) What has been the experience of other organizations with revenue generation? and (e) What are the costs necessary to begin revenue generation? The last question is particularly relevant as costs of marketing can quickly outstrip any potential revenue. Many staff development departments have excellent programs and good potential for marketing to audiences other than the organization. The decision to alter the focus of a department from internal to external has many consequences, including the perceived loss of an available service. This decision is crucial to the survival of the staff development program and should be made meticulously. Additional discussion about generating revenue is also found in Chapter 6.

How can we assure administrative support? The financial pressures in health care are felt directly in staff development departments. Interpretations of those pressures may be difficult. Rather than a response of fear and defensiveness, the staff development specialist can take a proactive position and be confident about the contribution the staff development effort makes to the organization. It is the responsibility of the specialist to teach administration about staff development and the contribution it makes toward helping meet goals and expectations. Listed below are some strategies that will help keep administration apprised of this contribution.

1. Provide routine reports on departmental activities. Base reports on contribution to nursing and organizational goal achievement. Help management see staff development as a proactive contributor to the success of the institution.
2. Develop a strategic plan or outline of the department's contribution to the organization's plan. Help management see staff development as a proactive contributor to the success of the institution.
3. Keep the Chief Nurse Executive apprised of standards set by regulatory agencies relative to education. There are many, and the staff

development program should include activities that help the organization meet these and other standards. These activities and their relation to regulatory body requirements should be reported.

4. Maintain contact with managers and be responsive and supportive of their goals. Help them see how staff development can assist with goal achievement.
5. Provide journal articles and position statements from other agencies that describe the necessary support. Don't assume management and administration know about the support needed to provide a quality staff development program.
6. Remember the mission of staff development as a service department. Assure that it contributes, and convey that assurance to others.

Summary

Nursing staff development is an essential component of any progressive nursing service department. Implementing the program to achieve the greatest good with available resources is a challenge to all staff development specialists. The changing environment has created unlimited potential for change, growth, new ideas, and creativity. Staff development specialists can be part of shaping the future of practice in the health care organization. Success depends on the mission, the strategies, the energy expended, and the flexibility and creativity demonstrated. The opportunities to do good and do well are endless.

SUGGESTED READINGS

Books

American Nurses' Association (1986). *Standards for continuing education in nursing.* Kansas City: Author.

Austin, E. K. (1981). *Guidelines for the development of continuing education offerings for nurses.* New York: Appleton-Lange.

Bille, D. A. (1982). *Staff development: A systems approach.* Thorofare, NJ: Slack.

Brookfield, S. B. (1987). *Understanding and facilitating adult learning.* San Francisco: Jossey-Bass.

Cooper, S. S. (1983). *The practice of continuing education in nursing.* Rockville, MD: Aspen.

Knowles, M. S. (1985) *Andragogy in action.* San Francisco: Jossey-Bass.

Knox, A. B. (1987). *Helping adults learn.* San Francisco: Jossey-Bass.

Puetz, B. E., & Peters, F. L. (1981). *Continuing education for nurses.* Rockville, MD: Aspen.

Articles

Barako, J., Reichert, A., & Nunez, A. (1989). The NYPEN method: Meeting learning needs and satisfying educational requirements. *Journal of Nursing Staff Development, 5*(3), 132–138.

Becker, J., Ellson, S. K. (1989). How to develop a competency-based head nurse orientation program. *Journal of Healthcare Education and Training, 4*(3), 32–36.

Blaney, D. R., Hobson, C. J., & McHenry, J. (1988). Improving the cost effectiveness of nursing practice in a hospital setting. *Journal of Continuing Education in Nursing, 19*(3), 113–117.

Boyer, V. M. (1986). The clinical nurse specialist: An underutilized staff development resource. *Journal of Nursing Staff Development, 2*(1), 23–27.

del Bueno, D. J. (1986). Nursing staff development: Critical times, critical issues. *Journal of Nursing Staff Development, 2*(3), 94–97.

Farmer, A. P. (1987). Costs and benefits of hospital education programs, Part 1. *Journal of Healthcare Education and Training, 2*(1), 32–39.

Farmer, A. P. (1987). Costs and benefits of hospital education program, Part 2. *Journal of Healthcare Education and Training, 2*(3), 17–19.

Farmer, M. L. (1988). I have to develop a program: Where do I begin? *Journal of Nursing Staff Development, 4*(3), 116–119.

Huegel, E. A. (1989). Utilizing an efficiency analysis in an educational department: Making an informed decision. *Journal of Continuing Education in Nursing, 4*(3), 81–21.

Joint Commission on Accreditation of Healthcare Organizations Quality Review Bulletin (1986). Monitoring and evaluation of quality and appropriateness of care: A hospital example. September, 326–330.

Kuramoto, A. M. (1988). Defining the image of your continuing education department. *Journal of Continuing Education in Nursing, 19*(6), 274–275.

Lewis, D. J., Saydak, S. J., & Robinson, J. A. (1987). Making the most of continuing education: A framework for developing programs. *Journal of Nursing Staff Development, 3*(3), 106– 109.

Puetz, B. E. (1989). Responding to changing times: Converting a seminar into self–study. *Journal of Healthcare Education and Training, 4*(3), 18–21.

Schoessler, M., & Conedera, F. (1987). Hiring nurse educators. *Journal of Nursing Staff Development, 3*(2), 61–64.

Stephens, D. J., & Dowling-Dols, J. (1988). The recipe for a successful workshop. *Journal of Nursing Staff Development, 4*(4),163–168.

Tobin, H. M., & Beeler, J. L. (1988). Roles and relationships of staff development educators: A critical component of impact. *Journal of Nursing Staff Development, 4*(3), 116–119.

Weeks, L. C., & Spor, K. M. (1987). Hospital nursing education: Dispelling the doomsday prophesies. *Journal of Nursing Administration, 17*(3), 34–38.

Chapter 8

Evaluation: Essential Skill for the Staff Development Specialist

Belinda E. Puetz

Evaluation skills are becoming an essential component of a nursing staff development specialist's repertoire. Because evaluation studies primarily are conducted to determine the worth or value of educational programs and processes, it is essential that nursing staff development specialists have the ability to plan and implement evaluation studies. Information obtained from an evaluation study can be used in making decisions about future operations, setting administrative priorities, and determining program directions.[1]

Information obtained from evaluation studies is invaluable, but must be offset by the resources, including staff and time, that are used in evaluation efforts. Decisions about the depth and scope of evaluation studies to be done must occur in the context of a realistic assessment of resources available to the nursing staff development specialist.

This chapter will discuss design and use of evaluation methods for individual educational offerings as well as the entire staff development department. Several models are offered which will help the nursing staff development specialist assess and document the value of the program. These evaluation studies can be used to demonstrate the outcomes of educational efforts, particularly with respect to nursing care,[2] as well as to show how effectively the staff development department activities coincide with the institution's mission, goals, and objectives.

Planning Evaluation Studies

Judicious use of existing resources occurs when the specialist plans an evaluation that meets information needs in a cost-effective, efficient manner.

While resources may not permit a formal evaluation study of the entire education department's effort, at the very least, each of the individual offerings sponsored by the department should be evaluated at its conclusion.

The evaluation of individual educational activities has been simplified by the American Nurses' Association's (ANA) recently revised Criteria for Accreditation as a Provider of Continuing Education in Nursing.[3] The criteria for accreditation of educational programs include specific standards that must be included in the evaluation of educational offerings. These measures include the learner's achievement of the offering objectives as well as their personal objectives for attending, the teaching effectiveness of each faculty, and, in general, relevance of content to objective, and the appropriateness of the facility.

A combination of quantitative and qualitative data can be collected to respond to these items. For example, participants can respond to the items on achievement of personal/course objectives by marking a number from 1 to 5 where 1 is "not achieved," and 5 is "achieved to a great extent." Then, they can be asked to amplify their ratings using a question such as, "Why?" or "Why Not?"

Teaching effectiveness of faculty can be addressed through a semantic differential, where the elements arrayed on the continuum reflect characteristics of effective teachers of adults.[1] Chart 8-1 presents a reaction form that measures these characteristics. Using characteristics of effective teaching allows participants to assess faculty effectiveness, rather than whether the instructor displayed good "platform skills" or was entertaining.

The results of an evaluation based on effective instructional skills also provides the staff development specialist with evidence that can be used to counsel and help faculty improve their ability to teach adults. Kirkpatrick[4] suggested a staff rating of the instructor that consists of assessment of faculty preparation, conduct of the session, suggestions for improvement, and potential topics. Combined with participant evaluations, the results of evaluation data from staff development specialists can be of value to teachers of adults.

Asking respondents to judge the teaching/learning environment is problematic for many nursing staff development specialists. Often, respondents are most critical of this aspect of the educational event. Many times, too, problems with the environment cannot be changed due to space limitations or other constraints on resources. While a common response is to delete this item on the evaluation form, a more prudent action is to frame the question in such a way as to allow the participant to express an opinion, yet maximize the usefulness of the information obtained. One way to approach this is to relate the environment directly and specifically to the teaching/learning process. Ask to what extent the environment was conducive to learning, rather than how satisfied the participant was with the milieu in which the educational event was held. While merely rephrasing the item may not eliminate all negative responses, it will focus the participant's attention on the teaching/learning activity instead of personal likes or dislikes about the setting.

In addition to the above items, participants should be asked to suggest modifications or changes in the educational offering before it is presented again. Participants are very knowledgeable about ways in which they learn best, and if asked for their candid comments will be likely to identify needed improvements. An open-ended item may elicit better information than asking participants to rate whether the ratio of lecture to discussion, for example, was "too much lecture," "about right," or "too much discussion."

An evaluation form can be designed to meet the ANA standards as well as include other evaluation items of interest to the nursing staff development specialist (see Chart 8-1). The form then can be used with each educational experience planned and implemented by the facility. Use of a standardized evaluation form is cost- and time-saving, provided, of course, that the questionnaire elicits information that is valid and reliable.

Additional information that is needed by the nursing staff development specialist can be added to the form, with the caution that unless the information actually will be used, it should not be requested. Information on an evaluation form should not duplicate information that can be obtained elsewhere. For example, demographic data on participants should be collected separately from evaluation of the educational offering. And, unless the demographic information will be used by the staff development specialist in some specific manner, it should not be requested at all.

Participants often are reluctant to spend time completing forms for which they cannot ascertain a worthwhile purpose. In order to assure that participants devote the necessary time to a thoughtful, complete evaluation of educational activities, staff development specialists should avoid the temptation to collect all kinds of information just because a captive audience is present.

The standard evaluation form developed by the staff development specialist also can be shortened for use with educational offerings such as inservice sessions of one or two hours. The essential five components identified by the ANA (1988), however, should be evaluated in each instance that an educational activity is conducted, regardless of its length.

Although a questionnaire is the most common method of evaluating an educational activity, there are other methods of evaluation that will allow the specialist to obtain the same information about educational activities. In addition, using other evaluation methods on occasion will provide variety for the participants in the programs.

Participant Evaluation Team

Instead of the traditional evaluation questionnaire, the staff development specialist may employ a participant evaluation team. A small number of randomly selected individuals who are scheduled to attend a particular class serve as the participant evaluation team. For example, if the registration list for a workshop has thirty nurses, choosing every tenth person would result in a participant evaluation team of three members.

The evaluation team members who agree to participate are introduced to the audience at the start of the educational activity. The evaluation team collects information about the educational activity throughout the course. The team focuses on responses to the evaluation criteria determined by the specialist, usually including the extent to which the objectives are being achieved, and participants' satisfaction with the learning experience.

Chart 8-1
Evaluation Form

*Please take the necessary time to respond to each item on this evalua-
tion. Your candid and complete responses are important so that we may
continue to satisfy quality control standards and improve these educational activities to better meet your learning needs! Thank you.*

Objectives

A. To what extent were the learning objectives for this session
achieved? (Please circle the appropriate number.)

	Not at all			To a great extent	
List Objective 1	1	2	3	4	5
List Objective 2	1	2	3	4	5
List Objective 3	1	2	3	4	5
List Objective 4	1	2	3	4	5
List Objective 5	1	2	3	4	5

Content

	Not at all			To a great extent	
B. To what extent was the content relevant to the learning objectives?	1	2	3	4	5
C. To what extent was the content relevant to your practice?	1	2	3	4	5
D. To what extent can you apply what you learned in your practice?	1	2	3	4	5

E. Identify specifically what
you intend to do in your
practice with what you
learned:

Faculty/Teaching Methods

F. Please rate the faculty on the following characteristics:

	Not descriptive			**Very descriptive**	
Demonstrated positive regard for learners	1	2	3	4	5
Showed respect for learners' questions and opinions	1	2	3	4	5
Used a variety of teaching methods	1	2	3	4	5
Facilitated learning through participation of learners	1	2	3	4	5

Additional comments:

G. To what extent were your personal objectives for this educational activity attained?

	Not at all			**To a great extent**	
	1	2	3	4	5

Why? Or, why not?

H. What changes, modifications, or improvements would you suggest before subsequent presentation of this educational activity?

I. Rate the appropriateness of the physical facilities in relation to the objectives, content, teaching methods, and learner comfort:

	Not at all appropriate			**Very appropriate**	
	1	2	3	4	5

J. Indicate other specific learning needs you have related to your practice:

K. Make any other comments:

The evaluation team obtains the information by talking with participants during breaks and meal times. Generally, the information is volunteered, although occasionally they may have to solicit comments about specific aspects of the course.

They should make themselves available during the course, by sitting in various places in the room rather than with each other. They should circulate at coffee break and meal times.

The participant evaluation team members record the information they receive anonymously, that is, an individual's comments are not identifiable. Precise details concerning data collection should be specified by the staff development specialist in advance.

The information collected by the team is reported verbally to the staff development specialist at the end of the program, or can be submitted in writing later. If the team is to meet after the program to report on their information, they should be informed beforehand. Participants in educational offerings generally are open to participant evaluation teams, and they may be more likely to give team members feedback that they would not share with a teacher or the staff development specialist. The participant evaluation team method can be supplemented by a brief questionnaire. The questionnaire should not duplicate the team's efforts, but can be used to elicit comments on items not covered by the evaluation team.

Group Discussion

In most educational activities, participants provide evaluation data in writing on an individual basis. This traditional approach overlooks the advantages of collecting evaluation data from groups of participants. In addition to providing some variety, group discussions serve as a learning method and result in information that may otherwise not be obtained from individual evaluation forms.

Group discussion should be scheduled rather than spontaneous. Groups composed of seven to ten people should be formed. Each group should identify a leader whose responsibility is to facilitate discussion. A recorder also should be selected. If small group reports are to be given, time must be allowed for that purpose.

The questions discussed by the group should include those related to the learning outcomes of the educational offering, satisfaction with the learning processes, and administration and organization of the course. If time permits, the groups also can discuss their learning needs. These needs then can be immediately validated with the audience.

Thirty to forty minutes is ample for group discussion. Another ten to twenty minutes will be required for small group reports (assuming one group does not repeat what another group already has reported) and discussion. This time frame can be shortened or lengthened, but more than an hour allotted to an evaluation group discussion is not advisable, or often feasible.

In a group discussion, there often are concerns that some individuals are withdrawing while others dominate. Instructions to the groups and the group leaders should include the need for all to participate. Responses to the evaluation questions can be elicited first from individuals and then followed by a group discussion, although more time generally is required. This approach, however, has the advantage of obtaining information from a group while maintaining the integrity of individual responses.

Tests

Although many adults do not like to take tests, they do provide a measure of learning that can be used for evaluation purposes. Being responsive to adults' discomfort with tests requires that the staff development specialist be judicious with their use, employing tests only when other methods of assessment are not preferable.

The staff development specialist also can avoid testing mistakes, such as relying on subjective rather than objective measures, and testing trivial rather than critical knowledge.[5] One way to avoid these common mistakes is to prepare a test blueprint.[6]

A test blueprint reflects the content and objectives of an educational activity and specifies the number of test items on each topic, based on the emphasis on the topic in the course. The blueprint also identifies whether the items refer to knowledge acquisition or to application. Only critical topics are tested, and the relative weight or importance of the course topics is reflected in the number of items included to test each topic.

In constructing a test blueprint, the staff development specialist first outlines the critical content to be tested. Next, the learning outcomes are specified in observable, measurable, and behavioral terms. The relationship between the content, observable behaviors, and number of test items per topic then is arrayed on a matrix. Finally, those test items that will measure desired behaviors are identified. For example, true/false items measure recall; multiple choice items measure knowledge, comprehension, and application; and essay questions can test application, analysis, and synthesis (see Chart 8-2).

In addition to constructing a test blueprint, the staff development specialist should write the test items, and then pilot test them to learn whether they "discriminate knowledgeable from less knowledgeable learners."[6] Once a variety of test items are written on a particular topic, they can be used indefinitely (as long as the content does not change). The staff development specialist simply selects a variety of items from a file, according to the topic to be tested and the level of the desired behavior, and designs the test.

The nursing staff development specialist may choose to use tests other than written ones. These measurement tools include performance check lists, competency models, preceptor ratings, simulations, games, and other similar means. Tests can be used at the conclusion of a staff development course, or in a pre-post test format, where knowledge is assessed both before and after a class. Assuming the pre post test is reliable and valid, the results can indicate the extent to which the course improved knowledge in a specific subject.

In any evaluation, the nursing staff development specialist considers using a variety of data collection methods. While a standardized evaluation form is simple to design and use, often the quality of data is affected when only a single measure is used. No one type of instrument can be relied upon to collect all of the information necessary to make decisions about the program, nor can conclusions and recommendations be based on limited data.[7]

Chart 8-2
Principles of Test Construction

Alternate Response Items (true/false; agree/disagree)

Confine the statement to one simple idea. Avoid specific words such as always, never, usually. Directions must be exact. There should be approximately equal numbers of false as true items.

For example:
1. The purpose of a needs assessment study is to assess the probability of attendance at specific programs.
   ....True
   ....False

Multiple Recognition

All alternatives (possible responses) should agree grammatically with the stem. Do not use "a" or "an" with the alternatives. Use at least four alternatives with each item. Avoid alternatives that may give clues to the correct response.

For example:
1. Multiple approaches to needs assessment are used to:
   (a) obtain additional information from the same population
   (b) validate the accuracy of the needs assessment data
   (c) discover which method results in the most information
   (d) experiment with various methods to find the best one

Completion Items

Blanks should be placed at the end of the sentence. Avoid using too many blanks in each sentence. Key words should be the ones omitted from the sentence. Only one answer should be possible for each blank.

For example:
1. Learning needs are best identified by...

Whether for an individual offering or an evaluation of the entire nursing staff development department, the specialist relies on a variety of sources. And, all of the data collection methods used must be valid and reliable ones.[7]

In addition to evaluating educational offerings at their completion, an evaluation of the nursing staff development program should be conducted at least every two years. Here, program refers to the educational, as well as administrative, efforts of the department.

While comfortable with evaluating individual offerings, many nursing staff development specialists are less comfortable with a total program evaluation. Some program evaluation methods exist that are simple to use, and the

Matching Items

More choices should be offered than can be matched. Terms should not give clues to the expected response. The matches should be unambiguous but not obvious.

Essay Questions

The nature of the task should be clearly stated ("discuss..." is not sufficient). The exact limits should be defined. The desired outcomes should be the basis for grading.

Situation Analysis

The situation should be geared toward the learner's knowledge and experience. Sufficient information should be included to assure clarity. The description should be of reasonable length. A variety of test items can be used to assess the analysis of the situation.

Critical Incident

The critical incident should be sharply focused. No extraneous information should be included. Questions should relate only to the information provided.

Decision Making

Criteria for judging the adequacy of decisions made should be specified in advance. A variety of test items can be used to assess competency in critical thinking.

Source: Puetz and Associates, Inc. © 1988. Reproduced with permission.

nursing staff development specialist can select one that best meets his/her current needs and available resources. The benefits of a total program evaluation far outweigh the additional effort. Nursing staff development directors can use the findings from an evaluation study as a basis for decisions about resource allocation, and to monitor the effectiveness of individual educational offerings as well as the entire educational effort.

Evaluation studies are useful in marketing an educational activity to prospective clients and within the organization. Positive results from a comprehensive evaluation study can be used to enhance the nursing staff development department's position within the organization.

Beyond the institutional focus, too, the results of an evaluation study may contribute to the existing knowledge base of the profession, if the study is published in the nursing literature. For these and other reasons, evaluation should be considered a worthwhile investment of nursing staff development resources.

Implementing an Evaluation Study

Once the decision has been made to implement an evaluation study of the total nursing staff development program, a framework for the study is chosen. A number of evaluation models may be used; these models are viewed as standards against which the program is measured.

Pattern Analysis Method

Perhaps the simplest means of assessing the educational efforts of a nursing staff development department can be called "pattern analysis." Adapted from qualitative inquiry methodology, this method describes a search for patterns or commonalities in a mass of data.[8]

To implement pattern analysis as an evaluation mechanism, the nursing staff development specialist accumulates evaluation data from each of the educational activities sponsored by the department in a period of time, generally one year. These evaluations are reviewed, and an attempt is made to elicit patterns or trends in the data. The review is best conducted by a pair of individuals, preferably not directly associated with the nursing staff development department, who review the data individually, discover similarities in responses, group these similarities, and then compare notes on the patterns they found. The resulting patterns can relate to achievement of objectives, effectiveness of faculty and/or teaching methods, and appropriateness of the educational environment. In addition, learning needs may be identified as a pattern.

While this method will provide useful information about the educational activities being sponsored by the nursing staff development department, it lacks depth and scope. Other evaluation approaches also consider administrative aspects as well as program planning. Among the evaluation models that take total nursing staff development efforts into consideration are the discrepancy model and transactional evaluation.

Discrepancy Evaluation Model

Of the many evaluation models from which to choose, perhaps the simplest to apply is Provus' discrepancy model.[9] This model involves a search for discrepancies or differences between two or more elements or variables that should be in agreement. Discrepancy evaluation usually focuses on inconsistencies between program design in comparison with established design criteria, projected and actual program operations, achievement of terminal objectives, or the program's cost in comparison with similar programs.

Most frequently, discrepancies involved in evaluating nursing staff development programs are those between program plans and actual program operations, or predicted and obtained program outcomes. In implementing this type of discrepancy evaluation, a determination is made as to whether what was planned was successfully implemented, or whether what was supposed to occur actually did happen.

Discrepancies that are found then are identified and analyzed. Should a discrepancy exist between what was anticipated and what was accomplished, the program is carefully analyzed to determine the cause of the discrepancy. Significant discrepancies between what was anticipated and what was accomplished indicate that changes in the program are needed.

Implementing discrepancy evaluation requires three steps.

1. Define standards for the program.
2. Search for discrepancies between the program and the standards.
3. Use the information about discrepancies for decision making about the program.[10]

Standards are the criteria used to describe effective programs in terms of resources, procedures, management, and outcomes. Typically, these criteria reflect the program's goals and objectives. The program's goals and objectives must be clear and unambiguous, concise, consistent with departmental policies and procedures, accurate in terms of the outcomes desired, and within the capability of the department to achieve. If the department goals and objectives are well written, a discrepancy evaluation can be implemented with ease.

Next, the means to measure the standards are selected; generally, a variety of data collection methods are appropriate. Once the data are collected, analysis occurs to determine if a discrepancy exists, and, if so, the extent of the discrepancy.

The final step requires that the evaluation information be used by the program's decision makers. Actions to continue, change, or end the program may result from the evaluation study.

Transactional Evaluation Model

This evaluation model works best in situations where there appears to be a system dysfunction.[11] In implementing this model, those involved in any way with the nursing staff development department (participants, faculty, instructors, administrators, etc.) submit their impressions in writing of what is wrong with the current system. Or, to avoid the emphasis on the negative, individuals can be asked to write down three positive observations, and three aspects of the program that need to be changed or improved.

These anonymous responses are used to construct the items on a questionnaire. Verbatim comments are used where possible. Similar comments can be combined into an item, but the meaning of the individual comments should not be lost in this process.

Everyone involved with the program then receives the questionnaire. The questionnaires are completed and returned for tabulation of the results. The results then are distributed to those involved in the study. Care should be taken to preserve anonymity at all stages of the evaluation.

After the collated summary of responses has been returned to the participants, a meeting is scheduled to discuss the issues raised by the evaluation. Both positive and negative aspects of the program should be discussed, but only those on which there was considerable agreement. In addition to talking about negative aspects of the program, time should be devoted to corrective actions.

Accreditation Evaluation Model

The ANA's (1988) continuing education accreditation process typifies the accreditation evaluation model. In this approach, known as the judgmental prototype of evaluation, an accrediting body reaches a conclusion about an organization's educational processes and thereby assists the organization to improve its program efforts.

The applicant organization first conducts an extensive self-study based on the criteria provided by the accrediting body. The self-study permits the institution to assess its strengths and weaknesses as well as areas that need improvement.

The applicant submits materials attesting to its ability to meet the established accreditation criteria. The application usually consists of the self-study narrative, plus whatever documentation is needed to substantiate that the criteria are met.

Experts then review the submitted materials in comparison with the established guidelines. A site visit to the applicant agency also may be conducted, during which experts confer with individuals involved in the program. The site visit team then determines whether the applicant meets the criteria or not, and transmits this information to the accrediting body.

The accreditation body, then, makes a decision regarding approval of the applicant institution. The primary focus of the judgmental approach to evaluation is the "application of presumed expertise to yield judgments about quality or effectiveness" of an educational program, and the accreditation system reflects this application of expertise.[12]

It should be noted that the current accreditation mechanism of the ANA focuses solely on the continuing education portion of the staff development program. The criteria on which the accreditation model is based, however, can easily be used to evaluate other components of the staff development department, including orientation programs, for example.

Countenance Evaluation Model

In this model, the evaluator collects, processes, and interprets descriptive data gathered from various audiences concerned with the program under study. After the descriptive phase of the evaluation, the evaluator derives a judgment about the value or worth of the program.[13]

The descriptive data collected on the program consists of antecedent, transaction, and outcome data. The evaluator's judgments consider the interactive nature of input characteristics, the curriculum and instructional processes, and output. Translated into Stake's terms, input characteristics are antecedents, the curriculum and instructional processes are transactions, and output is outcome.

Antecedent. An antecedent occurs prior to something else happening; in an educational setting, an antecedent is whatever exists before the teaching/learning process is initiated. According to this definition, the organizational structure, organizational philosophy, mission statement, and the nursing staff development department's goals and objectives all are considered antecedents.

Learner antecedents describe the individual coming to the educational experience in terms of age, sex, experience, education, motivation, reasons for attending, and other characteristics. Antecedent data also can be collected on faculty or planners or any other individuals involved in the program. The community and the institution in which the nursing staff development program is located should be included in the antecedent category.

Transactions. Transactions are interactions between learners and others in the program, such as the faculty, program planners, and other learners. Any interaction between people in the educational environment is considered a transaction.

In addition to human interactions, there are transactions between learners and the learning materials. Learners have handouts, audio-visuals are used, perhaps there is a pretest or posttest, or both, or a final examination: all of these are transactions. Learners also interact with the environment, so that transactions between learner and behavioral objectives, content outlines, the teaching methods used, and the evaluation methods also are included.

Outcomes. Outcomes result from the educational process. These outcomes can describe changes in learners' attitudes, or the impact of education on practice. The faculty and program planners also experience outcomes; perhaps the evaluation results were satisfying, and the faculty and planners felt good about the educational activity they planned and implemented.

Antecedents, transactions, and outcomes are assessed using existing data collection methods, or specific instruments are constructed for the purpose of the evaluation study. All of the descriptive data collected on a program are placed in a matrix. Comparisons between intended and actual antecedents, transactions, and outcomes of a program then are made.

In making a judgment about the program, the evaluator reviews relationships between intended and actual antecedents, transactions, and outcomes. Congruence between these aspects should be evident: transactions should depend on antecedents, and outcomes should result from transactions. Some outcomes may be contingent upon particular antecedents and/or specific transactions.

If there is not congruence between the intended and the observed, the evaluator determines whether the lack of congruence is significant. Obviously, it is a matter of opinion whether the lack of congruence is important; generally the nursing staff development specialist is in the best position to decide.

These decisions comprise the judgment component of Stake's model which also is comprised of antecedents, transactions, and outcomes. The evaluator makes judgments about the program, and again, these are arrayed in a matrix in which the two horizontal columns are "standards" and "judgments."

Standards are the basis for judgments about the program. Two types of standards are used: absolute or relative comparison. In absolute comparison, the program is judged against some standards of excellence, such as the ANA (1988) accreditation criteria. Relative comparison permits judgment of the program with respect to another program. The evaluation judgments involve which standards are the most important as well as which standards the program should meet.

As a result of the description and judgment components, a decision can be made about the merit of an educational program. Based on the determination of the worth of the program, recommendations for improvement of the program can follow.

While rather complex, this model has been used to evaluate a hospital staff development department[14] and a staff development program on lifting and moving patients.[15] One of the major constraints of Stake's model is that data often overlap, so that some distinctions are not clear. Because of its comprehensive nature, however, the model can be modified before being implemented, and the result still will be an evaluation of value to the program.

Goal-Free Evaluation Model

Michael Scriven's[16] model of evaluation, unlike the others previously described, does not rely heavily on the nursing staff development program's objectives as a basis for assessment. Accordingly, Scriven's model often is referred to as a "goal-free" evaluation model. Goal-free evaluation is the evaluation of "actual effects against....a profile of demonstrated needs."[16]

In implementing this model, the evaluator gathers data from a wide variety of sources, such as learners, members of the community, and representatives from the institution. These data reflect actual effects of the program, whether positive or negative, intended or not. Then, the program effects are objectively assigned weights to describe their relative importance. The weights are based on value judgments about various aspects of the program, including learner characteristics, the organization, and financial concerns. Information about each of these facets is weighted by the values assigned to it in order to arrive at an overall appraisal of the program.

Context, Input, Process, Product Evaluation Model

Decision-management evaluation models, typified by Stufflebeam's CIPP model, are for the purpose of describing programs, so that informed decisions can be made about the program.[17] Four types of evaluation—context, input, product, and process—are combined to form the CIPP model.

Context Evaluation. Context evaluation assesses the environment, including desired or ideal conditions, in comparison with existing conditions. Context evaluation also defines needs, particularly those that have not been met, and identifies problems that underlie the needs. Context evaluation provides information for decisions about program planning, such as those related to the environment or setting, the audience to be served, the goals of the program, and the specific objectives to be achieved.

Input Evaluation. Input evaluation assesses the program's capabilities, defines strategies for achieving the program's objectives, and identifies ways for implementing specific strategies. Assessment of a program's capabilities involves its internal and external resources. Strategies to implement program goals are identified, as are the costs and possible benefits of each of the strategies.

Input evaluation provides information about impediments to the implementation of the strategies. Input evaluation helps the nursing staff development specialist make decisions about the program's goals and the means necessary and available to reach them. It describes resources and suggests the best use of resources based on costs and benefits, resulting in a plan to achieve the program's goals.

Process Evaluation. Process evaluation provides information necessary to monitor the nursing staff development program and make day-to-day decisions about operations. In this phase of the evaluation, the focus is on complete and ongoing recordkeeping. These records should provide information about the program to describe program events over time, thus helping in drawing conclusions related to goal implementation.

Product Evaluation. Product evaluation measures and interprets program attainments. In addition, product evaluation data are related to the context, product, and process information. Product evaluation helps make decisions about whether to continue programs, based on whether the program actually accomplished its goals or not.

While the CIPP model is a holistic one that considers all aspects of the program being evaluated, there is little or no emphasis on value concerns. Information obtained from this evaluation will help the nursing staff development specialist make decisions and manage program operations, but not make a judgment about the worth or value of the nursing staff development program.

Audit Evaluation Model

Another evaluation approach that can assist the nursing staff development specialist in decision-making related to the program is the audit model, which quantifies the services offered by the nursing staff development program.[18] In this model, the evaluator gathers information to describe the learners attending educational offerings, the faculty planning and teaching these offerings, the number of programs produced, and the evaluations of the programs.

A combination of objective and subjective data, the model provides quantitative information about nursing staff development services offered. Within the overall data generated, specific information also is available to the institution and the nursing staff development specialist for decision-making purposes. Included in this particular information is faculty workload, who provides what program for what group of individuals, and other findings that can help in future planning.

While each of the models presented have advantages, they also have disadvantages, and so the nursing staff development specialist may be reluctant to embrace only one. Tiessen[19] echoed this concern in her presentation of an evaluation model that combined aspects of several others. The resulting model viewed input in the form of entry into the hospital system; throughput in the form of orientation, inservice, and continuing education; and output in the form of behavioral performance and improved patient care, as feedback mechanisms for the staff development department in making decisions about their educational activities. Similarly, models can be constructed by nursing staff development specialists to meet their needs in evaluating their programs or departments.

Impact Evaluation

Increasingly, attention is being addressed not only to the direct outcomes of an educational activity (change in participants' knowledge, skill, attitude), but to the translation of learning into practice. The nursing staff development specialist is being called upon to demonstrate that the educational activities provided actually do translate into changes in practice.

Evaluation studies of the impact of education on practice, particularly those that also assess changes in patient outcomes, involve sophisticated research design. Kirkpatrick[20] described several research studies in which evaluation of training programs was reflected in on-the-job behavior, primarily in industry, and cautioned that such evaluation is more difficult than assessing learning in the classroom setting. Further work reported by Kirkpatrick[21] described the outcomes of several training programs, again in industry. The results of the training program were reflected in decreased lost time due to accidents, and in fewer problems with mail following orientation of postal carriers. In health care settings, Rottet and Cervero[22] reported on a performance evaluation of an orientation program for professional nurses. The orientees' performance the first week and six months following orientation was rated on a concurrent audit tool used by members of the institution's quality assurance committee, and was assessed at high levels of transfer from the educational to the work setting.

Several simple methods of assessing the extent to which what has been learned has been translated into subsequent practice are available. Two of these methods involve self-reports of the participants. Self-reports, generally not considered sufficiently reliable, however, can be validated through other measures such as direct observation if desired.

In the first method, participants are asked to list on their program evaluation form a number of specific behaviors they intend to perform on the job as a result of what they have learned. This part must be identified with the learner's name, although the responses to the remainder of the questionnaire can remain anonymous if the two parts of the evaluation form are separated.

Some time after course completion, usually four to six weeks, the individual's statement is sent to him/her with a short form to complete. The form asks the individual to identify the extent to which he/she currently is performing the behaviors listed, and what helps or hinders the performance of the behaviors on the list. Results are tabulated, and can provide information regarding needed changes in the program as well as in the practice setting.

This approach has been formalized as The Participant Action Plan Approach (PAPA).[23] As defined, the PAPA involves five basic steps.

1. Planning: The staff development specialist decides what specifically is needed to implement PAPA based on the available resources and needs of the organization.

2. In-course activities: Participants are told they will be involved in preparing and implementing an action plan detailing what they plan to apply on the job as a result of what they learned in the class.

3. Follow-up activities: Usually occur several months after the training program, at which time participants are contacted and asked to describe what they have been able to do as a result of their training, and how effective their efforts have been. They also are queried about what problems they encountered when trying out new behaviors.

4. Analysis and conclusions: The data collected are examined to determine the extent and type of change that occurred.

5. Report: The results of the PAPA are summarized for key decision makers in the organization.

The PAPA can be used by the staff development specialist not only to evaluate the impact of education on subsequent performance, but also to assess other learning needs. A multipart form can be designed on which participants write the specific behaviors they intend to perform after the course. A copy can be given to the participant's manager for reinforcement of changed behavior, and one copy retained by the staff development specialist for follow up.

In another, somewhat more detailed, yet still relatively simple approach to impact evaluation, behavioral objectives for the course are written in measurable terms, at levels of application beyond comprehension. Following completion of the course, at three-, six-, nine-, and twelve-month intervals, the participants are sent the course objectives and asked to indicate their response to the following items on a scale of 1 to 5, where 1 is "to a minimal extent," and 5 is "to a great extent:"

1. To what extent is *[behavior]* appropriate and relevant in your current position?
2. To what extent are you expected to perform *[behavior]* on your job?
3. To what extent were you able to perform *[behavior]* before you attended the course?
4. To what extent are you now able to perform *[behavior]?*
5. To what extent did the course [name] help you in learning to perform *[behavior]?*

The effort required for busy individuals to complete even such a short questionnaire often is reflected in low return rates for such surveys. This discouraging rate of return can be offset somewhat by eliciting the cooperation of those involved.

Participants in courses that will be subject to follow-up evaluation should be notified at the outset of the course that they will be involve Supervisors can be recruited to distribute and collect forms. And, if c small, statistically significant numbers of courses and participants are cb for impact evaluation studies, the nursing staff development specialist's efforts can be targeted toward follow-up of nonreturned questionnaires from the entire sample in the study. The intent here is to obtain quality rather than quantity.

The nursing staff development specialist can use strategies designed to improve the transfer of learning into practice by ensuring that the courses offered are related to critical learning needs of staff. Courses also should be designed to anticipate potential problems that may occur in trying out new behaviors in practice. Accordingly, efforts should be made to allow participants to practice or rehearse what they will do when they return to their practice settings. Elements of change theory can be included in the course content, so that learners understand how to implement change in their settings. And, nursing staff development specialists can follow up on the nursing units to inquire how the educational program may have made a difference in a nurse's subsequent practice.

Impact evaluation studies require an extensive outlay of resources, so decisions have to be made about the value of the information received, based on the resources expended. Accordingly, follow up evaluation efforts should be targeted primarily toward critical courses. These critical courses are those in which the learning is expected to change practice, rather than those with the primary goal of transmitting knowledge. Obviously, courses in which skill rather than knowledge is the focus lend themselves more readily to impact evaluation efforts.

Summary

The evaluation of nursing staff development educational offerings and programs is an essential component of managing the education and training enterprise. Evaluation is useful for so many purposes in the educational setting that it is critical to plan, implement, and evaluate offerings and programs on an ongoing basis.

While many means of evaluation are complex and time consuming, many can be modified to fit specific situations and thus be greatly simplified. The models described in this chapter should be viewed as a framework or guide for evaluation efforts. The model used should be selected on the basis that it is the most appropriate one to address the specific needs of the nursing staff development department. Whichever approach is used should demonstrate conclusively that the nursing staff development program is meeting its goals and objectives, and, further, making an invaluable contribution to the institution.

References

1. Puetz, B. E. (1987). *Contemporary strategies for continuing education in nursing.* Rockville, MD: Aspen.
2. Hefferin, E. A., Kleinknecht, M. K., & Arndt, C. (1987). Trends in the evaluation

of nursing inservice education programs. *Journal of Nursing Staff Development, 3,* 28–40.

3. American Nurses' Association (1988). *Manual for accreditation as a provider of continuing education in nursing.* Kansas City, MO: Author.

4. Kirkpatrick, D. L. (1959). Techniques for evaluating training programs. Part 1: Reaction. *Journal of the ASTD, 3*(1–5).

5. Ebel, R. L. (1972). *Essentials of educational measurement.* Englewood Cliffs, NJ: Prentice-Hall, Inc.

6. Layton, J. M. (1986). Validity and reliability of teacher-made tests. *Journal of Nursing Staff Development, 2,* 105–109.

7. Puetz, B. E. (1985). *Evaluation in nursing staff development: Methods and models.* Rockville, MD: Aspen.

8. Miles, M. B., & Huberman, A.M. (1984). *Qualitative data analysis.* Beverly Hills, CA: Sage.

9. Provus, M. (1971). *Discrepancy evaluation.* Berkeley, CA: McCutchan.

10. Worthen, B. R., & Sanders, J. R. (1973). *Educational evaluation: Theory and practice.* Worthington, OH: Charles A. Jones Publishing Company.

11. Rippey, R. M. (Ed.) (1973). *Studies in transactional evaluation.* Berkeley, CA: McCutchan.

12. Worthen & Sanders, *Educational evaluation: Theory and practice,* p. 127.

13. Stake, R. E. (1967). The countenance of educational evaluation. *Teachers College Record, 68,* 523–540.

14. Fojtasek, G. (1985). A model for evaluating a staff development program. *The Journal of Continuing Education in Nursing, 15*(4), 58–62.

15. Tarcinale, M.A. (1988). The role of evaluation in instruction. *Journal of Nursing Staff Development, 4,* 97–103.

16. Scriven, M. (1976). Prose and cons about goal–free evaluation. *Evaluation Comment, 3*(4), 1–13.

17. Stufflebeam, D.L. (1971). *Educational evaluation and decision-making.* Bloomington, IN: Phi Delta Kappan National Study Committee on Education.

18. Posavac, E. J., & Carey, R. G. (1980). *Program evaluation: Methods and case studies.* Englewood Cliffs, NJ: Prentice-Hall.

19. Tiessen, J. B. (1987). Comprehensive staff development evaluation: The need to combine models. *Journal of Nursing Staff Development, 3,* 9–14.

20. Kirkpatrick, D. L. (1960). Techniques for evaluating training programs. Part 3: Behavior. *Journal of the ASTD, 4,* 10–13.

21. Kirkpatrick, D.L. (1960). Techniques for evaluating training programs. Part 4: Results. *Journal of the ASTD, 4,* 14– 17.

22. Rottet, S. M., & Cervero, R. M. (1986). Clinical evaluation of a nursing orientation program. *Journal of Nursing Staff Development, 2,* 110–114.

23. U.S. Office of Personnel Management (1980). *The participant action plan approach.* Washington, DC: Author.

chapter 9

Staff Development Programming to Meet Other Organizational Needs

Mary Cramer Simpson

In the real world of nursing staff development, educational programs and other activities do not always fit into neat and tidy frameworks. The work of staff development is driven by the needs and desires of the organization as represented by a variety of administrators, managers, and other individuals. There are occasions in which nursing staff development specialists may be asked or expected to function in capacities that may seem outside the role emphasized in this book. This chapter will discuss those situations and common responses. In addition, suggestions and advice about how to use those situations as opportunities for growth and political positioning will also be explored. Selected programs that do not fit into categories described in other chapters will be reviewed, including the new program area of unit development and team building. Finally, how to meet organizational needs within a politically savvy framework will be examined.

Facilitating Organizational Goals

A great deal of time, energy, and the resources of the staff development department will, at one time or another, be spent in activities that arise from organizational needs and priorities. Organizational priorities are reflected in a variety of activities, such as committee participation, project management, consultation with individuals or groups, and facilitation of organizational change.

At first glance, involvement in such activities may seem secondary to the "real work" of the staff development department—that of developing staff competencies through provision of orientation, inservice, and continuing education programs. In reality, aligning educational programs and services to organizational needs is central to the mission of the staff development department.

Because the scope of such activities is so diverse, it is important for the specialist to clearly understand the role of the staff development program and how it supports the goals of the organization. The primary mission of any health care organization is the provision of health care services to the client population it serves. Within nursing, goals are primarily related to patient outcomes, whereas educational goals are second-order goals that support the primary goals of patient care.[1]

The purpose of the staff development department is to provide educational programs and services that will enable staff to meet the performance expectations of their positions. However, the purpose of staff development is "not simply to provide education but promote the organization's service mission."[2] The role of staff development is to enable employees to utilize their knowledge and skills to accomplish the goals of the organization.

The relationship of the staff development department to the organization is one of a staff function versus a line relationship. Line relationships, such as those of administrators or managers, infer direct accountability for accomplishment of the organization's mission. Staff functions, such as those enacted by human resources, quality assurance, and nursing staff development departments, provide an advisory/supportive function to the organization. While services provided by staff departments contribute significantly to accomplishments of organizational goals, staff departments in and of themselves cannot directly set goals or bring about their achievement.[2] It is only when the staff function (education) is in partnership with line accountability (patient care outcomes) that the goals of the organization are realized. The administrator of the staff development department should enjoy equal rank and privilege to the clinical administrators in order to be effective; however, the role of the administrator and specialist does not include line authority over the nursing staff in most organizations.

The ability of a staff role to influence the achievement of organizational goals should not be underestimated. The staff development specialist is in a unique position to utilize both the educational expertise and inherent power of the staff development role in order to address organizational priorities.

A primary responsibility of the staff development specialist is to analyze organizational goals from an educational perspective. What competencies will be required by staff to achieve these goals? What levels of staff will be affected? What types of educational programming must be implemented to make that happen? What systems, either educational, administrative, or structural, need to be in place to ensure ongoing performance?

Attainment of organizational goals invariably requires some level of change; in turn, organizational change requires some level of educational support. Organizational change necessitates the need for acquisition of new knowledge and skills to implement the change, or "unlearning" or "relearning," from a previous way of doing things. The role of education is critical to the change process, whether it is with the organization, a group, or an individual.

The staff development specialist, operating from a staff role, interfaces with multiple departments and groups. This organizational mobility provides the specialist with a broad perspective of the total organization. An organizationally neutral position allows the staff development specialist to advocate staff needs to management and articulate management priorities to staff. With a "foot in both camps," options are viewed holistically and accomplishments of goals through result-oriented planning can be ensured.

The ability to access information and communicate it quickly and easily can assist the staff development specialist in promoting organizational priorities. By seeking information, researching the literature, and developing proposals and plans to address organizational needs, the staff development specialist assumes a proactive, versus reactive stance.[2,3]

Such proactivity can contribute to the avoidance of a common organizational practice—that of enacting change without sufficient time allocated to the planning and implementation of educational support that is needed to facilitate the change.[3] Without proactive involvement, the staff development specialist and the staff development department will fall victim to crisis management. The department's inability to facilitate organization priorities in a timely manner may be viewed as organizational liability, versus an asset.

Organizational goals, priorities, and needs should serve as the basis of the staff development department's annual planning. While the provision of educational services will be the primary focus, staff development specialists should not limit their ability to promote organizational goals to those activities that are solely educational in nature.

Several examples are provided to illustrate this approach:

- If a priority for the organization is to increase the market share through contractual agreements with other hospitals, the staff development department could contract educational services that would facilitate movement of patients from one institution to another.
- If an organizational priority is to increase sources of revenue, the staff development department might investigate and procure grant funding to offset the expenses of programs or projects.
- If an organizational priority is implementation of a clinical advancement program, the staff development department could offer their expertise in coordinating development and implementation of the program.

The degree to which the staff development department promotes attainment of organizational goals and priorities will be directly proportional to the perceived value of staff development to the organization.[2] Likewise, the overall effectiveness of the staff development effort will ultimately be measured by the ability of the employees and the organization to accomplish its stated mission.

Committee Involvement

Committee participation is an important responsibility of the nursing staff development specialist. Although business folklore contends that a camel is a horse that was designed by a committee, the work of an organization is planned and evaluated through its committee structures. Organizational goals, priorities, and needs are often first identified and addressed through committees.

Committees are used by organizations to define standards, problem solve, communicate, develop or maintain programs, and conduct short-term and long-range planning. Although the number and types of committees will vary from one institution to another, there are key nursing committees that warrant representation of nursing staff development resources. Chart 9-1 illustrates most of these committees and the general function of the committee within the organization.

Committee participation benefits the staff development department in numerous ways. Committee activities provide valuable sources of information that assist staff development specialists in planning, prioritizing, providing, and evaluating the effectiveness of their educational efforts. Several committees, for example, the Policy or Procedure Committee, define standards of practice that are expected of the nursing staff. Written standards, can serve as the basis to define the competencies and expected outcomes of orientation and skills training programs. Standard setting committees also provide needs assessment data from which to plan ongoing orientation, inservice, and continuing education offerings.

Chart 9-1
Organizational Committees Warranting Nursing Staff Development Representation

Committee	Function
Policy/Procedure Protocol Documentation/Forms Education Committees	Standard setting
Quality Assurance Safety/Risk Management Infection Control Product Evaluation Nursing Research	Monitoring and Evaluation
Nursing Practice Employee Relations Recruitment/Retention	Problem Solving
Task Forces Management/Executive Councils	Planning/Decision Making

Source: Mary Cramer Simpson, Ohio University Hospital, Columbus, OH. Reproduced with permission.

Committees such as Quality Assurance, Safety, or Risk Management, monitor and evaluate the organization's compliance to standards. They provide information that can be used by the staff development department to evaluate achievement of learning objectives, as well as the overall effectiveness of educational offerings. Such committees also provide an excellent vehicle for organizational problem-solving.

Failure to comply with established standards is usually the result of a knowledge problem, a performance problem, or a system problem. Nursing staff development resources assist these committees by analyzing data from an educational perspective and identifying which problems can and cannot be resolved through educational interventions.

Committees also provide a mechanism to ensure an organization's compliance to external accreditation or credentialing standards. Through active involvement in Safety or Infection Control Committees, for example, the staff development department can ensure the provision of educational programs that are required to comply with state or federal or other regulations. Participation in the Quality Assurance committee provides the staff development department with a mechanism to link educational programming to quality assurance findings—a standard required for agency accreditation by the Joint Commission on Accreditation of Health Care Organizations.[4]

Participation in committees provides opportunities for the staff development department to expand or develop new services. Issues related to employee satisfaction (or perhaps lack thereof) identified in Employee Relations or Recruitment and Retention committees, may be amenable to initiation of staff support groups or career development programming. Staff development specialists have the positional flexibility (staff relationships in the organization) and expertise to serve as facilitators or internal consultants to individuals and groups. Committee activities can guide the staff development department in knowing when and how to best utilize its expertise.

A final benefit of committee participation is the opportunity it affords the staff development department to increase visibility and be recognized as contributing to the mission of an organization. This is especially true of participation in task forces or decision-making committees, which focus on strategic planning, facilitation of organizational change, or policy making.

Staff development resources can help these committees understand the role education plays in effecting organizational change. Active staff development participation ensures that committee recommendations will be supported by timely and appropriate educational programming. Committee members can also be trained to assist with the dissemination of information that is generated by the group.

The staff development department cannot be effective or valued unless the department has full representation on the top administrative committee where nursing practice and policy decisions are made, such as a Nursing Executive Council. Full membership and voting power are essential components of an effective staff development program. Such committee responsibility is usually assumed by the leader of the staff development department. Participation with decision-making bodies provides an opportunity for management and education to work together to address organizational issues and to share equally in the accountability for outcomes.

The role responsibilities of the staff development specialist as a committee member are several. The primary responsibility of the staff development specialist is to determine the educational implications of committee actions and recommendations. When do committee actions warrant dissemination of information versus a need for in-depth educational program? What staff competencies need to be developed and within what time frames for committee actions to be realized? Analysis of the committee actions from an educational perspective assists both the committee and the staff development specialist in planning appropriate interventions to support committee recommendations.

The staff development specialist provides a communication link between the committee and the staff development department. The specialist maintains responsibility for communication of committee activities to other staff within the department, and for ensuring that information relevant to program planning or evaluation is shared.

By having access to information and a number of human and material resources within and outside the organization, the staff development specialist serves as a content resource to committees and their participants. As a liaison to multiple departments, the staff development specialist promotes consistent implementation of standards across the organization. There are few staff development specialists who have not experienced at one time or another the situation where what is written in policy is "not the way we do it on our unit." By tuning in to the realities of the practice environment, staff development specialists facilitate recommendations that are sensitive to both the realties of practice and the needs of the organization.

The staff development specialist also helps develop committee members through formal and informal actions. Committees are wonderful vehicles for developing people's skills. A recent study reported that 92% of nurses involved in committee work indicated learning occurred as a result of part of their committee participation.[5] Committees teach staff about organizational systems and group process, as well as the "how to's" of designing programs, analyzing data, conducting meetings, or defining standards. The specialist may teach the members how to analyze data, or how to organize and conduct a brief learning activity. The specialist may prepare background material for presentation to the committee or help a member organize a library search to find out about the latest information on a particular topic. These and other activities develop members and prepare them for future roles as active participants.

Educational programming that arises from committee involvement provides an opportunity for the staff development specialist to utilize creative educational strategies. Because education to support committee activities must be quickly accessible to multiple levels of staff, nontraditional educational approaches may be most effective. In some hospitals, staff education regarding changes in policy and procedure is accomplished through use of study guides. Questions or information that can only be obtained by review of a new policy are incorporated into the study guide. Nursing staff complete the guide, return it to the staff development department, and, upon successful completion, are awarded hospital contact hours.

At another hospital, educational programming to support implementation of a falls program was developed by the staff development specialist who served as a member of the Nursing Quality Assurance Committee. The educational program consisted of two traveling posters—one listing Fifteen Facts For Forecasting Falls, and the second, made of erasable china board, outlined the occurrence of falls by severity, type, time, and location. By writing in data specific to a unit's patient population, the staff development specialist was able to tailor the program to the learning needs of the staff on that particular unit. In addition, the confidentiality of quality assurance data was ensured.

Gaming is an effective teaching strategy that can be used to support committee activities. Word games, such as seek-and-find or crossword puzzles can be used as a teaching strategy to provide annual updates of fire, disaster, electrical safety, or other mandatory programs. Newsletters or fairs, such as equipment or new product fairs, are also strategies that can be used to disseminate information to large numbers of staff in a timely manner.

Although committee participation benefits the staff development department in many ways, it is not without drawbacks. Committee involvement takes time—time to prepare for meetings, attend meetings, and do committee work outside of established meeting times. Time allocated for committee participation ultimately results in fewer available man hours that can be allocated to accomplish the educational activities that are primarily associated with the staff development department.

Secondly, the demand for committee representation may exceed the available staff development resources. This is especially true of small or one-person staff development departments. Facing such situations, staff development specialists may need to seek pragmatic yet creative alternatives to full committee membership, such as

- Establishing informal coalitions with committee chairs to ensure ongoing communication
- Attending meetings at specific times when agenda items warrant their expertise or interventions
- Ensuring minutes of committees are received on a regular basis

A final concern is determining when committee involvement is critical to the staff development function, and when it is merely doing the work of the organization. Because much of the work of staff development is supportive in nature, staff development resources may erroneously be viewed as having the "most time" to devote to committee work. This is a common dilemma experienced by staff development specialists, especially those who are requested to serve as a committee chair. Assuming leadership responsibility for a committee may be an appropriate staff development role, given the nature of the intended outcomes or political implications of committee involvement. However, if staff development resources are used indiscriminately in activities that are not relevant to their educational function, the perception that staff development specialists have "nothing more important to do" will be reinforced.

Ultimately, decisions must be made by staff development departments regarding which committees and what degree of involvement is most critical to the staff development function. These are not easy choices to make—but, if made wisely, such decisions serve to benefit the staff development department greatly.

Clinical Ladder Programs

During the late 1970s, health care institutions began to implement clinical ladder programs as a way to recognize excellence in nursing practice and provide clinical advancement options for nursing staff. There has been a resurgence of clinical ladder programs in the last few years, as the nursing shortage has compelled organizations to create financial and professional practice environments that attract and retain nursing resources.

Regardless of their intended purpose, clinical ladder programs are a mechanism to promote professional development of the nursing staff. Clinical ladder programs provide organizations with the framework and structure to define, develop, evaluate, and reward various levels of expertise in nursing practice.

Although the design of clinical ladder programs vary, there are four elements central to most clinical ladder programs. First, there are *defined performance expectations* that differentiate levels of competency in practice. A nurse who is a beginning practitioner does not function at the same level of competency as does a nurse who is considered expert. Development of practice expertise is the result of both knowledge and experience. Levels of practice, as defined within clinical ladder programs, differentiate performance expectations among nurses and provide a pathway of progression as advanced competencies are acquired.

Secondly, *performance expectations* include competencies in the areas of nursing process, education, leadership, and research. Performance expectations in the nursing process include competencies related to advanced clinical knowledge and skills, care planning, patient care management, and clinical judgment/decision-making. Performance expectations in education encompass competencies related to the provision of patient, staff, and student education, as well as activities related to one's ongoing professional growth and development. Performance expectations related to leadership include competencies or activities associated with formal or informal leadership within a unit, the organization, and/or the community. Responsibility for development of projects/programs, participation in activities that support unit goals, committee work, problem solving, and working with groups are common performance expectations in this area. Performance expectations associated with research include competencies related to systematic analysis of clinical problems/issues, participation in quality assurance activities, and operationalizing nursing practice from a research base.

A third element of clinical ladder programs is a *formalized evaluation process*. Evaluation will include self-evaluation as well a management evaluation component. In addition, many clinical ladder programs include peer evaluation and a review process conducted by an external body, such as a committee or review panel, as part of the advancement process.

The fourth element of clinical ladder programs is requirement of some type of formalized *documentation* of competencies, activities, or individual accomplishments indicative of an identified level of practice. Documentation may include preparation and maintenance of a professional portfolio, summaries of specific activities, or submission of written materials that illustrate the individual's ability to demonstrate specific competencies, such as developing patient care plans or education plans.

In many organizations, management and coordination of clinical ladder programs are functions of the staff development department. Linking clinical ladder activities to staff development is consistent with the department goal of developing competence within the nursing staff. In addition, staff development programs and staff provide resources to the organization that promote the ongoing professional development of nursing staff.

Staff development specialists should be involved in the development and implementation of an organization's clinical ladder program. By participating in the creation and refinement of clinical programs, they assist in defining basic, intermediate, and advanced competencies associated with the different levels of practice. As an expert in education, they are content resources who identify educational competencies as well as the amount of time and experience that will be needed by staff to advance from one level to another.

A common temptation in developing clinical ladder programs is to establish stringent performance criteria, accompanied by short time frames for advancement. This often occurs because of a well-intentioned attempt to ensure that clinical ladder programs are meaningful, yet accessible and amenable to staff participation. In reality, establishing advanced practice options for nursing staff who may lack the knowledge and experience to enact them may set them up for failure and eventually reduce the professional growth options the program intended to achieve! The staff development specialist, as an educational expert, can identify appropriate time frames for competency development and assist in developing a clinical ladder program that is meaningful yet realistic.

Implementation of a clinical ladder program has several implications for educational program development. In order for a the ladder program to be successful, all members of the organization need to understand what the program is, how it works, and what roles they have in its operation. A massive educational effort addressing these issues must be provided throughout the nursing organization prior to initial program implementation.

Educational program requirements must be in place to support nurses who wish to pursue advancement through the program. Educational programs will need to be targeted in three areas:

- Education relevant to the design of the clinical ladder program
- Education to develop advanced practice competencies
- Education that provides opportunity for professional development

Education relevant to the design of a clinical ladder program includes those areas of knowledge and skill required by staff to support the elements of the clinical ladder's program design. For example, if peer evaluation is a component of the clinical ladder program, staff who have little or no experience with conducting formalized evaluations may need to learn how to describe, document, and objectively appraise the practice of their peers. The role of the nurse manager will shift from one of appraising performance to one of performance management—encompassing the need for skills in coaching, goal setting, and aligning advanced practice competencies to unit goals or priorities. Staff nurses who want to advance through the clinical ladder program may need to learn how to write a curriculum vitae or organize and develop a professional portfolio that documents their professional accomplishments.

Educational programs need to be provided that will enable nursing staff to develop advanced practice competencies. Sovie[6] describes three stages of a professional career pattern in nursing—professional identification (orientation), professional maturation (potential for development and expansion of competencies), and professional mastery (self-actualization of potential). Unfortunately, many staff development departments direct their educational efforts towards basic competency development of nurses in the professional identification stage. Implementation of a clinical ladder program necessitates redirection of educational efforts to provide programs relevant for nurses in the stages of professional maturation and professional mastery. Education relevant to group process skills, organizational dynamics, health care issues, nursing management of patients with complex care needs, or advanced skill development applicable to specific patient populations, should be provided.

Educational activities that promote nurses' ongoing professional development must also be available. These activities encompass a wide range of areas, such as how to

- Develop an inservice offering
- Develop patient education materials
- Organize a journal club
- Give a presentation
- Conduct a research study
- Develop a clinical protocol

Professional development programs provide a splendid opportunity for staff development specialists to share their expertise with other nurses. Professional development activities should not be limited to formal education programs. A working sabbatical in the staff development department to complete a project, mentoring of a staff nurse by a staff development specialist, individual consultation, or small group learning experiences are all effective strategies that can be used to support the professional development of nursing staff.

If the staff development department maintains the responsibility for the ongoing management of the clinical ladder program, they will assume an additional role of counseling and advising staff who wish to pursue clinical advancement options. Career counseling, assessment of performance competencies, and assisting individuals to establish plans that will position them for advancement are additional support services that are needed to implement a clinical advancement program successfully.

Unit and Group Development

The staff development department is frequently used as a resource to assist in the development of units or groups of staff. Unit/group development takes many forms—from designing educational interventions that address performance problems to assisting groups in problem solving, conflict management, or goal achievement.

Unit/group development activities often arise from a perceived need for educational support. Requests may come to the staff development department that "X" unit needs an inservice on "Y" topic because of "Z" reasons. The need for unit/group development, however, is usually the direct result of problems or issues that may be challenging a group or affecting a unit, or of interpersonal and group dynamic problems that may or may not be amenable to educational intervention alone.

When working with units/groups, the staff development specialist assumes the role of internal consultant as well as that of teacher/educator. An internal consultant analyzes situations from an organizational perspective and identifies interventions that facilitate change within the individual, the group, or the system. The focus of an internal consultant is to address organizational needs through a planned process that is directed towards facilitating the thinking, learning, or doing of others.[7]

In working with units/groups, the staff development specialist enacts a process not unlike the nursing process or the educational process, involving assessing, diagnosing, establishing plans, initiating interventions, and evaluating outcomes. These process skills, coupled with interpersonal and facilitation skills, objectivity, and a broad perspective of the total organization and its subsystems, can be adapted for use with units, groups of staff, or an entire organization.

As mentioned earlier, unit/group development needs are frequently camouflaged in educational requests. A nurse manager, perceiving a problem or a performance discrepancy on the unit, may conclude that the problem could be solved if staff "learned what they were supposed to do." Although defining such a solution is a well-intentioned attempt to deal with and resolve problems quickly, the problem may exist because of other reasons, such as lack of motivation or blocks within the system. Staff development specialists who respond with educational interventions prematurely and neglect to identify the true cause of a problem may find their actions ineffective. The problem will most likely continue to exist, the manager and staff development specialist will be frustrated by their efforts, and time and money will have been spent on activities that did not achieve the desired result.

The first step in meeting unit/group development needs is initiation of an assessment process that accurately defines the issues to be addressed. It is important that this analysis be done jointly by the staff development specialist and the manager or leader of the group, and include input from group members. Mager and Pipe[8] have developed a framework for analyzing performance problems that can be easily adapted to assessing unit/group needs. It is particularly helpful in differentiating the educational, management, or system interventions that will need to be implemented.

A discrepancy of some kind will be at the core of unit/group development needs. A discrepancy is the difference between what is actually happening and what you desire to happen. Discrepancies may be related to performance (the staff are not doing discharge planning) or to a desire to implement a change (a unit goal to implement a new care delivery model). Discrepancies are not necessarily negative in nature. They merely describe the difference between what is and what should be.

The first step in Mager and Pipe's framework is to identify the *nature* of the discrepancy. They pose several very specific questions, such as

- What is the difference between what is being done and what is supposed to be done?
- Why do I think there is an educational problem?
- Why do I want to initiate this change?
- What event causes me to think things aren't right?

These are questions that can help define a discrepancy as it currently exists.

The next step is to evaluate the *importance* of the discrepancy. What are the consequences of the discrepancy? What are the costs? What would happen if nothing was done? Would doing something change the outcome?

If a discrepancy exists and if it is important, the next step is to determine *why* the discrepancy exists. It is important to determine if the discrepancy exists because of a lack of knowledge or skill or for some other reason. Do the staff know what they are required to do? Could they do what is desired "if their life depended on it?"[8,9] Could a unit/group enact this change right now with their current knowledge and skills? If the answers to these questions are no, then an educational need exists and the discrepancy can be managed through educational interventions.

If the answers to the above questions are yes, then there may be other factors, internal or external to the system, that are causing the discrepancy. Is enacting a desired performance or behavior punishing? Is nonperformance rewarding? What are the benefits or drawbacks of doing something the way we are now, versus changing the way we are doing things? Does it matter if we do it or not? Are there obstacles that are preventing the desired behavior? Answers to these questions provide direction for initiating management or system interventions that can remove the existing discrepancy.

Once a unit/group development need has been assessed and analyzed, a plan can be developed that defines the course of action to be taken. The plan should clearly outline the intended outcomes to be achieved, the activities that will occur, within what time frames, the role expectations of all parties involved, and how results will be measured. Plans should be negotiated and agreed upon by the manager/group leader and the staff development specialist and shared with all group members prior to implementation.

It is important that plans be written. Written plans or agreements can assist the staff development specialist to establish a relationship with a group, define why certain interventions are proposed, and affix accountability for results. Even if the focus of unit/group development is primarily educational in nature, the accountability for outcomes is shared among the manager, the learner, and the educator. It is the manager's responsibility to support staff learning by providing release time for staff to attend the activity and by setting expectations for staff participation. It is the learner's responsibility to actively participate and the educator's responsibility to structure the learning situation so that the desired outcomes can be achieved. Written plans clarify expectations and provide a mechanism to ensure a clear understanding of everyone's responsibility in the process. Signatures of both the manager and staff development specialist provide a visible sign of commitment to the plan.

Once the plan has been defined, written, and agreed upon, the plan can be implemented, and interventions can proceed. In working with unit/groups, interventions provided by the staff development specialist can be quite diverse. Interventions may include assessment of existent competencies or provision of specific educational programs. Interventions may include serving as a process consultant for a group, by facilitating problem-solving activities among group members. Interventions may include providing objective feedback to a group on a regular basis, or addressing a need for policy or procedure change with nursing administration. Regardless of the interventions utilized, it should be appropriate to the problem or issue that has been identified.

Evaluation is the final phase of the process. At some point conclusions must be drawn about what has occurred, how effective the interventions have been, or if the plan has achieved its goals. This is a critical step needed to bring closure to an activity or to refocus action in another direction. Because it is not always easy or comfortable for a group to evaluate its own progress, it is important for staff development specialist to work with the group to design objective ways to measure results. The need for unit/group development does not always arise from the group itself or from a direct request for intervention. By being cognizant of the goals, priorities, changes, and stressors within an organization, the staff development department specialist can identify issues that are amenable to group development activities. Such organizational needs may be a catalyst for expanding traditional services offered by the staff development department to include those of internal consultation.

Ulschak and SnowAntle[9] similarly summarize these steps in their outline of eight steps of the consulting process. They list the following:

1. Precontracting
2. Contracting
3. Data collection
4. Data analysis
5. Presentation
6. Action planning
7. Evaluation
8. Termination

These steps provide a useful framework to organize the work of internal consulting as it relates to unit and group development in health care organizations. Ulschak and SnowAntle further emphasize the need to identify the client of this service and advocate for the person who is the decision maker of the unit as the client. This is consistent with the continued need of the nursing staff development specialist to establish sound working relationships with the clinical nurse managers.

One staff development specialist identified how she was able to initiate a service to nursing that involved team-building strategies.[10] Through analysis of the rapid changes that were occurring within the organization and assessment of common problems reported by managers, several needs were identified. These needs included a need for better team functioning, improved communication skills, assertiveness, stress reduction, improved morale, and an increased sense of professionalism. Team building strategies were selected as an appropriate intervention to address these problems.

The staff development specialist designed a plan to be piloted on one unit which included group process as well as educational interventions. An initial workshop was conducted, focusing on group process and cohesion, team work, and strengths and weaknesses of the group. Upon completion of the workshop, an action plan was developed which included monthly follow-up sessions with the staff and manager, and was facilitated by the staff development specialist. The meetings were used to conduct group problem solving, refine group process and team-building skills, continue education, and chart progress.

At the end of a year, both staff and the manager identified positive results that had been achieved. They reported an increase in group rapport and the ability to problem solve and manage conflict, and an increase in communication skills and positive changes in group morale. As the success of the interventions were realized, several other units requested similar assistance from the staff development department.

Through internal consulting, staff development specialists have a unique opportunity to apply their knowledge, talents, and skills to organizational needs. Twenty skills and behaviors have been identified as inherent in the internal consulting role:[11]

Personal	*Influence*	*Communication*
Adaptability	Leadership	Listening
Trust and Integrity	Influencing	Speaking and Informing
Results Orientation	Organizational savvy	
Service Orientation	Coaching and Advising	*Problem Solving*
		Diagnosing
Interpersonal	*Administrative*	Decision making
Relationship Building	Priority Management	Business knowledge
Facilitating Skills	Project Management	Technical (education)
Managing Conflict		Knowledge
Ability to give feedback		

Internal consultation requires staff development specialists to redirect these skills from a learner-oriented focus to a group or organizational focus. Internal consultation also requires staff development specialists to accept a different reward system than usually experienced within a traditional educator role,[7] that of recognition of staff development specialists as experts in the classroom. As internal consultants, efforts are behind the scenes, and recognition occurs as a result of their ability to facilitate the accomplishments of others.

Perhaps more important than recognition is success—success in helping units, groups, or organizations get to where they want to be. By serving as an internal consultant, staff development specialists provide a valuable service to the organization and can promote an environment where change occurs in a positive and supportive way.

Working with Other Hospital Departments

In addition to working with units and groups in nursing, staff development specialists collaborate with other departments within the organization. The focus of such collaboration may encompass direct provision of educational services to that department, provision of education to nursing that is in support of another department's goals and priorities, or cosponsorship of programs/projects of mutual benefit.

Institutions vary in how educational resources are structured, as well as to whom educational services are targeted. In small hospitals, for example, the staff development department may be the only formalized educational resource that exists. Other institutions centralize educational resources within one department, providing services on a hospital-wide basis. Larger hospitals, or highly decentralized organizations, may have designated educational units or resources within multiple departments. Regardless of the structure, it is likely that departments other than nursing will seek educational support from the staff development department or specialist at one time or another.

Staff development departments are often contacted by other hospital departments to assist in addressing a particular learning need that exists within their department. Programming primarily targeted to nursing staff may be quite applicable to employees within another area. Sharing information and materials and accommodating additional participants using existent programming are feasible ways the staff development department assists other departments to meet the educational needs of their staff.

Staff development specialists are viewed as clinical resources, as well as educational resources, within an organization. Other departments frequently request their assistance in meeting a staff education need associated with patient care issues. An example of this was experienced several years ago. As placement of central venous access devices became a more widespread practice within the institution, the radiology department began to see more patients who had central lines as their only venous access site. The staff, unfamiliar with the technology, had many questions related to how to safely manage these patients and troubleshoot the equipment. An additional issue was the degree to which these lines could be used to administer intravenous agents associated with completion of radiologic studies.

The staff development department was contacted with a request to provide inservice education for the staff on these issues. Through collaboration among the department manager, the medical director, and the staff development specialist, policies and procedures pertinent to the care of these patients while in the radiology department were developed, and education to increase the staff's knowledge and skill in these areas was provided. The involvement of the staff development specialist as an educational/clinical resource was most appropriate, given the nature of the situation.

The extent to which staff development resources can be allocated to provide direct educational support to other hospital departments is a sensitive issue. If the staff development department is organized as a unit within the nursing organization, then the primary focus of their efforts should be directed toward the educational support of nursing. Time, staff, and materials equal dollars—dollars that have been allocated by nursing to support the nursing function. On the other hand, nursing and all departments within the organization share the common mission of providing health care services to patients and their families. The relationship of nursing to other hospital departments is an interdependent one, and working together in support of each other's priorities is crucial.

An approach staff development departments can use to balance conflicting yet compatible demands for their services is to structure their activities so that other hospital departments will be in the best position to help themselves. Instead of staff development resources providing multiple inservice education programs for staff within a particular department, a core group of resources within another department could be prepared through a "train the trainer" approach, to provide the needed educational support. Staff development specialists can shift their focus from that of teacher to educational consultant, assisting other hospital departments with the design of educational programs, such as self-learning packets, that can be implemented without direct allocation of instructional resources. These are ways educational needs of other hospital departments can be managed while minimizing the impact on staff development personnel.

Other hospital departments may seek staff development assistance to help implement departmental changes or priorities that have educational implications for the nursing staff. A common problem encountered in working with other departments is their lack of understanding regarding the complexity of implementing a change throughout the nursing organization. Hospital departments, particularly those with small staffs or who do not provide 24-hour services, may fail to recognize the implications of their need to "inservice all the nursing staff within the next two weeks!"

Staff development specialists need to be involved early in the planning process when assisting other hospital departments with change implementation. Besides addressing educational issues, the staff development specialist serves as a link between the nursing organization and other departments, and can communicate the need for and impact of a change to both groups. Such involvement may require other hospital departments to carefully reconsider their priorities and time frames as originally proposed. In the long run, however, this may be invaluable with assisting them to accomplish their goals successfully.

Collaboration between staff development and other hospital departments may also involve working together on joint projects of mutual interest. In such activities, the focus of collaboration shifts, from one of direct service or support of another's goals, to one of shared responsibilities for the program or project. A common example of this would be cosponsorship of a continuing education program, which would be of benefit to both departments and their staff.

Cosponsorship of educational programming requires negotiation between each department to determine responsibilities. Written agreements, can be useful tools to assist the staff development specialist in planning a cosponsored activity. Cosponsored agreements should address the role each department will assume in the following activities:

- Program design
- Coordination of the program
- Marketing
- Selection of faculty
- Program management activities such as registration and/or materials duplication, record keeping, and evaluation

In addition, program costs and how expected revenues will be shared should be identified.

All of these points serve as a basis for negotiation in a cosponsored program. It is important that the staff development department maintain accountability to ensure that internal or external educational standards are met. With some approval bodies, such as the American Nurses' Association (ANA) Continuing Education Accreditation Program, this is a required element. In addition, if the program is one where contact hours are to be awarded, again, such as through the ANA continuing education approval system, there will be certain program responsibilities that may not be negotiable with another department—such as specific elements of record keeping or planning of the program with nursing participation. Negotiation of shared or individual responsibilities in a cosponsored arrangement, should always be made in consideration of time, resources, and potential benefit of the program to the staff development effort.

Working with other departments provides opportunities for staff development specialists to extend their influence within the system. Formal and informal networks with other departments keep them attuned to organizational priorities. By approaching collaboration with the attitude of "what can we do together to address issues," staff development specialists are viewed as committed, concerned, and helpful. This perception ultimately benefits both the staff development department and the nursing organization.

Using Education to Support Other Goals

Health care organizations are undergoing rapid change. Competition, economic constraints, a fluctuating labor force, and a consumer-oriented market place are all factors that are creating health care environments where priorities must be quickly identified and managed.

Staff development departments are also undergoing change. Programs and services, such as guest relations programs or professional outreach services, were rarely offered by the traditional staff development department of twenty years ago. In these times it is crucial for the department to be cognizant of the internal and external forces that are shaping organizational values and directing organizational priorities. It is equally important for the staff development department to do whatever it takes to support changing organizational needs.

The direction that an organization chooses to take in these changing times will have many implications for educational program development. An example of this has been the proliferation of guest relations initiatives in the past several years. Many hospitals, aware of the need to enhance their positions in a competitive market place, have created guest relations programs to promote patient satisfaction and create user-friendly, service-oriented environments that would attract patients to their institutions. Such programming usually includes an educational component for employees, addressing such topics as courtesy, patient rights, image, communication skills, confidentiality, and customer satisfaction. Staff development departments frequently participated in the development of these programs and have continued to provide them as part of their ongoing orientation and inservice programming for the nursing staff.

Specific organizational directives, be they guest relations, cost containment, or product line management, necessitate some level of educational support. It is critical for the staff development department to assess when these directives are an intermediary response of the organization to the specific need and when they reflect the core values of the organization. If the organizational need is an intermediate one, educational support will be time-limited until the goal is achieved. If the organizational need reflects a change or shift in the core values or mission of an organization, it will provide direction for ongoing programming or expansion of educational services.

An example of program development that reflects the changing values of organizations has been the development of revenue-generating capabilities within staff development departments. As health care dollars have decreased, organizations have become pressed to find new sources of revenue to support existing or new programs. In addition, costs associated with the ongoing operations of the organization are being critically scrutinized.

Many staff development departments, aware of these economic constraints, have become income-generating or revenue-producing departments. Revenue generation means that all or a portion of departmental costs related to salaries, benefits, materials, and overhead, are offset by fees that are charged for tuition, consultation, royalties, or sale of program products or services.[2] Revenue generation may be solely directed to those services provided by the staff development departments, or the department may function as a revenue generating arm of the nursing organization through coordination of professional outreach services of nursing to the community.

Revenue generation capability within staff development or nursing can do much to defray the notion that activities that are primarily supportive merely increase overhead and are a financial drain on an organization or have no direct impact on changing the bottom line. Revenue generation is a way for the staff development department to put a dollar value on their services and to be viewed as contributing to the economic goals of the organization.

Revenue generation activities, however, may be in direct conflict with other organizational needs. Programs and services provided to external sources will take time and resources away from activities that are needed within an organization to support staff in meeting other organizational goals, such as improved quality of care or the introduction of new technology. The degree to which the staff development department will direct their resources internally or externally will be dependent on the values of the organization, the defined mission of education within the organization, and, perhaps, the ability of the department to align their efforts to multiple priorities and values simultaneously.

A word of caution is in order to help staff development specialists avoid problems with a revenue generation effort. In addition to the dilution of services to other clients, the cost of generating revenue must be carefully considered. The most common approach to generating some income is to "market" selected staff development programs to nurses in the community or other health care agencies. A brochure is developed and a mailing is organized. The cost of postage, mailing labels, design and setup of attractive brochures, and the labor associated with these tasks can be significant. They may even outstrip the revenue generated! In addition, if the program does not deliver what was advertised in the brochure or expected by the paying participants, additional credibility problems may arise. The reputation of the organization may be placed at stake if these "products" are not sold in a manner conducive to consumers expectations. Strategic planning that includes all associated costs and potential income is a must. Expectations of all parties associated with the effort must be clarified and communicated.

Providing Additional Services

Staff development departments often provide other services to nursing or the organization that are not primarily educational in nature. Research, quality assurance, patient education, project management, and coordination of student educational affiliations within the organization are programs frequently included as a function of the staff development department. Such program responsibility may be placed within the staff development department because of the implications for development of staff, or because they have a parallel program coordination function, as do educational services. It is also possible that the staff development department is a logical choice because of their staff relationship and interactive function to the total organization.

Staff development departments should assume additional program responsibility with an attitude of being flexible but cautious. Many of these activities require similar knowledge and skills inherent in the staff development specialist role. Expertise in program planning, development, coordination, and evaluation are competencies applicable to the management of many other activities. In addition, staff development departments have the structural and system supports in place to operationalize these activities throughout the organization.

It is also important, however, to remember that coordinating a research program is coordinating research, not staff development. Coordinating quality assurance is doing quality assurance. Coordination of patient education is education for patients, not the nursing staff. At a time when staff development is becoming more clearly defined as a field of specialty practice in nursing, it is wise to give thought to the message we send throughout an organization when related but separate program responsibilities are taken on by the staff development department. When viewed as a jack-of-all-trades, it is just as easy to be seen as the master of none.

It is predicted that the health care organization of the 21st century will be quite different from the health care organization of today. Likewise, the staff development role will continue to evolve and expand in response to the demands of the organization and evaluation of the field. In these changing times, the staff development department needs to be open to new and different ways to structure their activities and align their services to the needs of the organization. Vision, risk taking, and sensitivity to the changes in health care will contribute much to the organization, as well as to the field of staff development practice.

Meeting Organizational Needs as a Political Strategy

Much of the discussion of the staff development department's programs directed towards meeting other organizational needs has focused on the specific activities that can be implemented by the department and their potential benefit to the nursing organization. But how and when do these efforts benefit the staff development department?

Organizations accomplish things because someone or something has power to make it happen. Power is an organizational necessity. Power is the *ability* to modify the conduct of others and influence them to do something you wish them to do.[1,12] Power comes from a variety of sources. It can come from the ability to sanction, reward, or coerce the actions of others, or it can be acquired through expertise, charisma, information, or association with powerful people or issues.[13] Having the power to do what you need to do is good.

Organizations are also political systems. Politics is the art of *attempting* to get what you want or need by influencing others to do something you wish them to do.[1,14] Being political is the ability to keep or get power through forming coalitions, taking advantage of opportunities, negotiation, using trade offs, compromising, lobbying, or posturing.[1,15] Being political to do what you need to do is good.

Political savvy is one's ability to analyze the power and political focus within an organization and use it to your advantage. Quite simply it means knowing who has power, why they have it, and what impact it has on what you want to accomplish. Having political savvy is not only good for the staff development department's continuing success, it's vital!

Meeting organizational needs is a political strategy the staff development department can employ to increase their value, power, and success within an organization. Aligning educational support to the right issues, valued by the right people, to deliver the right results gives the staff development department the "power" to integrate education as a necessary component of the business of organizations. In these days of economic instability, it can also keep the staff development department viable.

The importance of meeting organizational needs as a political strategy is best illustrated by a recent experience of a staff development specialist. Several years ago an organization was undergoing tremendous change. A period of downsizing and staff reductions was occurring across the board. The staff development department and the nursing division were not exempt from these cost-cutting strategies. The staff development department had experienced a 25% reduction in their allocated positions.

During the same period, the nursing organization also began to experience the effects of the nursing shortage. Nursing positions that were already reduced, were not being filled because of lack of applicants. The existing nursing staff were caught in the vise of having too few resources to do what needed to be done, while at the same time having more to do because of cuts in support services departments, such as dietary and pharmacy.

The effect of this situation began to become visible in participation in educational programming. Attendance at educational programs, previously valued and supported by management, dropped significantly because staff "were needed on the unit." Getting through the day became the prevalent survival mode.

The staff development department's director, recognizing both the vulnerability of the department and the need to be seen as productive, made a conscious decision to redirect departmental efforts to other organizational needs. When the need to strengthen the nursing quality assurance program arose, the director took this on as the staff development department's function. When the vacancy needed to be filled in chairing a key nursing committee, it became the responsibility of a staff development specialist. When the need arose for someone to coordinate preparation of an upcoming JCAHO visit, the director took on the responsibility. The political strategy was a simple one—make the staff development department so integral to the function of nursing that they would not be able to do without it.

Within a year and a half the organization stabilized. As the need to expand educational support arose, many of these activities were placed back within the nursing organization. In addition, the staff development department's positions were increased 30% to support new educational initiatives. The degree to which this scenario illustrates doing "staff development" is a debatable one. Were these actions reflective of the intended purpose of the staff development department? Probably not. Did the the staff development department's director use political savvy wisely in making such decisions? Maybe yes, maybe no. Did these actions keep the staff employed and the department intact? Absolutely.

Staff development specialists need to recognize the political advantages of their role within nursing and the organization. They also need to realize that the power of education, when directed to the needs of the organization, will not only do much for the system, but for themselves.

Balancing Work with the Work of the Organization

A consistent theme throughout this chapter has been the need to address organizational priorities while maintaining the educational focus of the the staff development department's function. To do so, the staff development specialists must weigh and balance their need to support the organization with their need to provide education to the nursing staff.

When one balances, one walks a fine line—as if on a tight rope. Going too far in any one direction will put one off center and consequently spell disaster. Like the tight rope artist, the staff development specialists must master the subtle shifts of moving in one direction and then another to keep themselves (and their department's) on target and moving forward.

The art of balancing the multiple priorities of the organization and the staff development department is not easy. What makes it particularly difficult is the time/priority dilemma it will create for the the staff development specialist. Inevitably, there will be more need for services than there will be resources to allocate to them. Time spent in one set of activities will ultimately take resources away from others.

How then can staff development specialists make good decisions about what should take priority and what should not? And, what strategies can they use to maintain the critical balance inherent in these issues?
These simple strategies may help.

- **Know your mission:** A clearly defined mission for the staff development department within the organization will provide direction for decision making. Not only must the the staff development department know, understand, and value its purpose, so must administration, management, and the nursing staff. It is easier to negotiate what actions can and cannot be taken, when everyone is clear about the underlying principles that direct them.
- **Get administrative support:** Having administrative support means having clear direction regarding the goals, priorities, and objectives of the organization. It also means knowing what is expected of your department. The staff development department must be prepared to clearly define how education can and cannot contribute to the objectives of the organization, as well as be accountable for the outcomes of their actions.
- **Plan and replan:** Staff development specialists must be prepared to change their focus when needed. Needs and priorities within an organization will change, and a plan once devised is only effective when it meets the purpose it is intended to achieve. Time should be taken on a regular basis to review plans and priorities, and to determine if they are still on target.
- **Be realistic:** Never promise what you can't deliver. When faced with more demands than can be managed, the staff development specialist has the responsibility to clearly define for decision makers what can be done and what cannot, as well as what trade-offs will occur. Prepare them to make choices. Providing accurate information for decision-making is more beneficial to you and the organization than

being willing to help but letting them down in the long run. Be honest.

- **Weigh the benefits with the costs:** Be willing to evaluate the benefits of taking action against the costs of not doing so. Know which customer you ultimately serve—is it the learner, or is it the decision maker? Who ultimately decides your fate?
- **Be flexible:** Flexibility is being willing to bend without getting all out of shape. It is tolerating ambiguity. It is being willing to adapt. It is seeing crisis and chaos as interpreted in Chinese script—opportunity as well as threat. Be open to possibilities.

Meeting organizational needs will provide tremendous opportunity for staff development specialists to test, refine, and maximize their special talents. It will be one of the most demanding aspects of their role, but will also be one of the most challenging and rewarding aspects of their position.

Summary

This chapter has described some of the other responsibilities commonly associated with the role of the staff development specialist. Other roles will emerge in the future. Some may seem appropriate, some may not. Each will be decided based on many variables, including the political, financial, and cultural climate of the organization. There are no right or wrong roles for the nursing staff development specialist. However, it is up to the specialist to communicate the ideal role and benefits of that role to the organization's decision-makers. The contribution of the staff development specialist to the organization, in identifiable and measured outcomes, is the most significant message.

REFERENCES

1. Stevens, B. (1985). *The nurse as executive* (3rd ed.). Rockville, Md: Aspen.
2. del Bueno, D. (1986). Nursing staff development: Critical issues, critical times. *Journal of Nursing Staff Development, 2*(3): 94–97.
3. Tobin, H., & Beeler, J. (1988). Roles and relationships of staff development educators. *Journal of Nursing Staff Development, 4*(3): 91–95.
4. Joint Commission (1989). *1990 Accreditation manual for hospitals.* Chicago, Ill: Joint Commission on Accreditation of Healthcare Organizations.
5. Beyerman, K. (1990). Committee work: Serendipitous teaching and learning. *Journal of Continuing Education in Nursing, (1)*18–22.
6. Sovie, M. (1983). Fostering professional nursing careers in hospitals: The role of nursing staff development Part II. *Nurse Educator, 8*(1): 15–18.
7. Ulschak, F. M. (1988). *Creating the future of health care education.* Chicago, Ill: American Hospitals Publishing Company.
8. Mager, R., & Pipe P. (1984). *Analyzing performance problems* (2nd ed). Belmont, CA: Pitmann Learning.

9. Ulschak, F. M., & SnowAntle, S. M. (1990). *Consulting skills for health care professionals.* San Francisco: Jossey-Bass.
10. Miller, P. (1988). Enhancing organizational effectiveness. *Journal of Healthcare Education and Training, 3*(2): 36–37.
11. Gebelein, S. (1989). Profile of an internal consultant: Roles and skills for building client confidence. *Training and Development Journal. March, 43*(3): 52–58.
12. McMurray, R. (1973). Power and the ambitious executive. *Harvard Business Review, 52*(6): 69–74.
13. Willey, E. (1987). Acquiring and using power effectively. *Journal of Continuing Education in Nursing, 18*(1): 25–30.
14. Ehrat, K. (1983). A model for politically astute planning and decision making. *Journal of Nursing Administration, 13*(9): 29–35.
15. del Bueno, D., & Freund, C. (1986). *Power and politics in nursing administration.* Owings Mill, MD: National Publishing Company–Rand Communications.

SUGGESTED READINGS

del Bueno, D., & Dixon, J. (1989). A cost effective educational response to an organizational need. *Critical Care Nursing, 43*(3): 52–58.

Fisher, R., & Ury, W. (1981). *Getting to yes: Negotiating without giving in.* Boston, Mass: Houghton Mifflin Company.

Garity, J. (1989). Trends in OR education: Is it an educational issue or a management problem. *OR Manager, 5* (8):8.

Huse, E., & Cummings T.(1985). Organizational development and change. (3rd ed) St. Paul, MN: West Publishing.

Jones, W., et al. (1988). Clinical career ladder development in nursing: Concepts and issues. *Journal of Health and Human Resources Administration, 10*(4): 361–377.

Lomurno, A., & Dowling-Jones, T. (1990). Retaining expert nurses through clinical ladder alternatives. *Journal of Continuing Education in Nursing, 21*(2): 5–10.

Scully, R. (1983). The staff educator as a process consultant. *Nurse Educator, 8*(1): 39–42.

Steel, F. (1982). *The role of internal consultant: Effective role shaping for staff positions.* Boston: CBI Publishing.

Weeks, L., & Spor, K. (1987). Hospital nursing education: dispelling the doomsday prophesies. *Journal of Nursing Administration, 172*(3): 34–38.

chapter **10**

Administration of the Staff Development Department

Karen J. Kelly

Most health care organizations today have an individual responsible for nursing staff development. This nurse may have staff development responsibilities only, or, more commonly, they may be part of several responsibilities. The size, complexity, and development of the nursing department often dictates the size, complexity, and status of the staff development program. In some agencies, the staff development process may be organized as a department with its own leader, staff, space, budget, and programs. In others, the process may be integrated into the role of nurse managers with one staff development specialist coordinating selected activities. This chapter addresses the staff development program that is organized within a department dedicated primarily to the staff development function. Specifically, the leadership, direction, administration, structure, and formation of the staff development program are discussed.

Leadership to Transform Nursing Practice

The role of the staff development director as a leader with others in the transformation of nursing practice continues to emerge. Some organizations recognize the integrated position of nursing staff development in achieving goals, others need help with understanding this role. The tumultuous health care environment requires nurse leaders who are able to create and communicate a vision of nursing, in addition to possessing refined decision-making and problem-resolution skills. The staff development leader should be part of the creation of this vision and assist with communicating it through staff development activities.

Transformational leaders have characteristics such as change agency, courtesy, belief in people, and the ability to deal with complexity, ambiguity, and uncertainty.[1] In addition, life-long learning is another characteristic of the transformational leader. Staff development leaders possess many of these traits and can use them to enliven the work of nursing within organizations.

The ability of nurse leaders to inspire others with the vision of what can be accomplished and empower staff members to do their best through a shared vision was investigated by Dunham and Klafehn.[2] Transformational nurse leaders were found to be charismatic, able to give individualized consideration, and provide intellectual stimulation. These findings provide useful information for the staff development administrator who is mentoring and developing specialists and other nurse managers as they develop their transformational skills. Through the refinement of transformational leadership skills, the staff development administrator will influence nursing practice.

One Best Way?

Plurality and diversity are the positive benefits to the current organizational status of staff development departments within nursing departments. Efforts to define "one best way" to organize a staff development department are generally fruitless, since the environment in which the work occurs must be taken into consideration. However, certain factors must be considered in structuring any department responsible for the staff development of a group of nursing personnel. This chapter is arranged using the following organizational elements:

- A theoretical framework to assist in the organization and administration the department
- Human resource management
- Environmental management
- Positioning, policies, and procedures
- Records, reports, and automated systems
- Resource allocation analysis and productivity
- Regulatory bodies

Quality management is another significant element of the staff development administrator's responsibility. Due to the specific applications of quality concepts to nursing staff development, this topic is examined in the following chapter.

The leader of the staff development program will find this chapter helpful. In addition, departments in the self-evaluation process may find some concepts worthwhile for consideration. As the fields of nursing administration and nursing staff development continues to evolve, so too will the evolution of methods and strategies to improve the practice of these two disciplines of nursing. In time, the integration of selected practices from the administration and staff development disciplines, as well as other fields, will be common and will strengthen the field.

Theoretical Framework

Many theories are available to assist the staff development leader in managing and administering the department. Classic theories relating to systems, roles, bureaucracies, and leadership have been described, researched, and applied to a variety of nursing organizational situations. Few investigations have been completed to test theories regarding the organization and management of nursing staff development departments. This does not mean theoretical models are not used in practice. To provide the full spectrum of staff development services, some form of organization, task specialization, and decision-making arrangement must exist.

As staff development administrators become more sophisticated in their designs of programs and departments, more will use organization and management theories to assist with their efforts. One organizing theory is proposed here. Others will and should be proposed to meet the continually changing needs of health care organizations. To help organizations and, in particular, nursing personnel effectively accommodate change, it is useful to adopt open systems concepts. Contingency theory is a systems theory that is useful for the staff development administrator.

Critical Concepts of Contingency Theory

Classical theorists generally believe there is one best way to organize. Proponents of contingency theory believe that the integration of the environment, technology, and structure of organizations will lead to success and advocate a variety of structures to meet goals. Woodward,[3] a British researcher, first proposed this theory when she studied the relationship between organizational structure and success. She found no relationship between these two concepts during her investigation of English manufacturing firms. As a result of this work, she concluded that different technologies imposed different kinds of demands on individuals and organizations. Woodward also determined that successful organizations will have a structure appropriate to meet these demands. Burns and Stalker[4] specifically focused on the environment and studied internal management practices and that the relationship to rates of change in scientific techniques and marketing. They found that each system was appropriate to its own specific set of conditions. Again, another challenge to the "one best way" approach was advanced. Burns and Stalker also suggested that organizational structure is contingent on the nature of the organizational environment, both internal and external.

Charns and Schaefer[5] advanced a contingency model for health care organizations. They defined the work of organizations as two types, direct and managerial, and were two of the first to blend these concepts in this way. They further defined this direct and managerial work into three elements—structure, coordination, and people. Hence, Charns and Schaefer modified contingency theory to include people, a feature not specifically addressed by previous authors. In addition, they saw managerial and direct work as organizational work. Previous investigators saw management as something done to accomplish work or output. This important distinction is one of the appealing concepts of the Charns and Schaefer model, as it recognizes the integration of management work and direct work, rather than management as directing and controlling work. This integration is also congruent with current nursing practice delineations; that is, nursing practice embraces clinical, administrative, and research practitioners who are all considered to practice nursing in various roles.

Charns and Schaefer also emphasize environment as the most important element in their framework. In their application of contingency theory to health care, they define the direct work of organizations as the provisions of services to patients. Managerial work includes the strategies and technologies used to accomplish the purposes and objectives of the organization. To extend this concept to nursing staff development, direct work is the provision of nursing services to patients, and staff development work is one managerial strategy used to accomplish the purpose of quality care and the objective of delivering care by competent staff.

This model of contingency theory blends many of the concepts of other contingency theorists and adds new elements that further refine the theory. While contingency theory is one of the newer management theories, it seems to have wide appeal. Experience teaches us that there is no single, best way to organize a staff development department. Various structures exist with success in various organizations. However, the concepts proposed by contingency theory have application to the design of staff development services and departments. As departments continue to improve their structure and organization of services, contingency theory can be used to guide that process.

Application to Staff Development

Charns and Schaefer[5] also propose a model that illustrates the distinct interrelatedness and interaction of all elements (see Figure 10-1). This model of organization and management provides a framework for decision making and administration within nursing staff development. The staff development program administrator may find definitions of the elements and concepts useful when designing or redesigning the structure and organization of the department. The following list defines the elements and concepts of this model within a staff development context.

Environment. Staff development program administrators would consider the organizational environment to determine programs and projects. In addition to patients as clients, consumers of education programs, as represented primarily by nurse managers, would also be considered an important source to describe the environment. In addition to government bodies such as the health department, other regulatory bodies like the Joint Commission on Accreditation of Health Care Organizations (JCAHO) should be considered. Professional associations and their published standards of practice would be considered part of the influencing environment. Finally, another

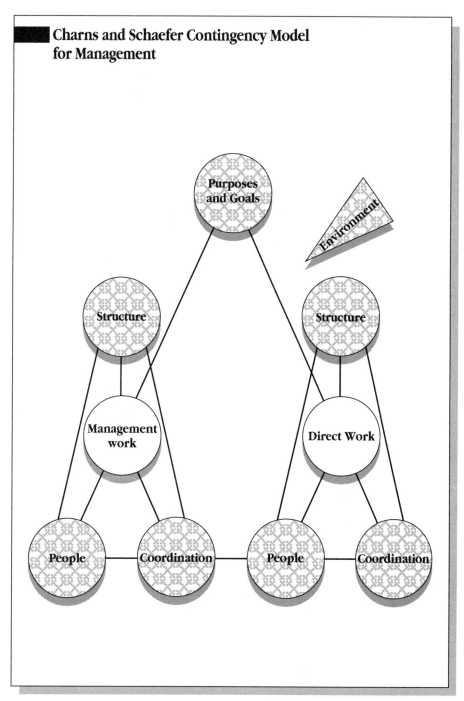

Charns and Schaefer Contingency Model for Management

Figure 10-1 *Charns and Schaefer contingency model for management. (Source: Charns, M. P., & Schaefer, M. J. [1983]. Health care organizations: A model for management. Englewood Cliffs, NJ: Prentice-Hall. Reproduced with permission.)*

internal environmental element that should be considered by the staff development program administrator is anticipated or planned changes in services and expectations of departments within the nursing division, particularly those that clearly indicate a need for educational programming to meet identified goals. Most changing organizations would benefit from the use of staff development services to assist with the changes. This includes changes in competency expectations (nurses will perform a new procedure) as well as changes in structure and care delivery systems (nurses must learn how to organize their care within new systems).

Purposes and Goals. The staff development administrator should verify clearly with other nurse administrators their purposes and goals for their assigned areas of responsibility. Only then can the administrator design a staff development program that will address the scope of expected services and the purpose and goals of the educational effort. Successful staff development administrators are those who can link programs intimately with organizational goals and objectives.

Work. Staff development work has been defined as a process that assesses, maintains, and develops nursing competencies. Work associated with this process includes programs such as orientation, inservice education, continuing education, leadership development, skills training, and competency assessment. Several of these work assignments have evolved over the past decade and are frequently designed in response to particular needs of the organization. Past successes with staff development efforts designed to bring about change are more likely to yield creative and flexible responses to organizational needs. The direct work of staff development is defined as the service delivery mechanisms such as direct provision of education, coordination, consultation, and collaboration. Other staff development work can be defined using the competencies proposed by McLagan, discussed in Chapter 1.

Structure. Staff development organizational charts should recognize the talents and skills of individuals. In addition, the chart should be fluid enough to allow for new or different assignments to emerge. The chart should be reviewed and updated regularly. Program reassignments are made based on the changing needs of the organization. Formal communication lines of staff development personnel to the administrator and clients should also be specified through this structure.

Coordination. The staff development administrator should play a significant role in setting up systems to coordinate activities with the many consumers and clients of staff development services. Structure will also dictate who will typically be involved in most staff development transactions.

People. Staff development is a service provided for people by people. The skills, abilities, perceptions, motivations, and satisfactions of staff development personnel should be integrated into job design to reach high levels of productivity. Staff development specialists also need role development. One of the most important elements of this role development is the ability to remain flexible in the changing environment with a refined ability to respond to changing needs.

The staff development administrator who uses these elements to refine the staff development program should then define indicators of success. One indicator of success is the positive effect of the staff development program on the organization's accomplishment of purposes and goals. Structure, people, and coordination can be redefined as needed to continue to help the organization effect its mission.

There is some evidence that this theory, or selected elements, is already in use by staff development directors. The various structures and forms of staff development programs and departments are indicators that the environment of the organization is already the primary factor in designing staff development programs. Other elements in this model should also be addressed by administrators.

The use of contingency theory as a potential framework for the administration, organization, and design of the staff development program and department will contribute to the success of this effort. Organizations are dynamic. Units such as staff development must maintain a high degree of flexibility and tolerance for ambiguity in order to contribute effectively to the organization's success. This theory encourages those characteristics.

Managing Human Resources

Recruiting and retaining staff development specialists is a significant challenge for the staff development administrator. Using the elements of contingency theory defined above, the administrator would define the work, organize a structure, develop coordination activities, and select people to accomplish the goals and purposes of the staff development unit within the organizational environment.

Defining the Roles

The department director generally inherits or hires individuals in staff development roles that may be well- or ill-defined. The selection of nurses to fulfill the staff development specialist's role is one of the most important aspects of an administrator's job. Furthermore, these individuals are a reflection of the department. Position descriptions and performance standards are used to guide the selection and development of individuals in the department. Dynamic in nature, the position descriptions should be reviewed and updated annually to reflect the current expectations of the role.

Position descriptions can be developed or revised by individuals in the role. One helpful approach is the use of already available competency statements from other sources that have similar responsibilities. For example, the work of the Task Force on Competencies and Standards of the American Society for Training and Development (ASTD) serves as a superior exemplar.[6] Their continuing research identified 74 key work dimensions for the human resource development field. The list of key work dimensions or outputs is not exhaustive, but does include the most critical roles. The task force further grouped the work dimensions by role. Roles included

- Administrator
- Manager
- Materials developer

- Individual career development advisor
- Instructor or facilitator
- Marketer
- Needs analyst
- Organization change agent
- Program designer
- Researcher

Selected key work dimensions could be used from this model to structure or restructure a position description that captures the essence of the role. For example, the staff development specialist within a large department is often expected to manage all program aspects such as faculty confirmations, room and equipment reservations, and registration processes. The specialist in a staff role still retains management responsibility, even though the individual may not manage other people. A second example of the use of these work dimensions is the role of the specialist as an organization change agent. In those organizations with a defined organization development (OD) program and staff, the nursing staff development specialist may not have a significant role in this type of work. In other organizations, the staff development administrator may fulfill this role through work with committees and councils.

Performance standards and expectations are defined and used for role definition, performance evaluation, and development. The format of these documents vary but usually include primary functions with discrete, measurable subtasks delineated. Some organizations arrange this information on a document that can also be used as an evaluation form. Chart 10-1 is an example of this approach. Additional discussion about these work dimensions can be found in Chapter 1.

The role of the performance technologist as described by Mager[7] also seems to have some relevance to a typical staff development role description. Elements of the Mager model include

- Analyst
- Designer/developer
- Course manager
- Evaluator
- Manager

Each of these activities is defined with associated tasks. For example, during analysis the performance technologist/staff development specialist will extract boundary statements from decision makers, detect restrictions, reconcile conflicts, perform job and task analyses, conduct performance and goal analyses, and so forth. This approach to the description of the work of the nursing staff development specialist is congruent with the expectations of many organizations. Others may need to be helped to understand this approach.

The job description serves as an important document in the selection, appraisal, and continuing development of specialists in this field of nursing practice. Sample position descriptions for an education specialist in a large urban community hospital can be found in Appendix A. Additional samples can also be found in Chapter 3, Charts 3-2 and 3-3.

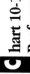 **hart 10-1**
Performance Standards Framework with Annual Objectives and Outcomes

Major Function I: Collaborates with nursing managers and staff to assess learning needs

Performance is satisfactory when the education specialist:

	Objectives	Comments
1. Develops and utilizes a mechanism for ongoing needs assessment for designated areas.	Continue using network of staff to provide input for ongoing needs assessment	Continued to use staff meetings as well as informal task forces to plan content of continuing educational offerings.
2. Participates in department-wide needs assessment.	Assist in needs assessment as indicated by Director.	
3. Meets with staff and management as necessary to validate needs assessment of future needs.	Meet with assigned contact persons at least annually to identify needs of staff.	Done—used information to plan CE offerings as well as other inservices.
4. Responds appropriately to perceived needs with learning activities or other recommendations of assist change.		
5. Collaborates with Associate Director–Nursing Education and Research, to establish priority needs based on organizational and departmental goals.		

The roles of other staff assigned to the staff development department can also be defined using a similar process. For example, if a role such as that of an enterostomal therapist or diabetic educator is assigned to the staff development department, the administrator can review available job descriptions, performance standards of the professional associations, and the needs of the organization to verify or document the accuracy of the description.

Staff development support personnel also require the same approach to role definition and development. Though the needs of the staff development department are unique when compared with those of clinical services, the support needs are similar to those of other service departments. For example, clerical and secretarial work is a component of any department responsible for delivering a service. Records and files must be maintained, phones must be answered, and systems supported. Advances in word processing systems have allowed some staff development departments to redefine the support needed to keep the department running well.

As automated systems are integrated into staff development work, the roles and expectations of support personnel and specialists will change. For example, if word processing is available to the staff development specialist, typing support is no longer required, but the need for an individual to assist with aspects of automation and systems management is required. Staff development departments with various accreditations and certifications, such as ANA accreditation for continuing education programs and American Heart Association CPR Certifying Agency approval, will need support to maintain the records required for these accreditations. The key to the integration of support personnel into the staff development department lies in role expectation and in distinguishing between what the specialist does and what the support person is does. The assumption that the staff development specialist must be able to perform the function of the support person is not valid. Role distinctions should be clear and observed in actions. If not, the administrator will have difficulty justifying differences in salary structure.

Collecting, reviewing, and describing performance expectations, particularly those that deal with the interpersonal skills required for interaction with managers, are an essential aspect of the administrator's job. Each department has unique needs that are driven by the services provided. Roles are often defined based on these services. For example, a department that has taken on the responsibility of centralized, educational records and transcripts will find it necessary to identify an individual who will provide the necessary reports to nurse managers for their monitoring responsibilities. A sample job description of a person assigned to this role can be found in Chapter 7. Other support roles may include administrative and clerical personnel, audio-visual support personnel, and instructors assigned to implement specific programs.

Staff development administrators will find a significant amount of time consumed with assigning programs and projects to available personnel. It is the judicious and creative use of available personnel in these projects that provides an important challenge to the administrator. The success, satisfaction, and continued growth experienced by the staff development department personnel as a result of these assignments is a reflection of the skill of the administrator. Subsequent success of the program is linked closely to this administrative skill.

Personnel Selection

The staff development director with the opportunity to select and hire an individual for a staff development role is confronted with several questions:

- Should this opportunity be used to redefine the role?
- Are there other activities that need to be included in this position?
- Why did the individual vacate the role? Were job stress, low morale, or poor job design factors? If so, what needs to be changed to enhance the role?
- How involved should other department members and users of services be in the selection of the new person?
- How should services be structured during the selection process in order to cause the least disruption?
- How current is the job description and performance standards?
- What characteristics should the incumbent have to best meet the demands of the role?
- How long will it take to fill this vacancy?

None of the above questions can be answered in a linear fashion, as each affects the answer to other questions. However, the staff development administrator should use the vacancy as an opportunity to review contingency theory elements and determine what improvements might be experienced if changes were made in structure, people, and coordination activities.

The staff development administrator should define some general characteristics that will enhance the individual's ability to perform the role. Characteristics of successful staff development specialists identified in Chapter 1 may provide some information in this area. Using the job description and the identified characteristics, and consultations with the personnel department, recruitment strategies are developed to attract candidates to the department and organization.

Each organization has internal recruitment policies and policies mandated by law. The administrator should review these policies and work with the appropriate departments to follow these policies and internal practices. Forms may be a part of the process, and approval for certain levels of recruitment may be necessary. For example, approval to advertise vacancies in national journals may require additional approval, particularly in areas where a large pool of individuals who are qualified for the role already exists. However, the decision to run an ad in local papers may be the joint decision of the staff development administrator and the recruitment professional.

The staff development director should be prepared to justify the expense related to any recruitment effort. An average of $3000 to $5000 is estimated to recruit a staff nurse, this cost is proportionately increased depending on resources used and the amount of time and effort needed to fill the position. Once a recruitment plan is approved and implemented, and depending on the job market, many or a few may respond.

The request for a resume or curriculum vitae is standard. These are reviewed and screened to determine if identified qualifications are met. It is generally helpful to look for some management background, as this experience is useful in preparing the nurse for the broad organizational perspective necessary in staff development. In addition, for the novice staff development applicant, specific actions and examples of experience that support the desire to help others learn are essential. Such activities as preceptoring, teaching unit-based inservice education sessions, and serving as faculty for seminars and other related activities are testimonials to the incumbents inclination to perform in a staff development role.

Several candidates are selected from the applicants for an interview. Resumes can be ranked in order of most wanted for an interview to least qualified. Commonly, the top three candidates are interviewed. The interview process must also be guided by a framework that will yield data about the candidate and recognize legalities. Chart 10-2 illustrates questions that may *not* be asked in employment interviews.

When scheduling interviews with prospective candidates, several details must be considered:

- How long should the candidate plan for the interview process?
- Does the candidate know how to get to the department and/or organization?
- What advice should the administrator give the candidate to prepare for the interview?
- What is the plan for a selection decision?
- Will others be involved in the selection process, and if so, whom?

If the candidate will be interviewed by several individuals or groups, this should be communicated. The applicant who is not informed of this plan may be frightened and justifiably annoyed if this plan is discovered during the first few moments of the interview.

Other departmental or organizational personnel used to assist the administrator with the interview process should be briefed on expectations about the interview process. Will a standard list of questions be provided by the administrator, or will each interviewer come up with his/her own? What particular areas of strengths and limitations are of interest? How long will each interview take and how many are planned? A list of questions that may not be asked may also warrant a review.

Data gathered during the interview will yield interesting perspectives and perceptions about nursing staff development. The candidate's viewpoint about nursing staff development is a key perspective to explore. A nurse's experiences with staff development departments and programs may also yield perceptions that may not correspond with the department and role under consideration. Careful examination of these viewpoints by the administrator and staff will give insight into the ability of the candidate to fulfill role expectations and adopt the culture of the department.

A final consideration for the staff development administrator is how each interviewer or group should communicate their findings about each candidate. For example, if a panel of nurse managers is convened to assist with the selection of the specialist, is the group expected to come to consensus or report individually? Should each candidate be ranked against the others, or should strengths and limitations be identified? Careful attention to the

C hart 10-2
Questions That Cannot Be Asked During Interviews

Employment interviewers are forbidden by law to ask the following questions:

1. Your age
2. Your date of birth
3. The length of time you have resided at your present address
4. Your previous address
5. Your religion; the church you attend; your spiritual advisor
6. Your father's surname
7. Your maiden name (of women)
8. Your marital status
9. Your residence mates
10. The number and ages of your children; who will care for them while you work
11. How you will get to work, unless a car is a job requirement
12. Residence of spouse or parent
13. Whether you own or rent your residence
15. The name of your bank; information on outstanding loans
16. Whether wages were ever garnished
17. Whether you ever declared bankruptcy
18. Whether you were ever arrested
19. Whether you were convicted, unless this is a job-related necessity (for example, in jobs requiring a security clearance)
20. Hobbies, off-duty interests, clubs
21. Foreign languages you can read, write, or speak, unless this is a job requirement

Source: Adapted from conference with Paula Andrews, personnel director, University of South Alabama Medical Center, Mobile, AL, 1983. Reproduced with permission.

expectations of those assisting with the selection process will provide guidance to those assisting and give credence to the outcome. The staff development administrator always retains the final decision and responsibility for the selection of the successful candidate.

A final detail that may be forgotten is worth mentioning here. Nurses apply for positions for many reasons. The interview process is an investment on the part of both parties. While the staff development administrator may have devoted a great deal of time to this process, the applicant is also a stakeholder. Opportunities for the applicant to explore concerns and issues about employment in the staff development department and organization should be provided. Materials that describe the department and the organization should be given to the candidate. Phone numbers for follow-up questions and clarification should be exchanged. The habit of acknowledging the investment made by both parties in this process will serve the administrator well and may help create an environment of mutual respect that is precisely what an applicant is seeking.

Depending on the outcome of these interviews, the administrator may have an easy or difficult choice. These choices include

- Selecting a clearly outstanding candidate with no reservations
- Selecting a candidate with reservations and a plan to address those reservations
- Not selecting any interviewed candidates and continuing the recruitment process

Each choice has inherent advantages and disadvantages. Some administrators may be willing to take risks with candidates, and others may not. Much depends on what needs to be accomplished. The staff development administrator is in the position to make the best judgment about the issues confronting the department and how the selection of a candidate will affect those issues.

Development of the Specialist

Depending on the experience of the staff development specialist, an orientation plan is established that will begin the formation of the individual in the assigned role. Using the job description and performance standards, a plan is developed for the first year or two of staff development practice. If the incumbent has been employed within the organization and knows the practices and climate of the agency, this area will not need to be included in depth. If the incumbent has nursing staff development experience, that experience should be factored into the plan. This individual may only need to learn about specific systems and practices of the new organization or, in some cases, may need to expand and enhance already acquired skills.

However, if the specialist is new to the organization and staff development, a plan should be detailed that will include specific activities and skill acquisition recommendations. The plan may be incremental, in three- to six-month blocks for example, to make it more manageable, or it may outline activities for a longer period of time. Chapter 1 details a skill acquisition plan using Benner's novice to expert framework and Chapters 3 and 7 include other recommendations to help formulate this plan.

Another approach to the orientation and development of specialists and other personnel is the creation of a self-directed learning contract as described by Knowles.[8] The approach is based on the accepted premise that adults are highly motivated to learn naturally (rather than being taught) and will learn more in depth and breadth concerning a particular subject if given the opportunity to develop their own plan. The fact that the specialist must acquire and develop prescribed skills can be reconciled with the adults motivation to learn through the use of a learning contract.

To develop a learning contract with a new staff development specialist, the administrator develops and provides a document that includes

- Performance expectations or job objectives derived from the job descriptions
- Available resources and strategies that may be used for the continuing inquiry
- "Inquiry units" specifying the questions that need to be answered to demonstrate skill acquisition and evidence of accomplishment of objectives
- Criteria and means for validating evidence

This document is reviewed with the neophyte specialist and refined based on input and feedback from the specialist about preferred strategies. Evidence of accomplishment of objectives may also be negotiated. The administrator may prioritize selected items based on the needs of the organization and the talents of the individual. Time frames and evaluation methods are established, and the contract is begun. As the contract is fulfilled and evaluation data is observed, the specialist continues with other parts of the contract. New skills may be added to the contract as competency is gained.

The advantage of this method is the eventual ownership of the learning contract process by the specialist. Individual desires are recognized and supported for inquiry within the context of expected performance standards. This self-directed learning contract process also recognizes knowledge and skills acquired through a variety of experiences, rather than limiting the specialist's learning activities to one specific project, such as reading an article or interviewing an individual. For example, if the specialist has to organize a new product learning activity before the opportunity to read about the process is available, the successful implementation of the activity serves as evidence of competence, and the need to read articles about the item no longer exists. Outcomes are emphasized in this process and provide direction for the development plan. This approach can be used on an ongoing basis and provide structure for the specialist who has moved beyond the orientation phase.

Learning resources and inquiry units can also be developed collaboratively by the administrator and the specialist. The key to success with this method is the freedom of the learner/specialist, with the guidance of the administrator, to identify and discover knowledge needed to perform the job. Chart 10-3 illustrates a sample learning contract for a staff development specialist with one area of skill identified and placed in this framework.

This approach can be used with other personnel in the staff development department. Skills to include in a "standard learning contract," used to structure orientation and the first year or two of development, are obtained directly from the job description and performance standards. Skills and knowledge related to competent, proficient and expert practice, and the desire for continued growth, are obtained from other sources such as the professional literature, theory and research, and new practice exemplars and expectations as they evolve.

Coaching for Performance

Success of the specialist and the staff development program can be clearly associated with the skills of the administrator. Advanced program

Chart 10-3
Sample Learning Contract

Name _____ Employee I.D. no. _____

Date Initiated _____ Page _____ of _____

Learning Need(s)	Priority	Action(s)	Outcome(s)	Date

Reviewed on Initiation: _____ Reviewed on Completion: _____

                                    Employee   *Employee*

                        _____   _____

                        Head Nurse or Designate   *Head Nurse*

White Copy—Head Nurse   *Pink Copy—Employee*   *Yellow Copy—*

development skills are essential and are acquired through academic preparation, experience, and continued professional development. The modeling of these skills by the administrator and other senior specialists is integral to the acquisition of the skills by the neophyte specialist. Careful planning for this modeling and mentoring is a basic factor of any performance coaching plan. The specialist's development plan should include verification and expansion of skills related to program development. A systematic approach to investigating problems and proposing solutions is an essential element to the success of the specialist.

Coaching for performance assumes a certain strategy and mindset adaptation. Often identified with sports, coaches provide guidelines and instruction to players who then try the instructions out in a supervised situation. Feedback is exchanged about the experience—how it felt to the player and how it looked to the coach. Feedback provided by the coach is specifically based on observed behaviors. Continued improvement is planned from that point. Fournies[9] described a process that included the following steps:

1. Reach agreement that a problem exists.
2. Mutually discuss alternative solutions.
3. Mutually agree on action to be taken to solve problem.
4. Follow up to assure agreed upon action has been taken.
5. Recognize any achievement.

The staff development specialist as a knowledge worker must be given the latitude and autonomy to develop the role in a manner consistent with personal and organizational expectations. The staff development administrator who creates an environment of mutual respect and continued reflection on how to improve services and skills will enjoy success as a leader. With each experience comes an opportunity to reflect on a paradigm that will develop maturity and continued growth. That paradigm includes thoughtful regard to

- What happened?
- What was learned as a result of the experience?
- What will be done differently in the future to improve the service?

The key concern of the staff development administrator related to the continued growth of departmental staff is their ability to do their assigned jobs. While elements of the positions may change over time, core competencies generally remain the same. The identification of those core competencies will guide the administrator in this work. The document that provides that guidance is the job description and associated performance standards—hence, the primacy of current, relevant, and accurate job descriptions.

Appraisal Strategies

The performance of the specialist and other staff as it relates to expected standards can be evaluated by the staff development administrator through various systems and frameworks. Some organizations have prescribed mechanisms and forms to assist this process. Other organizations have required forms but expect administrators to add documents to support adequate performance.

Van Ort[10] described five models used to document the effectiveness of faculty of schools of nursing. With some modification, these models can be used to evaluate staff development personnel:

1. **Developmental model:** Collects data on an ongoing basis for both specialist growth and decision making.
2. **Personnel decision model:** Provides for data collection only as needed for personnel decisions. Data in this model are used to compare specialists with each other and with predetermined evaluative criteria.
3. **Personal growth model:** Formative data are used to indicate growth with the focus of the model on change to meet individual goals.
4. **Criterion-based model:** Sets standards by which staff members are judged.
5. **Objective-based model:** In contrast to the criterion-based model, this is predictive and outcome-oriented as staff develop individuals' contracts for growth.

From this list, it is possible to design an approach using elements from several models that will support the needs of the organization, the administrator, and the staff. Most personnel evaluation systems use an eclectic approach that attempts to meet many needs. The major functions of performance evaluations have been described[11] as observation and identification of job behaviors, measurement, and development. While the intent of most users of performance appraisal systems is comprehensive and with good intent, Fombrun[12] found that appraisal systems in most organizations do not fulfill the major functions described.

As long ago as 1957, McGregor[13] discussed the problems associated with performance appraisal and the resistance of managers toward using prescribed programs. This resistance has been related to a normal dislike of criticizing a subordinate, a lack of skill with interviews, a dislike of the procedure, and mistrust of the validity of the prescribed system. Despite these issues, staff development administrators must use systems that will assist them in finding out about and documenting the development of their staff.

Whether comparative procedures, absolute standards, direct indices, or objective accomplishments are used to appraise performance, the administrator must develop and share the performance appraisal system used within the staff development department. Individuals who may be providing input to the performance appraisal system are also identified. These may include consumers such as nurse managers and other learners. Instruments used to measure and document performance are also shared with staff to give them the opportunity to acknowledge expectations and perform accordingly, or negotiate different expectations.

Systems that use peer review as a component of the appraisal process are emerging and used with increasing popularity. Peer review processes require structure and format for success. Peers asked to provide data generally need to be briefed to fulfill expectations and need to be informed about how information will be used. Issues that may emerge relate to confidentiality and allocation of scarce resources (peers) to collect and provide the data. In addition, the peer's desire to do no harm and be overly kind in the appraisal must be considered by the administrator. The time used for this process may not yield the benefits to make it a cost-effective system. However, a well-defined process of peer review that addresses these issues may make a significant contribution to the continuing development and professionalism of the specialist.

Problems of judgment involved in any of these approaches are the nemesis of any administrator. This is not unique to staff development. The solution to many of these issues may be found in placing the responsibility of performance appraisal, goal achievement, and progress with the staff development specialist.

Managing the Environment

The environment of an organization's staff development program emanates from the department and its staff. The staff development administrator can create and maintain an environment with elements that will contribute to continued professional growth. Naisbett and Aburdene[14] describe the three most important qualities that individuals offer an organization as information, knowledge, and creativity. In order to allow knowledge workers in the health care system to reach their potential and make a contribution to the organization, administrators must create an environment which recognizes that potential.

An environment that promotes learning is one which facilitates physical comfort, privacy, informality, and a lack of distractions.[15] As with any systems model, the environment provides input and affects the throughput and eventual output of the staff development program and nursing practice. Administrative actions necessary to create and maintain a learning environment include

- Establishing an atmosphere of respect and trust
- Verifying helpfulness as the basic response to requests
- Initiating freedom of expression in the classroom and during other idea exchange opportunities
- Recognizing the four precepts of adult learning theory related to the adult's self-concept as a learner, the role of experience and learning, the adult's readiness to learn, and their orientation to learning
- Accepting differences among learners
- Establishing expectations about the frequent use of creative and innovative responses to requests for service
- Most importantly, setting these maxims as operational precepts for the department

Staff development specialists should be expected to create a physical environment that is conducive to learning and to attend to the interpersonal aspects and characteristics of the adult learner. The use of these principles in the day-to-day procedures of nursing staff development will create an environment that provides satisfaction and challenge to the knowledge worker.

The staff development administrator has an extended role in the creation of an environment that is contributory to continued professional growth and development of the individual and the organization. The administrator can use role and personal power to influence the continued progress of nursing practice within the organization. The environment needed for continuous improvement is similar to that of an environment that is conducive to learning.

Staff development is considered a strategic management component that is a factor in organizational success.[16] Using the example of the health care organization's need to respond to the change in reimbursement systems to a prospective payment, staff development found itself in a pivotal role, able to help (or not help) all hospital staff understand the relevant issues. In addition, staff development had the opportunity to facilitate an environment that expected nurses and others to discover ways each could contribute to the organization's response to the significant problems associated with this change.

Through the use of strategic planning processes, the staff development administrator may discover a variety of issues related to the strengths, limitations, and the internal and external environment that may affect the ability of nurses and staff development specialists to make progress toward identified goals. The processes used in strategic planning and the data collected as a result of these processes may provide information to help the staff development administrator and other nursing administrators adjust and improve the environment for greater goal achievement. Discussed in detail in the final chapter of this book, strategic planning is a powerful process which can help the administrator understand the dynamics of organizational change and development. With this understanding comes the ability to effect needed improvements which will create an environment instrumental in continuing professional development.

Several seemingly mundane aspects of environmental management will be discussed in the following section. While each aspect alone may not seem significant, taken in the aggregate they may overwhelm the specialist's ability to perform expected duties. The staff development administrator is in the unique position to analyze the cumulative effect of these aspects on the functional capacity of the staff development department.

Physical Space

Staff development departments are often relegated to space that has no logical connection with services provided. For example, services are provided on clinical units and in classrooms, yet staff development offices are often located at the furthest possible point from the provision of services. Specialist must haul bulky instructional equipment to the site planned for instruction. Storage space for this equipment is limited as is work space for the production of instructional programs.

Reasons for this often lie in the evolution of the health care organization. Space planning for all eventualities remains one of the most significant challenges for hospital administrators. As organizational goals change and new services are developed, space needs change. Logical placement of most services and departments within organizations is lost after ten years, as the need to revise space to accommodate new services and departments creates new logic. The nursing staff development department, as a traditional department, may be moved about to house new departments. Staff development administrators can look on these experiences as opportunities to redesign space to adjust to new staff development services. The opportunity can also be used to negotiate for learning centers and space dedicated to clinical skill development labs.

Ideally, staff development specialists would have classroom, office, and storage space under the control of the department. In reality, space may be shared with other departments, and access to various classroom space controlled by several parties. Occasionally, the staff development department is assigned its own adequate space. But the department, like all others in the health care organization, is always at risk of new space allocations. The frequent and functional use of any space may mitigate against change.

The organization may adopt a space standard for office work. Some use 150 square feet per person. Others cannot afford this space allocation and assign as little as 50 square feet. Storage space is also at a premium. Conference and classroom space is often adapted from areas not in use. Dedicated classroom space should be protected through frequent use. The staff development administrator may accept space located in a distant building due to the available square footage. This judgment must be weighed against the potential loss of access to departmental personnel.

Creativity, flexibility, tolerance, and good negotiating skills are characteristics that will serve the staff development administrator well as efforts to design good work space are in process. A joint effort by all members of the department, fashioned to make the most of any available space, will also contribute to an environment designed to stimulate creativity and tolerance.

Support Equipment

The staff development core curriculum will dictate the requisite training aids needed to implement the program. Training aids are those items that assist the staff development specialist with simulating learning experiences that closely replicate the actual performance of a particular skill. Simulation aids commonly used in staff development programs include

- CPR manikins
- Intravenous arms
- Intravenous pumps and controllers
- Enteral feeding pumps
- Dysrhythmia simulators
- Resuscitation carts
- Other disposable items used during demonstration exercises

Manufacturers of these devices usually provide care and maintenance instructions. Most devices are expected to last about five years with usual and customary use. Cost justification of these devices should be spread over five years and include an estimated number of users. Devices that no longer provide a relatively realistic simulation should be discarded.

Audio-visual equipment is another common tool used by staff development specialists to assist their work. Common equipment includes

- Overhead projectors
- Slide projectors
- Video tape players and monitors

Less commonly used equipment includes opaque projectors, laser disc players and monitors, and computers for simulation and instruction.

The complexity of the equipment will dictate the maintenance plan. The simpler the device, the less need for assistance. A supply of light bulbs for replacement should be maintained. Staff development specialists should be able to change bulbs in overhead and slide projectors, but this skill will need to be demonstrated. Other equipment, such as video players, will likely require assistance from the biomedical department or an outside vendor. Audio-visual equipment requires dedicated and secure storage space to prevent loss through theft.

The proficient use of these devices is a learned behavior. The staff development administrator will need to plan activities to develop this skill for specialists. Sources to guide this plan can be located in the media section in libraries.

Decisions by the staff development administrator to acquire training aids and support equipment must be grounded in the program plan. For example, if dysrhythmia interpretation is a new skill for a selected group of nurses, the teaching strategy may include the interpretation of rhythms as they appear on the cardiac monitor. The skill required for this interpretation is different than that required to interpret a static rhythm from a rhythm strip. This justification may be used to acquire the necessary rhythm simulator. Support from nurse managers can also be garnered to assist in this acquisition.

Equipment can also be acquired from other departments. For example, the biomedical department may retire a defibrillator or monitor from the patient care area as new technology becomes available. This equipment may still be serviceable for educational purposes and may be acquired by the staff development department with the assistance of biomedical personnel. The equipment must be safe for this purpose. The administrator must also consider the likelihood that this equipment will provide an adequate simulation for the learner. If the equipment is so outdated that an adequate simulation cannot be created, an alternative is to borrow a defibrillator or monitor from a nursing unit for the actual session.

Workbooks and Texts

Staff development activities of short duration usually do not include a required text; those of longer duration may do so. For example, a critical care course may use a single text for the readings and reference. Likewise, a management development course that extends over a period of time may include a book recommendation. The expense of these texts must be a factor in the decision-making process of the staff development administrator. Questions about who will pay, the learner or the organization, must also be answered. In some self-directed programs of several months duration, for example, head nurse orientation, an optional text may be recommended as an initial reference for the neophyte head nurse.

Staff development specialists and administrators have a role in the selection of reference texts and additions to the organization's library collection. Despite the fact that few texts may be used to support staff development coursework, the administrator should maintain a working knowledge of current reference texts and should update professional collections regularly.

It is common to organize collections of articles to support selected coursework. These articles may be bound into a workbook or distributed separately to support selected topics. Caution must be exercised regarding copyright infringements in these cases. Generally, permission to provide a copy for each learner is given readily by the copyright holder.

Films and Videos

As the scope of nursing knowledge expands, more packaged learning activities are used. Many excellent films, videos, and slide or filmstrip with sound programs exist to support this effort. The media must be reviewed carefully by the administrator or specialist and selected based on the congruence of the message of the media and the message of the staff development program.

Media may be purchased, rented, or obtained for no charge. Product vendors will often supply a video of their product for use in training. Film and video companies usually have preview, rental, and purchase policies that vary from company to company. Preview fees are frequently applied to the full purchase of the film. Questions to assist the staff development administrator in determining the selection of media to support programs are

- Is the information in the media accurate and current?
- Is the message in the media consistent with the staff development program objectives?
- Is the cost of the media efficient if compared with other options for presentation of the information?
- Will the program get adequate use to justify the outlay of scarce resources?

Some organizations have sophisticated media production capability. Before a decision is made to produce an in-house program, the staff development administrator must again make a decision that satisfactorily answers the following questions:

- Is this the best method for presenting this information?
- Do the staff have the expertise to get messages across through this media? If not, how much training of staff will be necessary?
- What support is available to organize this production?
- How much will the production cost, particularly what is the cost of salaries of those involved in the production?

- How many people will be reached with this production?
- Is there a more efficient strategy to transmit this information?

The decision to organize an in-house video or slide production is a difficult one because of the costs involved. However, the product may well justify the cost, and subsequent similar efforts may cost less due to the staff's experience with production.

Departmental Policies and Practices

Administrators rely on policies to guide practice. These policies should be in writing and readily available. It is common to organize departmental policies into a manual. The format of the departmental manual is usually guided by organizational standards. The titles in the table of contents of a staff development practice manual are quite different from clinical manuals. Topics covered in the manual should reflect common practices.

The process of generating staff development policies includes the following:

1. Identify a standard of practice or topic that requires consistency and guidelines.
2. Discuss with staff development specialists and others, such as nurse managers and executives, how the policy should be developed.
3. Use a consistent approach in the writing of the policy.
4. Circulate a draft copy of the policy to others for comment and feedback, ask for the effect the policy may have on practice.
5. Finalize the policy and gain appropriate endorsements.
6. Practice and enforce the policy.

Specialists may be assigned to develop selected policies, particularly those that primarily affect the members of the staff development department. Other policies may require more careful handling. In particular, those policies that affect the entire nursing division will require additional consideration and management as they are developed.

Most staff development practice manuals also include a description of the overall program and plan, the scope of service, and the providers of those services. Organizational charts and structures are included. Policies such as attendance at educational offerings, contact hour accrual, confidentiality, and consequences of failure to attend a program are common topics that will require endorsement and support of the whole nursing division.

Practice manuals evolve over time and can become cumbersome. A regular review of the contents is the responsibility of the staff development administrator. This review includes accuracy, appropriateness, and continued need for the policy. Updating with the date noted on the policy should also take place during these reviews. A table of contents from one practice manual can be found in Appendix B. This list can be used to initiate a practice manual or to add to an existing one.

Budget Planning and Control

The staff development program requires a budget. The budget is a plan for use and allocation of resources. Most budgets have three broad categories: (1) salaries, (2) operations, and (3) capital items. The staff development program budget has commonalities and differences in comparison to other nursing unit budgets. The most significant commonality is the ratio of salaries to total budget. About 65% to 80% of the budget is commonly dedicated to salaries. The most significant difference is the use and structure of the operational budget. Unlike a clinical nursing unit budget which would list many medical surgical supplies for patient care and treatments, the staff development budget would list expenses for faculty honorariums, program materials, office supplies, and other costs related to program implementation.

Staff development programs that are new may require a year or two of experience with expenses before the operational budget is accurately planned. To begin this process, a list of common program expenses is made. This list is then structured to allow the recording of expenses for each program offered over a specified period of time. This matrix approach assists the staff development administrator with sufficiently capturing minor expenses associated with various programs. Chart 10-4 illustrates this matrix approach to budget planning.

Tracking systems for budget control may be provided by the organization. If not, the director must develop a recordkeeping system that tracks the flow of funds in and out of the budget plan. Only through this approach can decisions be made about continuing allocation of future funds. The budget plan is like any other and serves as a guide to assist the administrator with goal accomplishment. A simple tracking form for individual programs is illustrated in Figure 6-3 in Chapter 6. Use of this form will help the administrator keep track of expenses related to single programs for comparative, as well as cumulative purposes.

Generating Funds

Staff development programs are a service to the organization, and, therefore have costs associated with them. During time of financial stress, the staff development department may be expected to generate funds. This effort must be strategically and realistically planned. Funds are commonly generated from registration fees and the sale of staff development work products. However, costs associated with generating these funds may outstrip the actual funds generated. For example, the development of an attractive brochure and mailing it to 2000 nurses in the community may easily cost more than $1000. If only ten nurses register and pay a $65 registration fee, a clear loss of $350 is observed. This conservative estimate does not include the additional salary cost of individuals involved in the development and mailing of the brochure, or the cost of purchasing the mailing list needed for a large mailing.

It is not appropriate for the staff development department to focus on the generation of funds. If efforts to generate funds can be combined with other endeavors such as recruitment and retention, and costs are shared, then these enterprises may be worthwhile to the organization as a whole.

Health care organizations in general are experiencing extreme economical duress. This duress is passed on to all member departments of the organization. The cost of health care is the major issue of concern among most Americans. Reductions in cost have been attempted through various programs, the most significant of which is the Prospective Payment System (PPS) for Medicare recipients. The most profound effect of this system is the reduction in available health care dollars to conduct the business of health care delivery. Staff development programs also have experienced pressure as a result of changes in reimbursement patterns.

C hart 10-4
Matrix for Budget Planning

Item	Program								
	A	B	C	D	E	F	G	H	I
Faculty Fee									
Faculty Travel									
Program Site Rental									
Catering									
Promotion									
Program Materials									
AV Rental									
Miscellaneous									
Anticipated Registrants									
Projected Fee									
Anticipated Revenue									
Totals									

Financial management is a key skill of the staff development administrator. This includes obtaining funds, optimizing the use of those funds to support the staff development program, and ensuring that outcomes are in line with goals. The development of these skills requires concerted effort on the part of the administrator. In addition, accounting procedures, productivity measures, analysis of the cost-effectiveness, and cost-benefit of programs are skills required of the staff development administrator. Financial management competencies include behaviors that establish control and effective use of resources, including personnel, supplies, and equipment. The bibliography includes a variety of current references for the staff development administrator interested in developing these competencies. Though some are specifically applied to staff development practice, others will require adaptation.

Records and Reports

The staff development administrator also provides a variety of records and reports for various consumers and stakeholders of the program. Records of staff development activities include

- **Program files:** Program title, date/time/place of offering, objectives, faculty, coordinator, teaching strategy, evaluation method, evaluation, and attendance roster.
- **Employee transcripts:** A list of staff development activities, dates, and contact hours. These records may be kept centrally, in the staff development office or decentrally, on the nursing units. The transcript may or may not include grades. Chart 10-5 shows a sample staff development record used in a small community hospital to track learning activities and other factors required by regulatory agencies. It is designed to be used by the employee and assessed by the nurse manager responsible for the employee.
- **Faculty qualifications:** The curriculum vitae or resume of faculty who teach in the staff development program. A standard form may or may not be used. Minimal data include the current title and position of the individual, academic and other educational preparation that qualifies the faculty and relevant experience. Publications and research may or may not be included.

These files represent a minimal standard for staff development recordkeeping. Programs with several hundred activities each year may find a coding system useful. Chart 10-6 illustrates a simple system in which codes are self-generated and organized in a classic staff development model. Other methods include chronological recordkeeping and alphabetical filing. Whatever system is used, these records represent the work products of the department and serve as valuable sources of data for analysis and reports. These records should be maintained for a specified period of time, usually five years.

Common reports generated by the staff development administrator include

Chart 10-5
Staff Development Record for Employees

Name:_____ Entry Date: _____

Title: _____ Dept./Unit: _____

Employee no.:_____

Do Not Write in This Box

Orientation 3-month Assessment Date: _____

6-month Assessment Date: _____

CPR Date(s) _____, _____, _____, _____, _____

Fire Safety Date(s) _____, _____, _____, _____, _____

Electrical Safety Date(s) _____, _____, _____, _____, _____

Infection Control Date(s) _____, _____, _____, _____, _____

Current Licensure Date(s) _____, _____, _____, _____, _____

Performance Appraisal Date(s) _____, _____, _____, _____, _____

Other Assessments *(Specify Skill and Date Assessment Done)*:

_____

_____

_____

_____

Record Assessment by Clinical Coordinator *(Date and Signature)*:

_____, _____, _____

_____, _____, _____

_____, _____, _____

Staff Development Activity

Please record participation in any staff development activities such as classes, courses, workshops, patient care conferences, unit meetings, committee meeting attendance. Self-Learning Package (SLPs) and Study Guide (SG) will be recorded (after post-test is assessed) by authorized individual. Comment column also reserved for assessor.

Program/Topic/Meeting	Code	Date	Contact Hours	Comment (Date and Initials)

Source: Fort Washington Medical Center, Fort Washington, MD. Reproduced with permission.

Program/Topic/Meeting	Code	Date	Contact Hours	Comment (Date and Initials)

Chart 10-6
Program Code Number Generator
Staff Development Program

Inservices

Page _____

Code Number	Contact Hours	Program Title	Date(s)	No. Partic.	Inst./ Coord.	Record Assmt.
201-91						
202-91						
203-91						
204-91						
205-91						
206-91						
207-91						
208-91						
209-91						
210-91						

Source: Greater Southeast Community Hospital, Washington, D.C. Reproduced with permission.

- **Annual report:** A listing of all educational programs implemented. May include additional data such as dates, number of participants, instructors, and number of contact hours awarded. May or may not include an analysis of effectiveness or outcomes.
- **Focused report:** An analysis of a single or series of offerings that includes dates, participants, contact hours, and an in-depth evaluation of the program. Focus is on outcomes. Cost-effectiveness analysis is often included.
- **Compliance reports:** Reports showing compliance of employees participation to selected required programs such as CPR, Fire Safety, Infection Control. For certain departments this may also include other competency assessment measures such as electrical safety, equipment orientation, blood products management, chemotherapy administration, and other similar topics. These reports vary from agency to agency and often depend on regulatory body requirements for licensure and accreditation.
- **Progress reports:** Periodic reports for long term projects that require communication about progress toward goals. These may be for internal use or to meet external requirements. Programs and projects receiving funds from grants often require periodic progress reports.

The administrator may choose to organize information in a report to communicate and describe the work of the department. The decision to develop a report should be based on the need to organize and communicate information for a purpose. Reports should not be written unless they will be read! Reports are written with the reader and the purpose of the report as the primary focus. Reports longer than three pages should be accompanied by a brief (no more than one page) executive summary.

Some organizations find a regular reporting system is useful, others find them unnecessary. Reporting systems may require the staff of the department to submit identified documentation regarding programs, consultations, collaboration, and other activities on a monthly or quarterly basis. This information is compiled into a report and often used in the annual report. It may also be used to monitor and measure productivity of the department and staff.

Automating the Department

The decision to automate features of the staff development department is based on need and available resources. If the organization expects educational transcripts to be maintained centrally by the department, and the organization has more than a few hundred nursing staff members, an automated system is warranted. Several software packages are available to assist with this process. The administrator should expect to devote a significant amount of time to initiating and implementing an automation effort. Roles regarding data entry and report generation must also be clarified.

Software programs to track registration, class attendance, completion of competency requirements, and budget exist. Most can be modified and adapted to meet specific departmental needs. Spreadsheet software packages can also be used to track selected aspects of staff development practice. The common availability of these systems makes their appeal even greater to the administrator interested in organizing large amounts of data into useful information.

The health care industry is late in joining the information management systems movement. It is appropriate for staff development departments to acquire and use automated systems for efficiency. The use of a word processing system is a skill developed by individuals in graduate schools since the mid eighties. These same individuals employed as staff development specialists should be given the equipment to perform their job efficiently and effectively. Documentation is an integral part of the specialist's role; therefore, it is up to the administrator to acquire hardware and software to facilitate this role. This will be easier in organizations that value automation and provide support services for developing this capacity.

Resource Allocation Analysis

The administrator is responsible for using resources efficiently and effectively within a plan or framework. Decisions about which resources to allot for which program or project can be difficult and require the staff development administrator to consider financial and personnel management processes as well as ethical and legal issues.

The systematic budgeting process used by the organization will help prepare the administrator for this role. Budget preparation requires a classification of costs into systematic categories such as

- Personnel salaries and benefits
- Personnel travel and incidentals
- Personnel tuition and registration fees
- Office supplies
- Program materials and supplies
- Printing, graphics, and reproduction
- Faculty fees and honoraria
- Faculty travel, lodging, and incidentals
- Equipment expense allocation
- Equipment rental
- Equipment maintenance
- Miscellaneous

These categories and the associated budget for each line item are the first step to resource allocation analysis.

At periodic (often monthly) intervals, the administrator should analyze budget reports to determine if expenses are congruent with allocated resources. Similar to the decreasing balance in a checkbook, each line item should be evaluated to determine if it is

- Adequately funded
- Efficiently spent
- Appropriately used

Experience will help the administrator gain confidence with projecting costs for new programs with no track record of expenses. Using similar program expense records is helpful.

The administrator should be realistic about resource allocation and analysis. The highest expense related to any staff development effort is the loss of patient care hours related to learner time. Analyses of any staff development offering will consistently show 80% to 98% of the cost of the staff development experience is learner salary. Attention to this fact will do more to contribute to the efficiency of the operation than any other detail. The time spent by staff in a staff development activity must be tightly planned; time must be used well. In addition, measurable outcomes to demonstrate outcomes of learning will contribute to the efficiency of the staff development department.

Advanced resource allocation analysis techniques, such as cost-benefit analysis and cost-effectiveness analysis may be required by some organizations. One formula that has proven worthy was developed by del Bueno.[17] This formula requires the assignment of a value for the actual outcome or effectiveness of the program which is placed in ratio to the associated costs. To calculate the costs, the usual expenses related to supplies and equipment are determined. The cost of the learner salary is also calculated and a value is assigned to the final costs. This formula illustrates the high cost of learner salary and gives insight about how an administrator can achieve more cost-effectiveness. This is generally accomplished by reducing the costs (learner time) or raising expected outcomes. Administrators who recognize the high cost of lost patient care hours will make concerted efforts to use time spent in staff development activities efficiently. Raising outcome measurement to assure learning is one way to accomplish this task.

Cost-benefit analysis techniques have also been described to assist staff development managers.[18] These strategies are less common but may have some value for the administrator attempting to determine additional benefits of staff development activities for the organization and patient care.

There is no single, correct, and simple efficiency analysis formula. Many formulas are used, each with its strengths and limitations, biases, and assumptions. Some are reasonable, others comprehensive, still others seem superficial, and others are quite unbelievable. Disparity exists between the definitions as well. In general, the broad definitions provided by Rossi and Freeman[19] are the most useful.

- **Cost-benefit analysis:** Requires the economic efficiency of a program expressed as the relationship between costs and outcomes *usually expressed in monetary terms.*
- **Cost-effectiveness analysis:** Measures the efficacy of a program in achieving given intervention outcomes in relation to program costs, *usually expressed as cost per unit of outcomes achieved.*

Staff development administrators should select programs for resource allocation analysis. This analysis will yield data useful in the continuing management of the overall program.

Productivity Measures

Methods and measures to determine adequate productivity measures for nursing staff development are evolving. These formulas and the results are used to demonstrate the quantitative contribution of the staff development program. Most efforts to define productivity begin with a measure of the efficiency with which labor, materials, and goods are converted into goods and services.[20] Linear time standards are often used to express the productivity of nursing staff development specialists[21] and others use automated systems to accumulate data about staff development productivity.[22] Ulschak[23] conducted a survey of productivity measures used in hospital training departments and found the following to be most commonly used:

- Achievement of goals and objectives
- Number of participants multiplied by hours in class
- Number of hours per program per instructor
- Set standards based on work units
- Number of programs offered
- Number of contact hours awarded
- Monthly or quarterly reports
- Daily activity logs

Each of these measures has advantages and disadvantages. The single disadvantage common to all is the lack of comparison with an expected productivity. Kelly[24] attempted to address this issue and developed a formula that calculated a ratio of expected instructional hours to actual instructional hours given in a calendar year. The expected hours of instruction were calculated based on the number of employees who were expected to accumulate a specified amount of hours each year, and modified with an average attendance. The actual hours of instruction were calculated using program records and modified with an average attendance. Hours of instruction were used rather than contact hours because orientation consumed resources as well. Each year the final figure is compared with the expected figure to determine overall departmental productivity. This formula, used in several organizations during development, is a comprehensive and efficient approach which can be used by staff development administrators to determine departmental productivity.

The perceived value of nursing staff development to the organization is often subjective. The collection of data and outcomes measures to support this perceived value is an important component of the staff development administrator's role.

Performance of the Administrator

The demonstration of competency by the staff development administrator is essential to the continuing evolution of this service to organizations. Competencies have not been consistently defined or accepted by practitioners. Blending standards of performance from a variety of sources may assist the staff development director with continued development of competencies. Appendix C illustrates performance standards of a staff development administrator in an urban community hospital. Modifications to accommodate expectations of other types of organizations will make this document useful. Nurses engaged in multiple roles that include staff development administration will also find that these performance standards instruct them about expectations of practitioners.

Summary

Staff development administration is unfolding as a field of practice along with the field of nursing administration. There is no question that the specialty field of practice within staff development is nursing practice. This chapter offers a beginning attempt to organize the staff development program through the application of contingency theory as a framework. Though no single "best way" has emerged to organize and structure staff development programs and services, nurse executives must attend to the structure and process of this essential service. The chapter has addressed common administration themes such as personnel selection and development, and appraisal strategies. In addition, other functions, such as managing the environment, maintaining records, budgeting, and resource allocation analyses, are presented as they relate to staff development administration. Nurses engaged in the role of nursing staff development will define the field and blend concepts from various sources, theories, and frameworks. This will add strength and value to this practice and assist others as they learn how to conduct themselves in a way that makes a contribution to nursing and patient care.

References

1. Tichy, N. M., & DeVanna, M. A. (1986). *The transformational leader.* New York: Wiley.
2. Dunham, J., & Klafehn, K. A. (1990). Transformational leadership and the nurse executive. *Journal of Nursing Administration, 20* (4), 28–33.
3. Woodard, J. (1958). *Management and technology.* London: Her Majesty's Stationary Office.
4. Burns, T., & Stalker, G. (1961). *The management of innovation.* London: Tavistock.
5. Charns, M.P., & Schaefer, M.J. (1983). *Health care organizations: A model for management.* Englewood Cliffs, N.J.: Prentice-Hall.
6. McLagan, P.A. (1989). Models for HRD practice. *Training and Development Journal.* September, 49–59.
7. Mager, R. F. (1985). *What performance technologists do.* Mager Associates, Inc. P.O. Box 1233, Carefree, AZ 85377.
8. Knowles, M. S. (1980). *The modern practice of adult education: From andragogy to pedagogy.* Chicago: Association Press.

9. Fournies, F. F. (1978). *Coaching for improved work performance.* New York: Van Nostrand Reinhold.
10. Van Ort, S., Noyes, A., Longman, A. (1986). Developing and implementing a model for evaluating teaching effectiveness. *Image, 18* (3), 114–117.
11. Szilagyi, A. (1988). Performance evaluation. In *Management and performance.* Glenview, Illinois: Scott, Foresman.
12. Fombrun, C. J., & Laud, R. L. (Nov/Dec 1983). Strategic issues in performance appraisal: Theory and practice. *Personnel, 33–38.*
13. McGregor, D. M. (May/June 1957). An uneasy look at performance appraisal. *Harvard Business Review,* 4–8.
14. Naisbett, J., & Aburdene, P. (1985). *Reinventing the corporation.* New York: Warner.
15. Knowles, M. S. (1984). *Andragogy in action: Applying modern principles of adult education.* San Francisco: Jossey-Bass.
16. Smith, H. L., & Smith, N. F. (1986). The health care supervisor's guide to staff development. Rockville, MD: Aspen.
17. del Bueno, D., & Kelly, K. J. (1980). How cost-effective is your staff development program? *Journal of Nursing Administration, 10*(4), 31–36.
18. Kelly, K. J. (1985). Cost-benefit and cost-effectiveness analysis: Tools for the staff development manager. *Journal of Nursing Staff Development, 1*(1), 9–15.
19. Rossi, P. H., & Freeman, H. E. (1990). *Evaluation: A systematic approach* (4th ed.). Beverly Hills, CA: Sage.
20. Edwardson, H. R. (1985). Measuring nursing productivity. *Nursing Economics, 3*(1), 9–14.
21. Haynes, P. R. (1983). The evolution of a model to measure productivity: Implications for the hospital education department. *Proceedings of the 1983 Annual Conference of the American Society for Healthcare Education and Training. Chicago: American Hospital Association.*
22. Dombro, M. (1985). Using a computer data management system to measure hospital staff development productivity. *Journal of Nursing Staff Development, 1*(2), 52–60.
23. Ulschak, F. (1988). *Creating the future of healthcare education.* Chicago: American Hospital Association.
24. Kelly, K. J. (1990). A productivity measure for nursing staff development. *Journal of Nursing Staff Development, 6*(2), 65–70.

Appendix A: Performance Standards for Staff Development Specialists

POSITION DESCRIPTION

Position Title:

Education Specialist

Reports To:

Associate Director, NER

Main Function:

The Education Specialist serves as a role model, consultant, change agent, and facilitator in assessing learning needs and in planning, implementing, and evaluating educational activities for the nursing staff.

Major Functions:

1. Collaborates with nursing managers and staff to assess learning needs.
2. Plans and implements educational activities to meet identified learning needs, utilizing adult education principles.
3. Develops and utilizes appropriate evaluative systems to determine effectiveness of educational activities.
4. Promotes collaborative relationships among health care professionals.
5. Participates in committees, task forces, meetings and activities to assist in the development of staff, ultimately resulting in improved patient care.
6. Participates in activities that promote professional development through education and other activities that enhance the practice of nursing and education.

Qualifications:

1. Eligible for licensure as a Registered Nurse in the District of Columbia.
2. Baccalaureate degree required.
3. Graduate preparation in adult education desirable.
4. Three years experience in clinical nursing practice.
5. Previous experience in nurse-peer teaching.
6. Ability to communicate effectively with all levels of staff.

General Responsibilities:

The Education Specialist functions as an analyst, designer and developer, instructor, evaluator, and manager in a broad range of activities that lead to development and implementation of instruction, job aids, practice, feedback systems, as well as other solutions to problems of performances, clinical competencies, and professional development. The procedures/techniques that constitute the substance of these activities include those of problem definition, analysis, solution development, and implementation.

Tasks Performed:

1. Needs Analysis—extracts boundary statements from decision makers, performs job and task analyses as they relate to competencies and learning needs, analyzes critical incidents and performance for learning deficiencies, derives skills from task analysis for instructional designs.

2. Course Development—determines major competencies; interprets target population's needs; designs learning environment; writes pre-tests, and post-test; writes instructional programs including objectives, scripts, learner exercises, instructional content, audiovisual media mix; develops and uses course control documents such as performance checklists and other related forms; designs promotional materials; interacts with information sources and content experts; creates feedback systems to validate course content and impact on performance.

3. Research—participates in the hospital-based research program, as a proposal reviewer, support person and committee member; uses the research process in own research.

4. Course Manager/Supervisor—arranges learning environment; prepares learners; analyzes student performance; replenishes/orders materials; records learner progress; compares student performance with criteria; diagnoses performance weaknesses; selects remedial activities; selects and arranges AV equipment; solicits suggestions for improvement.

5. Course Delivery—delivers background, introductory and content material; uses presentation media, models sophisticated platform skills; performs tasks being taught; interacts with students; recognizes and minimizes obstacles to learning; interprets questions and formulates answers; makes self available to students.

6. Supervision of Course/Class Development—supervises clinical nurses during development of learning activities; approves learning activity records; advises their instructors on necessary improvements; serves as an advisor to instructors during course developments; acts as a consultant to staff on the educational process; writes proposals; prepares course budgets.

7. Evaluation—selects evaluation formats; develops and uses evaluation instruments including reaction forms, tests, surveys and criterion-referenced performance sheets; conducts evaluation; analyzes and interprets results; communicates results to appropriate leaders.

8. Committee and Task Force Membership/Leadership—chairs committees and task forces as requested; prepares project schedules; writes proposals and reports; assigns personnel to tasks; coordinates and monitors work of members; develops evaluation reports; acquires services, supplies and materials as needed.

9. Own Professional Development—participates in continuing education and professional association activities to continue competency development role.

10. Community Outreach—represents hospital in community and professional development activities to showcase the organization's good works and provide basic health education to community members.

PERFORMANCE STANDARDS FOR EDUCATION SPECIALIST

Major Function I:

Collaborates with nursing managers and staff to assess learning needs.
Performance is satisfactory when the education specialist:
1. Develops and utilizes a mechanism for ongoing needs assessment for designated areas.
2. Participates in department-wide needs assessment.
3. Meets with staff and management as necessary to validate needs and assessment of future needs.
4. Responds appropriately to perceived needs with learning activities or other recommendations to assist change.
5. Collaborates with Associate Director, Nursing Education and Research to prioritize needs based on organizational and departmental goals.

Major Function II:

Plans and implements educational activities to meet identified learning needs, utilizing adult education principles.
Performance is satisfactory when the education specialist:
1. Plans learning activities based on needs assessment.
2. Collaborates with selected members of target audience in planning program content.
3. Conducts program planning within appropriate time frame.
4. Functions within the guidelines of Center for Nursing Education Practice Manual.
5. Utilizes adult education principles in conducting programming.

Major Function III:

Develops and utilizes appropriate evaluative systems to determine effectiv ness of educational activities.
Performance is satisfactory when the education specialist:
1. Develops and utilizes an appropriate evaluative tool for each educational activity.
2. Provides feedback regarding program evaluation to the learner and other appropriate individuals.
3. Provides feedback regarding participant performance to the participant and immediate supervisor, when appropriate.
4. Revises educational programming based on compiled evaluative data.

Major Function IV:

Promotes collaborative relationships among health care professional.
Performance is satisfactory when the education specialist:
1. Assist in the identification of appropriate resource people to promote collaboration.
2. Promotes collaboration among nursing professionals and with other health care disciplines.
3. Works in conjunction with clinical specialists in assessing and meeting the needs of staff.
4. Works in conjunction with other education specialists to establish and maintain standards of educational programming throughout the hospital.

Major Function V:

Participates in committees, task forces, meetings and activities to assist in the development of staff, ultimately resulting in improved care.

Performance is satisfactory when the education specialist:

1. Participates in the development and attainment of goals and objectives for Patient Care Services.
2. Participates as an active member in at least one Patient Care Services/hospital committee.
3. Participates, as an active member in the Nursing Education and Research Committee.
4. Participates in additional meeting and task force activities as appropriate.

Major Function VI:

Participates in activities that promote professional development through ed cation and other activities that enhance the practice of nursing and education.

Performance is satisfactory when the education specialist:

1. Attends continuing education offerings and other activities to meet identified learning needs.
2. Collaborates with other education specialists for purposes of seeking validation of professional effectiveness.
3. Develops annual goals and objectives to guide professional performance.
4. Serves as a consultant to health care providers in regard to health care issues.
5. Actively participates in the research program of Patient Care Services Department.

Source: Greater Southeast Community Hospital, Washington, D.C. Reproduced with permission.

Performance Standards for Associate Director
Nursing Education and Research/Patient Care Services

Standards	Tasks
Determines nursing practice and management standards and reviews/revises annually.	

Conceptualizes and interprets nursing and nursing services.	Conceptualizes nursing and nursing services by:
	  a. defining nursing
	  b. identifying philosophy of PCS
	  c. identifying the philosophy of administration
	  d. determining Patient Care Services purpose and objectives
	  e. determining nursing care standards
	Ensures that objectives and goals are relevant and consistent with goals and objectives of the institution.

Devises formal communication system to support:
  Divisional meetings
  CNE staff meetings
  Other communication meetings
	Designs and implements essential records and reporting systems.

Provides communication liaison between first line administrator and executive.	
Attends regularly and participates in Nursing Executive Council, Departmental Meeting and other meetings as appropriate.	Summarizes educational activities and presents information to Vice President on an ongoing basis.
Participates with the appropriate Departmental Chairman in coordinating educational activities.	Writes an annual report summarizing and evaluating educational programs.

(continued)

Performance Standards for Associate Director *(cont'd)*

Standards	Tasks
Reflects knowledge base and clinical competence by direct involvement in the nursing care process or indirectly by planning and guiding care with other health team members.	Assists in designing and instruction about nursing care delivery systems in conjunction with head nurses.
Coordinates and utilizes clinical resources for maximum efficiency and effectiveness in the delivery and promotion of health care.	Responds to crisis and/or emergency situations as needed.
Maintains communication at staff level by routinely collaborating with CNE staff regarding the delivery of patient care and educational programming to support same.	
Plans and participates in the evaluation of patient care and educational programs.	Evaluates quality of educational programs not less than 6 times a year.
Promotes compliance with hospital Quality Assurance Program.	Approves new and/or revised department/division policies and procedures.
Establishes policies and procedures consistent with the requirements of accreditation agencies and ensures compliance.	Serves as a consultant in disciplinary action.
Functions as a liaison among the health care providers to maintain optimum working relationships.	
Evaluates recruitment efforts and analyzes and supports retention.	Monitors effect of educational programming on recruitment and retention efforts.
Provides administrative coverage on a scheduled basis for Patient Care Services.	Participates in the organization of Patient Care Services through input in the structuring of the department.
Contributes and ensures implementation of organizational charge.	Meets with each CNE staff members on a regularly scheduled basis to provide direct ongoing feedback with regard to job performance.
Utilizes performance standards in developing the educational specialists and the nurse clinicians fn the role of nurse educators.	

Standards	Tasks
Clarifies and refines CNE staff roles	Completes performance appraisals of all CNE staff in timely manner.
	Reviews and approves job description, performance standards and staff assignments.
Maintains an atmosphere conducive to ongoing educational and professional motivation.	
Maintains an active involvement in the educational development of CNE staff fn a formal and/or informal teaching capacity.	Develops goals and objectives for performance appraisal with CNE staff.
Identifies strengths and weaknesses related to professional performance and utilizes available resources to enhance and promote growth and development.	Completes leadership assessments and reports developmental plans to Vice President.
Continues with own educational enrichment to maintain a current knowledge base and clinical/management/educational expertise.	Establishes with Vice President a learning contract annually.
Promotes economical utilization of human and material resources.	Reviews and submits divisional budget on an annual basis to the Vice President.
	Ensures appropriate budgetary planning for educational goals and objectives.
	Monitors budgetary compliance for the division.
	Monitors personnel work schedule.
Administers the Nursing Clinical Ladder Program.	Chairs Clinical Ladder Committee.
	Revises Program.
	Monitors compliance of all program participants.
Encourages and supports individuality and creativity in the change process	Reviews findings of research projects with other Associate Directors.
Facilitates research in areas of nursing care and management systems.	Utilizes an external consultant to guide the development of a research project within PCS as necessary.

(continued)

269

Performance Standards for Associate Director *(cont'd)*

Standards	Tasks
Participates in the planning of clinical nursing experiences for schools of nursing.	Monitors school affiliation program and policies and communicates changes/recommendations to other ADs.
Participates in at least one professional organization.	Keeps current with national patient care trends and developments.
Establishes and maintains a network with other health care professionals.	
Establishes and maintains community outreach programs.	
Assesses, plans, implements and evaluates educational programs based on (1) a position-oriented core curriculum and (2) goals and objectives of the Vice President.	Prepares and submits CNE goals and objectives to Vice President.
Serves as resource for the educational process and curriculum development for educational programs.	Establishes systems to assist PCS staff develop instructional abilities.
	Establishes systems to assure the use of sound educational strategies.
Administers nursing education department	Maintains educational record keeping systems that support data retrieval.
	Maintains ANA accreditation for nursing continuing education Program.
	Maintains AHA Certifying Agency status for the CPR program.
Approved By:	
Vice President, Patient Care/Services	
Date:	
Reviewed:	
Reviewed:	
Reviewed:	

Source: Greater Southeast Community Hospital, Washington, D.C. Reproduced with permission.

Appendix B: Staff Development Practice Manual Index
Center for Nursing Education/Practice Manual

CNE 164.0   Workshop Fees
CNE 165.0   Registration Fees for Retired Nurses
CNE 166.0   Brochure Content
CNE 168.0   Program Cancellation/Refunds
CNE 169.0   Program Cancellation/Inclement Weather
CNE 170.0   Catering
CNE 172.0   Parking
CNE 173.0   Needs Assessment
CNE 174.0   Target Audience Identification
CNE 175.0   Program Evaluation
CNE 176.0   Budget Planning for Individual Program
CNE 175.0   Program Evaluation
CNE 178.0   Measuring Participant Reaction
CNE 182.0   Developing Course Outlines
CNE 190.0   Awarding ANA Continuing Education Contact Hours
CNE 192.0   Co-Providership of Continuing Education Activities
CNE 193.0   Co-Sponsorship of Programs with HRD
CNE 194.0   Product Evaluation—Guidelines for Implementation of Study

Section IV: Nursing Education Programs and Services

CNE 200.0   Inservice Education
CNE 300.0   CPR Program Policies and Guidelines
CNE 500.0   Nursing Continuing Education Program
CNE 700.0   Specialty Staff Development—Critical Care

Section V: Forms Index

CNE 001.0   Learning Activity Record
CNE 002.0   Program Approval Record
CNE 003.0   Permanent Transcript—Non-GSCH Employees
CNE 004.0   Permanent Transcript—GSCH Employees
CNE 005.0   Vitae Sheet for Instructors
CNE 006.0   Checklist for Quantitative Review
CNE 007.0   Budget Planning Worksheet
CNE 008.0   Program Planning Guide
CNE 009.0   Participant Reactionnaire
CNE 010.0   Evaluation
CNE 011.0   Education Attendance Sheet
CNE 012.0   Education Attendance Verification
CNE 013.1   Certificate of Course Completion (ANA)
CNE 013.2   Certificate of Course Completion (GSCH)
CNE 014.0   Faculty Agreement—Out-of-State
CNE 015.0   Faculty Faculty Agreement—Local Faculty
CNE 016.0   CNE Registration Form
CNE 018.0   PCS Learning Plan
CNE 019.0   Participant Action Plan
CNE 020.0   SDL Learning Activity Record
CNE 021.0   Course E—CPR Form Letter
CNE 022.0   Co-Providership of Continuing Education Activities

Section VI: Use of Conference Facility

Appendix C: Position Description for Administrator of Nursing Staff Development Department

Position Title:

Associate Director of Nursing for Education, Research, and Development

Reports to:

Vice President, Patient Care Services

Functional Statement:

The Associate Director is responsible for assessing, planning, implementing, and evaluating nursing education and staff development activities within the Department of Patient Care Services in accordance with the established philosophy of Nursing. In addition, incumbent is responsible for facilitating the nursing research process with the Patient Care Services Research Committee.

Qualifications:

- Registered Nurse with current District of Columbia license.
- Master's degree required.
- Progressive experience and responsibility in clinical area and nursing education required. Nursing management experience desirable.
- Ability to communicate effectively with varied levels of staff.
- Ability to design and implement education activities.
- Ability to teach in small and large group settings.
- Minimum of four years clinical nursing practice, two years nursing management experience, and one year formal and informal teaching experience.

Purpose:

The Associate Director is responsible for directing the Center for Nursing Education (CNE). In accordance with the established philosophy of Nursing, the incumbent assesses, plans, implements, and evaluates nursing education and staff development activities within the Department of Patient Care Services. The incumbent also facilitates the nursing research program with the Patient Care Services Research Committee. In addition, the incumbent acts as consultant to educational programs other than Patient Care Services for selected programs.

Dimensions:

The incumbent supervises four (4) Nursing Education Specialists, one and one-half (1½) Enterostomal Therapists, one (1) Health Educator, one (1) Nutrition Support Nurse, and one (1) Systems Manager.

Position Location:

The incumbent reports directly to the Vice President for Patient Care Services along with seven (7) Associate Directors, six (6) Nursing Supervisors, one (1) Administrative Assistant, and one (1) Administrative Secretary II. The Vice President for Patient Care Services, in turn, reports to the Hospital President.

Environment:

The incumbent functions in an organization located in an urban setting with a mixed ethnic, social, and economic population. In addition, the incumbent operates within a highly clinical and educational environment which interacts largely with clinical and professional individuals.

Position Function:

The incumbent determines nursing practice and management standards and reviews/revises annually. In addition, the incumbent devises a formal communication system to support Divisional, CNE staff, and other communication meetings. The incumbent writes an annual report summarizing and evaluating educational programs. In addition, the incumbent meets with CNE staff members on a regularly scheduled basis to provide direct ongoing feedback with regard to job performance, complete performance appraisals, and review and approve job descriptions, performance standards and staff assignments. The incumbent develops goals and objectives for performance appraisal with CNE staff. In addition, the incumbent completes leadership assessments, developmental plans, divisional budget, and reports on each to the Vice President for Patient Care Services. The Vice President for Patient Care Services develops a learning contract on an annual basis with the incumbent. The incumbent ensures appropriate budgetary planning for educational goals and objectives as well as monitoring budgetary compliance and personnel work schedule for the division. The incumbent also assists in designing and instruction about nursing care delivery systems in conjunction with the head nurses. The incumbent assesses, plans, implements, and evaluates educational programs based on position-oriented core curriculum and goals and objectives of the Patient Care Services Department, as well as monitoring the effect of educational programming on recruitment and retention efforts. In addition, the incumbent facilitates research in areas of nursing care and management systems. *The incumbent maintains educational record keeping systems that support data retrieval and ANA accreditation for nursing continuing education Programs. The incumbent approves new and/or revised Center for Nursing Education Department policies and procedures.* The incumbent also participates in the organization of Patient Care Services through input in the structuring of the department and active membership in the Patient Care Services Executive Council. The incumbent serves as a consultant in disciplinary action. In addition, the incumbent establishes systems to assist Patient Care Services staff and others within the hospital develop instructional abilities and to assure the use of sound educational strategies. Finally, the incumbent administers the Nursing Clinical Ladder Program.

Subordinate Activities:

The incumbent receives all information adhering to Personnel Policies and Procedures and current departmental activities from the Nursing Education Specialists, Enterostomal Therapists, the Health Educator, the Nutrition Support Nurse, and the Secretary/Registrar.

Major Challenges:

The incumbent handles multiple and complex situations associated with the development of educational programs, budgets, and the evaluation of staff. In addition, the incumbent remains current on national patient care trends and developments. The incumbent is challenged to manage a safe and effective department by adhering to all established guidelines established by Patient Care Services and the Hospital and other regulatory bodies.

Latitude:

The incumbent has authority to hire, fire, and take appropriate disciplinary actions for all subordinate staff members. In addition, the incumbent has the responsibility to change salaries, titles, and job responsibilities and assignments of staff members according to established Personnel Policies and Procedures with final approval coming from the Vice President for Patient Care Services. The incumbent approves new and/or revised Center for Nursing Education Department policies and procedures.

Performance Measures:

The effectiveness of performance is measured by the incumbent's ability to assist in designing and instructing in the areas of nursing care delivery systems in conjunction with the staff nurses, head nurses, members of Patient Care Services Executive Council, and other members of the Patient Care Services division. In addition, performance is measured by the ability to effectively manage the department within the established guidelines, budget, and procedures of Patient Care Services. The incumbent must be able to respond to crisis and/or emergency situations as needed.

Contacts Inside and Outside the Organization:

Internal contacts include: attends regular meetings of the Nursing Executive Council; daily interactions with hospital department heads in coordinating educational activities as well as Vice President for Patient Care Services, Management Council, and Center for Nursing Education.

External contacts include: monitors and participates in school nursing affiliation programs; establishes and maintains a network with other health care professionals and community outreach programs; functions as a liaison among the health care providers to maintain optimum working relationships; participates in at least one professional organization.

Knowledge and Skills:

The incumbent must have progressive experience and responsibility in the clinical area, nursing management, and nursing education. The incumbent should have the ability to communicate effectively with all staff. In addition, the incumbent must be able to design, implement, teach, and evaluate education activities for small and large groups.

The incumbent must have a baccalaureate degree in Nursing and must have a current R.N. license in the District of Columbia. A Master's degree in

Nursing or Adult Education is required. A minimum of four (4) years clinical nursing practice, two (2) years nursing management, experience, and one (1) year formal and informal teaching experience is required.

Approved by:
Vice President Patient Care Services
Date:
Reviewed:
Revised:

chapter **11**

uality Management Within Staff Development

Karen J. Kelly

Quality management is an integral component of the staff development program. Total quality improvement is a philosophy that has been adopted by many specialists. This approach, to assure consumers that staff development services are continually scrutinized and improved, has benefit for many. This chapter will discuss the relationship of staff development and quality assurance, the use of standards for monitoring and evaluation, the technical aspects of monitoring and evaluation, the use of data to drive improvements, and the concept of continuous improvement as an underlying theme of quality management. Staff development specialists who adopt these beliefs and practices will demonstrate their professionalism and commitment to the continuing development of the field.

The Relationship of Quality Management and Staff Development

Relating the word "quality" to products and services has become a popular notion. The actual use of quality improvement strategies within staff development has also received attention recently. The concepts of quality improvement are used by specialists whenever program evaluation methods are used. However, the use of data derived from these evaluations is often not organized in a way that allows for quality monitoring or systematic improvement. To strengthen the quality management of the staff development program, specialists should consider using different approaches. This will require the adoption of new belief systems and the integration of that belief system into new evaluation practices.

Common Evaluation Methods

Evaluation practices commonly used by staff development specialists include those described by Kirkpatrick:[1]

Reaction. Evaluations that measure the reaction of participants to the learning activity. The reaction of faculty may also be measured. Reactions may be measured through verbal polls or using a tool completed by the participants. Sometimes referred to as a "happiness index," carefully constructed forms to measure reaction yield good data that can be used to improve programs. Chart 11-1 is one example of a form that will yield data for analysis.

Learning. Evaluations that objectively measure learning, usually using a written or performance test. This level of evaluation is commonly used to measure learning that is required to meet performance standards. Tests administered to critical care nurses to measure skill with dysrhythmia interpretation are a common example of evaluation of learning in this model. Performance tests given at the completion of skills training or revalidation sessions fit into this category. CPR is a good example of this. Another example of evaluation of learning acquired in the classroom is a case study presented at the completion of a lecture on a disease entity in which the nurse is expected to answer a series of questions related to the care and management of a hypothetical patient with the disease or health care problem discussed in the lecture.

Behavior. Evaluations conducted to gather data about behavior are those that occur outside the classroom and are often referred to as "follow-up" evaluations. Measures of performance, identified as specific behaviors that can be observed as a result of a training session, fit into this category. Less frequently conducted, these evaluations are costly and yield data that may be considered unreliable. The reason for this is the difficulty in measuring a specific behavior and relating it to classroom learning. For example, the behavior of a nurse is measured as she performs a chemotherapy procedure taught three months earlier in class—is that behavior directly related to classroom learning (or nonlearning), or is it related to experience? It may not matter if the competency assessment is satisfactory. However, if the performance is unsatisfactory, was it because of poor classroom instruction, inadequate learning by the nurse, or lack of experience with the skill? Evaluations conducted to measure behaviors must recognize these limitations.

Impact. Measures of impact evaluate the effect of a learning activity on an outcome. For example, if a nurse is taught to assess breath sounds of patients at specified times after surgery to prevent complications, is there a reduction of post-surgical respiratory complications in the group of patients cared for by those nurses who received the training? A common impact measure is the infection control education program. The anticipated effect of these learning activities is a reduction (or maintenance at a certain level) of nosocomial infection. The inherent difficulty is the strength of the correlation of the two variables, nosocomial infection and learning activities. Many other variables also have an effect on these outcomes, and the specialist must recognize the limitations and strengths of these measures.

These evaluation methods lend themselves to quality management. Staff development specialists have used data gathered from these evaluation activities to improve programs. It is the extension of this activity that will strengthen the management of quality within staff development.

The Natural Relationship

Quality management and staff development have a natural relationship. The goal of quality management and staff development is the improvement of the quality of patient care. Quality is defined by the JCAHO[2] as "the degree to which patient care services *increases* the probability of desired patient outcomes and *reduces* the probability of undesirable outcomes, given the current state of knowledge." The role of staff development in organizations is to assess, maintain, and develop nursing competencies that *increase* the probability of desired patient outcomes and *reduce* the probability of undesired outcomes. Nursing competencies can be further defined as the use of knowledge and skills in the provision of patient care services.

Staff development is an organizational quality improvement activity. The challenge to specialists is the integration of these concepts into staff development practice. The greatest challenge is the integration of the central component of quality management, that is the monitoring and evaluation process. Other challenges include the need to clarify terms and the use of data to improve practice. Differences in organizations have also precluded the use of quality management data across organizations. The future will generate new quality management approaches that will yield data to *rationally* compare nursing staff development practice across organizations. These comparisons and subsequent recommendations will cause natural improvements in staff development services.

Staff development specialists will also define future standards of practice and accepted monitoring and evaluation activities. The monitoring and evaluation activities will yield data that will drive the improvement process. It is the role of the nursing staff development specialist to define quality for the program and services provided. The role also includes the development or adaptation of monitoring and evaluation activities that will yield data to improve practice. This process can be learned and integrated into staff development practice.

Forces and Motivators

A quality evolution has occurred in health care.[3] This evolution is the result of many factors. The expectations of the health care consumer, the desire of health care providers to improve quality, and the quality management practices of other industries are just a few of these factors. External motivators also include the expectation by the Joint Commission on Accreditation of Healthcare Organizations (JCAHO) that certain forms of quality management are evident within the health care agency.

Chart 11-1
Sample Reactionnaire to Yield Data
for Analysis Program Title

Program Title
Code No.
Date

Reactionnaire

Please check the appropriate column to indicate your reaction and return this form. Thank you!

KEY: **E** = Excellent   **A** = Adequate   **U** = Unsatisfactory

Session	Value of Presentation			Delivery of Presentation		
	E	A	U	E	A	U
Topic/Presenter						

Please Rate the Following Statements:

KEY: **1** = Not at all   **2** = A little   **3** = Some/Sort of
             4 = A lot   **5** = Very much so

	1	2	3	4	5
1. Regarding objectives, I feel that I can: a. b. c. d. e. f.					

	1	2	3	4	5
2. This program content matched the stated objectives.					
3. The teaching methods used were appropriate for type of content presented.					
4. The conference facilities were conducive helping me learn.					
5. This program is pertinent to my personal needs and interests.					
6. This program is pertinent to my current area of practice.					
7. I learned what I expected to learn from this program.					
8. The content presented had adequate detail to give me new information.					
9. The level of presentation of this program was appropriate for me.					

10. This program failed to satisfy my expectations in the following ways:

11. My suggestions for modifying this program are:

12. My suggestions for other continuing nursing education courses are:

13. Specifically, I plan to do the following as a result of my learning during this program:

14. I would also like to comment:

Date of Origin:
Reviewed:
Revised:

Source: Greater Southeast Community Hospital, Washington, D.C. Reproduced with permission.

Quality assurance has had a narrow, negative definition.[4] Chart audits and meeting report expectations of others was the common practice. Results of these audits were shared, but little was done to improve results. Nor did a comprehensive program of wide and substantive activities for quality management exist. This has changed in most organizations. Health care organizations have established programs with ongoing studies that have effectively improved patient care services and systems.

Health care professionals have always been oriented toward giving the "best" care possible to patients. But what does that mean? What can the patient expect when they receive services from a provider? Staff development specialists have also delivered their best when providing services. But, again, what does that mean? What can the organization (represented by the nurse manager) and individual consumer (represented by the nurse learner) expect from the staff development program. The monitoring and evaluation activities of quality management will yield data that will help define those expectations. Philip Crosby[5] defines quality as conformance to requirements, not goodness. This definition fits with the tradition of setting standards for practice within nursing and nursing staff development and provides us with a framework to improve our approach to standards. As an emerging field of practice, we can provide seminal work with the use of standards as a document that provides information for all interested parties about conformance to requirements. What are the requirements for a nursing staff development program, and what evidence do we have that we are conforming to those requirements? How can we cause quality through our conformance to requirements?

Standards for Nursing Staff Development

A standard of practice is simply an acknowledged measure of comparison. It can also be viewed as a requirement for quality. Standards serve as norms or criteria to determine how an observed behavior or result compares with a defined behavior or result. Is there conformance to requirements? The staff development specialist can define professional standards for practice within a particular organization. These standards describe the behaviors that can be observed as the specialist goes about staff development work. These standards are often defined as performance standards or a job description.

Performance standards have been suggested for the human resource development role.[6] Competencies are organized into four categories: technical, business, interpersonal, and intellectual. Key work dimensions were also identified such as administrator, evaluator, materials developer, instructor, facilitator, marketer, needs analyst, organization change agent, program designer, and researcher. These work dimensions also describe the functions of the staff development specialist and can be used to modify or improve performance standards (and job descriptions) of the individual specialist.

The Council of Continuing Education and Staff Development of the American Nurses' Association[7] has also defined standards. These standards help define the structure, process, and outcomes of staff development practice and can be used to model a staff development department. Eleven standards have been defined related to

- Organization and administration
- Human resources
- Learners
- Educational design
- Material resources and facilities
- Records and reports
- Evaluation
- Climate
- Program planning
- Consultation
- Systematic inquiry

Standards of practice in nursing staff development focus on the field of practice and clarify measures that will lead to a quality staff development program. Standards of performance specify behaviors of the specialist within the organization that can be observed as the staff development program is planned, delivered, and evaluated. Quality management monitoring and evaluation activities are used to determine if practice and performance standards are met, if there is conformance to requirements.

These sources provide excellent background for the staff development specialist to begin to define or improve standards of performance and standards of practice for nursing staff development within health care organizations.

Continuous Improvement

Berwick[8] differentiated the current approaches to quality management from past QA practices. He described the antiquated "theory of bad apples" as one that relied on inspection. He designated the new approaches as a "theory of continuous improvement" and described current efforts to understand and revise systems based on data as a refreshing change from the past. He also emphasized the importance of using all workers to participate in the process to reduce waste, rework, and complexity. Health care systems are increasingly complex and often defeat the purpose, that is, care of the patient that they are designed to help. The application of these principles to health care will improve quality. The application of these same principles to nursing staff development will improve the quality of programs and activities.

Staff development specialists who integrate a quality management approach to their work will find an increase in customer satisfaction along with job security. The contribution of staff development to the organization continues to be challenged in some sectors. Outcome measurements are few and often considered unreliable evidence of the effect of staff development interventions. The integration of quality management principles will address these issues and provide data which support the contribution of staff development. The work of Wolgin[9] which attempts to organize and demonstrate outcome measures used in various organizations will contribute to this effort. Staff development specialists who are able to demonstrate outcome measurements resulting from quality monitoring activities will make a meaningful endowment to the field of practice.

Quality Management Principles

Several charismatic, quality leaders have emerged in the past decade. The work of Crosby, Juran, Deming, and Shewhart are well-referenced in the quality management literature. Their principles guide most quality improvement efforts. Crosby defines "four quality absolutes" and says the ingredients include the following:

1. Quality is defined as conformance to requirements, not goodness.
2. Quality is achieved through prevention, not appraisal.
3. The quality performance standard is zero defects, not acceptable quality levels.
4. Quality is measured by the price of nonconformance, not indexes.

Juran was using a "fitness to use" approach and had much success with his strategies in Japan before he was rediscovered by American industries. Juran defined a "quality trilogy" as quality planning, quality control, and quality improvement.

Deming also experienced success in Japan before his principles were accepted in the United States. Deming is a statistician and was influenced by Shewhart in his early work with sampling techniques. Over time, Deming has improved his quality management principles and adapted several to be more closely aligned to his belief system. He currently advocates a total quality management approach based on this philosophy. He advocates 14 quality management principles. The basic assumptions in the Deming philosophy are

- Workers are trying their best to do a good job.
- Fear (of reprisal or bad evaluations) must be reduced, as they interfere with improvement efforts.
- The systems used for service delivery and production are the root of poor quality most of the time, and efforts to improve *systems* must be the focus of any quality improvement efforts.

Many of these apply to nursing staff development. Chart 11-2 illustrates an adaptation of Deming's 14 principles to a nursing staff development quality management philosophy. Deming also exhorts people to create a constancy of purpose for the improvement of service and product. This underlying principle also pervades many health care organization quality improvement programs. Training and development is also an integral component of the Deming approach to quality management. Organizations that have a quality imperative define the role of staff development as one which assists transformations that must occur to accomplish quality service initiatives.

Quality Management Models

Many models exist that incorporate these principles and provide a framework to organize the quality improvement efforts. The American

Chart 11-2
**Quality Management Philosophy for Nursing Staff
Development Based on Deming's Fourteen Points**

Based on the Deming principles of quality management, the nursing staff development department is committed to strive constantly (Point 5) toward improvement of our services (Points 1 and 2). Within this new philosophy, we will monitor and evaluate our processes (Point 3) and work toward the efficient use of resources for the best quality program (Point 4). Continued learning activities will be designed to help nursing personnel learn to do their jobs and develop professionally (Point 6). Staff development specialists will help employees learn how to learn (Point 8) and assist with intradepartmental and interdepartmental team building (Point 9). Staff development specialists will help nursing personnel develop professional pride and assist with the removal of system barriers to quality nursing care (Point 12). To that end, this department will provide a vigorous staff development program (Points 13 and 14).

Source: Kelly Thomas Associates, Alexandria, VA. Reproduced with permission.

Nurses' Association (ANA) model[10] identifies seven components to review nursing care. They are

1. Identify values.
2. Identify structure, process, and outcome standards and criteria.
3. Measurements needed to determine degree of attachment of standards and criteria.
4. Make interpretations about strengths and weaknesses based on measurements.
5. Identify possible courses of action.
6. Choose course of action.
7. Take action.

This framework was used for many years on a voluntary basis by nurses in various health care settings. Schroeder[11] extended this model and developed a unit-based quality assurance model. This model proposed eleven steps to the process used by nurses at the clinical unit level:

1. Develop standards of practice and criteria based on identified values and scientific knowledge.
2. Identify pertinent problems or issues.
3. Prioritize topics, and select one with which to deal.
4. Refine question.
5. Identify criteria relevant to the issue.
6. Select appropriate methodology for dealing with the issue or problem.

7. Collect data.
8. Analyze data.
9. Plan and implement corrective action.
10. Reevaluate issue.
11. Report results

Schroeder's model was adopted by many organizations, and other models often reflect these steps.

The JCAHO[12] also advocates a quality management model for monitoring and evaluation. Health care organizations seeking accreditation are required to produce evidence that the components are in place. The ten steps involved in this model are presented in Chart 11-3. This model integrates several of the steps defined in the Schroeder model and uses language that attempts to clarify the steps. This model can be used on individual nursing care units and to guide an entire organizational effort. The model can also be used to direct a multidisciplinary quality monitoring and evaluation effort. The monitoring and evaluation process of this model (Steps 2 through 9) is illustrated in Chart 11-3. Katz[13] applied the JCAHO model to nursing staff development and provided additional insight for specialists. Lewis and White[14] extended this work and advocated a comprehensive QA plan to monitor the outcome of educational activities.

Commonalities exist among all of these models. They include values identification, a definition of quality, standards or requirements development, measurement and appraisal, and action and reappraisal. These commonalities

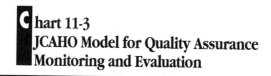

Chart 11-3
JCAHO Model for Quality Assurance
Monitoring and Evaluation

Monitoring and Evaluation 1988 Model

1. Assign Responsibility
2. Delineate the Scope of Care or Service
3. Identify Important Aspects of Care or Service
4. Identify Indicators
5. Establish Thresholds for Evaluation
6. Collect and Organize Data
7. Evaluate
8. Take Action to Resolve Identified Problems
9. Assess the Actions and Document Improvement
10. Communicate to Organizational QA Process

Source: Joint Commission on Accreditation of Healthcare Organizations, Chicago, IL. Reproduced with permission.

can be used to develop new and innovative approaches to quality management or to refine current models.

Monitoring and Evaluation

Monitoring and evaluation processes remains the weakest link in these models. The remainder of this chapter will apply the JCAHO ten-step model to staff development practice and provide examples to assist staff development specialists with this process. Through individual and innovative use of these ten steps, specialists will meet the challenge of data-driven improvements for quality management.

Data-driven improvements are those in which facts and figures are measured and analyzed for potential refinements. There are many available sources of count data in nursing staff development. Those sources include attendance records, test scores, reactionnaire scores, checklist performances, scores on other measurement tools used for teacher effectiveness, and learner acquisition of knowledge and skill. These sources of data can be used in quality monitoring and evaluation activities to improve the staff development program. As specialists gain skill and experience with the use of data to improve programs, more sophisticated measures will be attempted, and further improvements will be made.

Assign Responsibility

The decision process used to assign responsibility for quality monitoring and evaluation should involve all members of the staff development department. In cases of small or single person departments, the responsibility may be shared or integrated into current responsibilities. To achieve the commitment and clarification of values related to a quality improvement program, discussion about roles and responsibilities is essential. If it is viewed as "one more thing that has to be done" without an understanding of the need for a commitment to the process, then the program will not be successful. During this first step, staff development specialists should engage in discussions about quality and what quality means to each individual. These discussions will yield many feelings about expectations. Confusion about the quality improvement program can be clarified, and old beliefs about the "inspection for bad apples" can be dispelled. A document should define the results of these discussions and assign roles and responsibilities for this effort. Chart 11-4 represents one example of such a document.

Delineate Scope of Service

The roles and responsibility discussion described above should be continued and should include a delineation of the scope of service. Depending on past documentation and practice patterns, this discussion may be brief or prolonged. If members of the staff development department are very clear about their services, and documents exist that describe those services, this discussion may simply include a clarification and update of already developed materials. However, if the department is unclear about expectations, or has recently undergone some change, this discussion may provide the ideal opportunity to specify and clarify the scope of services. Agreement among all members of the department is again an essential component of this step of the ten-step process.

Chart 11-4
Assignment of Quality Assurance Statement

Responsibility for Quality Assurance in the Nursing Education Department

The Associate Director of Nursing for Education and Research is ultimately responsible for quality assurance within the nursing education department. A senior education specialist is assigned to the QA Central Committee and is primarily responsible for coordinating monitoring and evaluating activities within CNE using the guidelines and advice of the Central Committee. In addition, this education specialist provides some educational programming for the committee as requested.

The entire CNE department serves on the department's QA committee and is involved in the development of the QA program. QA development plans take place within the regularly scheduled CNE staff meetings. As necessary, selected staff are involved in data collection activities. However, all staff are involved in identifying indicators, evaluating data, and the development of action plans.

The CNE department consults on a regular basis with the QA Coordinator to affirm the direction and progress of the department's QA program. In addition, the QA Central Committee member also consults with the Committee and provides feedback to the CNE.

Communication of QA goals are shared through the usual channels defined in the PCS departments QA Program Plan. That is, study ideas are shared for input with the PCS Executive Council, the Head Nurse Council (if needed), and the QA Central Committee. Once the monitoring or evaluation activity is completed results and actions plans are shared with the same groups for feedback and improvement.

Finally, since many departments' action plans include education, the department also has a responsibility to provide advice and consultation to action planners and help them select appropriate educational interventions. The education specialist who serves on the QA Central Committee fulfills this responsibility primarily through suggestions during the presentation of action plans during regular committee meetings. However, any education specialist may serve in this capacity.

Source: Greater Southeast Community Hospital, Washington, D.C. Reproduced with permission.

To delineate the scope of a staff development service, staff development specialists should ask, "What programs do we offer, what services do we provide, and what is done by this department?" Answers to these questions will provide a tally of the many programs and services provided. This list must be organized and, in some cases, generalized.

In departments which have a variety of services, including some clinical services, a general statement of those clinical services should be developed. For example, if the department includes a diabetic educator, the statement may read, "Care consultation, knowledge assessment, and instruction for patients with diabetes."

Staff development departments that include clinical specialists may choose to include a statement like, "Clinical specialist consultation and case management services for patients with cardiovascular disease."

A scope of service statement can be crafted from answers to the following questions:

What types of staff members are served by the staff development program? If the staff development program provides services to only selected members of a single department, then this should be specified. More commonly, the department is expected to provide services to all members of the nursing department. In addition, selected programs are provided for other members of the organization. A review of these facts may yield valuable data for subsequent monitoring and evaluation activities.

What are the common services provided? The department that includes many individuals in many roles will develop a list of services provided by each of these departmental members. To generate this list, staff members could be asked to list the three (or more) most common services provided. Services are different from programs, though they may overlap. Common services may include those mentioned above by clinical specialists and diabetes educators. In addition, staff development specialists may provide an assessment and resolution service for difficult patient situations that includes the facilitation of a group problem-solving process. Also, specialists may provide an assessment service for a nurse or other staff member who is having difficulty meeting performance expectations. Finally, the department may also provide a registration service, an attendance transcript, and other tracking services for individuals and department managers. These examples of services are not comprehensive. Each staff department must carefully consider how they spend their time and what services are delivered during that time.

What are the common activities performed? Activities include such items as program planning and design, program implementation, program evaluation, lecture preparation, skills session preparation, and other common daily activities of staff development specialists. In addition, activities such as collaboration for program development, consultation, coordination, and delivery of instruction are commonplace in the work of staff development.

What are the common programs offered? The inventory generated to answer this question should be organized under common headings. Most departments have common programs offered on a routine basis. These generally include orientation, new graduate transition programs, and other competency development activities. Programs can be grouped by specialty service, such as critical care nursing, maternal-child health nursing, medical-surgical nursing, or in some other way. The common headings of orientation, inservice education, continuing education, leadership development and skills training can also be used, though the overlap between each may cause some difficulty in using these categories. An efficient approach may be to categorize programs as they are provided by each specialist. Many organizations assign programs to specialists based on experience and expertise, and these specialists can individually and easily answer the question of the most common programs offered.

What types of practitioners are offering the service? The answer to this question should be quite evident from the members present. It is necessary to specify the roles of the practitioners providing the staff development services.

The answers to these questions provide the data for choosing important aspects of the service and other subsequent steps in the monitoring and evaluation process. The lists generated as a result of these activities may be quite long and unwieldy. The organization and editing of staff development consumers, activities, services, programs, and practitioners will provide a comprehensive and satisfying statement of the scope of service of the department as it exists. A sample scope of service for a nursing staff development department may be found in Chapter 7, Chart 7-1.

Identify Important Aspects of the Service

The next step of the ten-step process is more difficult. The specification of the *most* important items from the scope of service should lead to the identification of important aspects of service. These aspects are used to develop monitoring and evaluation activities. It is unreasonable to expect that all aspects of a service will be evaluated. This impossible task is not necessary to the management of quality within a program or department. However, samples of common programs should be monitored and evaluated on an ongoing basis. Those samples selected for monitoring and evaluation should have some importance to the overall delivery of service. While difficult to specify what is *most* important (after all, isn't everything important), this task can be facilitated using the following guidelines:

1. Review the scope of service statement.
2. Identify those activities, services, and programs that have a high volume.
3. Identify any activities, services, and programs that may be high risk. For example, those that consume a great deal of resources yet have difficulty measuring outcomes, should be considered high risk.
4. Identify any activities, services, and programs that are problem prone.

This task may have to be exercised several times before there is satisfaction that the list includes the important aspects of service. There is no rule about how many important aspects of service except one of rationality. These aspects serve as the basis of monitoring and evaluation. If the list includes an excessive number of aspects, the resources necessary to monitor these aspects will rarely be available. Common sense must prevail in this effort.

Beginning attempts to develop a sound quality management program may perish at this point. It is strongly suggested that the staff development specialist selects only one or two important aspects of service at this point for a monitoring and evaluation activity. The aspect may also change over time as the requirements for staff competency development change. Those aspects identified as important should represent a certain priority for the monitoring and evaluation activity.

The development of language to specify the important aspect of service is the next step. Clinical aspects of service consider a patient and a nurse in this language. A sample statement for an important aspect of service for an intensive care unit is, "The nurse manages patients requiring ventilator support." Using this same approach for nursing staff development, a broad, general statement for an important aspect of service considers a staff development specialist and a learner. The statement may read, "The staff development specialist teaches nurses effectively." To specify an important program taught by the specialist, the statement may read, "The staff development specialist teaches nurses to interpret dysrhythmias accurately."

The learning objectives specified in program files can be used effectively to help use appropriate language for the important aspect of service. If the behavioral objectives specify the outcome anticipated for the learner, then they can also be used for quality monitoring. This should also be considered as program objectives are developed. What objectives might serve as a quality monitor? The use of this approach to program development may also improve statements of objectives and link quality monitoring activities to the usual delivery of services.

Other aspects of service that relate to the administration of the staff development program and can be considered for quality monitoring and evaluation include

- Management of the orientation process for new nursing employees
- Provision of adequate opportunities for staff to maintain and develop relevant competencies
- Provision of pertinent topics, particularly those required for continued licensure or to meet regulatory body requirements
- Management of records and reports

These topics and others provide the staff development administrator with a variety of opportunities to collect data that can be used to continue to improve the staff development program. The priority set for any aspect can be determined through a consensus process or a simple judgment call.

Identify Indicators

An indicator is a quality-related variable that can be easily and reliable measured.[13] Clear indicator statements are important because they drive the data collection process. A sample indicator statement for the important aspects identified above is,

The staff development specialist teaches nurses to interpret dysrhythmias accurately, as evidenced by scores on written tests.

The integration of the evaluation component commonly used in program design helps with the development of clear indicator statements. Another sample indicator statement for the reaction level of evaluation is,

The staff development specialist organizes learning activities in conformance to requirements (or effectively), as evidenced by scores on learner satisfaction surveys completed at the end of the session.

This indicator statement provides data regarding the satisfaction of the learner with the learning experience and, once data is available through the data collection process, can be used to improve programming or support the current approach as a quality approach.

If adults are reliable reporters of their ability to perform specified behavioral objectives, the staff development specialists may also use an indicator statement such as,

The staff development specialist teaches effectively, as evidenced by scores on learning objectives accomplishment scales.

It is common practice to distribute reaction surveys at the close of seminars and programs. Carefully constructed behavioral objectives presented with a Likert scale for data collection can also provide valuable data for the specialist to use for program improvement efforts.

An indicator statement that demonstrates the regulatory body requirement is

The staff development specialist assesses nurses conformance to the requirement for knowledge about the protocol for blood component transfusion, as evidenced by scores on the test included in the Blood Component Transfusion Study Guide.

Development of indicators for important aspects of service is a deliberative process. Indicators for measurement may be changed, refined, and improved over time. This developmental aspect of the monitoring and evaluation process is typical and should be expected by specialists engaging in the ten-step process for the first several years. Satisfaction with well-stated aspects and indicators occurs after trial and error, testing and experimentation with statements and data collection. With time, experience will generate common aspects and indicators that can be used in many settings by all staff development specialists. The next step in this process defines a level of conformance that represents quality for the individual.

Establish Thresholds for Evaluation

The data that will be collected is designated in the indicator statement. This step defines a point in the cumulative data that will trigger an in-depth evaluation. Thresholds for evaluation are usually stated in a ratio or percentage statement and are based on observed or experimental evidence, or judgment from experience.

It is common for clinical nurses to set a 90% or 95% threshold for evaluation. This is often due to discomfort with setting thresholds that are lower because they may imply that a "low standard" of care is acceptable. This is disconcerting, as the threshold is often an arbitrary number, based on limited experience with the aspect and indicator under observation. It is not bad to set high thresholds. However, when results are below the threshold, and an in depth evaluation is indicated, this evaluation is often not done. Rather, some changes are made, results are communicated, perhaps, education is provided, and the monitor is repeated at a later date.

An alternative to this approach, particularly for those areas where it is difficult to judge where to set a threshold, no threshold should be set for the initial monitor. Once the monitor is completed, the results are analyzed and judged for acceptability. Using the continuous improvement principle, a higher threshold can be set for subsequent monitors on the same important aspects.

Special consideration should be made for setting low thresholds. An example of an appropriately low threshold is nosocomial infection rates. One would expect that rate to be low and, if the rate increases, an in-depth evaluation would be done. This differentiation between setting high and low thresholds for evaluation has caused some confusion in the quality literature. The use of clear language in establishing the threshold for evaluation is essential. Sample statements include

> Nurses will achieve a passing score of 80% of a possible 100% on the written test in 85% of the cases.
>
> *or*
>
> Seminar satisfaction scores will average at least 4.0 on a scale of 5 in 100% of the cases.
>
> *or*
>
> Nurses will achieve a score of at least 7 of a possible 10 on the chemotherapy performance test in 95% of the cases.

The question of whether or not this is "good enough" is a question each staff development specialist must answer. Judgments based on risk to patients and the organization, confidence in measurement tools, and available resources are relevant.

The key point in quality monitoring activities is conformance to requirements. If a staff development specialist chooses to set a threshold of a 100% written test score in 100% of the cases, this is not wrong, particularly if the organization agrees that the nurses must demonstrate this level of knowledge, and the test instrument is valid and reliable. It is more common to accept some human frailties and work toward continuous improvement of the teaching and the test instrument for a period of time. Once this has been established, it may be reasonable, based on this experience, to set those thresholds. Remember, thresholds *trigger* in-depth evaluations.

The first five steps of the process set-up or design the monitor. The next few steps implement the design.

Collect and Organize Data

The data collection step includes the development of a method to aggregate and arrange the data so that it can be analyzed. To guide this process, consider the following questions:

What are the sources of data? Who or what will serve as the primary source of data? Is it already available in the record or is there a need to develop a tool? Common sources of data include educational transcripts, program files, educational records and reports, participant reactions forms, test scores, participants themselves, managers, patients, infection control reports, performance checklists, incident reports, direct observation, formal evaluation studies, and other assessments performed as an ongoing component of the staff development program.

What will be the data collection method? Will the data be collected retrospectively or concurrently? Will it be collected all at once or over time?

How much data is needed? What is the population of interest? How many are in the population or what is the N? Is it necessary to collect data about the entire population, or is sampling appropriate? The JCAHO recommends a sample size of 5% of the population but not less than 20. How long will it take to get an adequate accumulation of data for analysis?

How often will data be collected? Will this be a one-time data collection, or will it be spread over several intervals? If spread over intervals, what are those intervals—daily, weekly, monthly? For how long?

How should the data be displayed so that analysis can occur? Data collection forms are often developed within organizations that may or may not be helpful. If the form does not work, develop something that will help you see trends and occurrences. This may take some trial and error. If a form developed for a monitor is found to not be useful, nurse researchers or other data analysts may provide some help. Software programs with spreadsheets may also be useful in guiding the development of a data collection tool that will yield data useful for analysis.

Data collection tools should be set up with simplicity. A tool designed to collect data about test scores should list the participants by letter or number, their individual test score, and a judgement (Y = yes or N = no) if the threshold of 80% was met. The number of Y's are tallied, and an average is calculated. If the calculated score is less than the set threshold of 85%, then an in-depth evaluation may be warranted. The next step discusses this in more detail. However, if the data indicates that 85% of the scores are 80% or greater, then that data is used as evidence of conformance to requirements. Data is available to indicate quality that exists within the staff development program.

Data can be collected on an ongoing basis and aggregated annually to support the continuing quality of a particular aspect of the staff development program. By continuing to use the test score data collection tool, quality monitoring becomes integrated into staff development practice.

Another example of a data collection tool that is designed to collect data over time is one that measures the nurses demonstration of a particular skill. This skill should be identified as an important aspect of a particular clinical service. For example, the oncology department requires nurses to administer chemotherapy for selected cancer patients. During the new nurses' orientation, instructions and opportunity to practice are provided in a structured setting. Within a specified time frame, the nurse is expected to demonstrate competency as specified in performance checklists and perhaps in written tests. A quality monitor can be conducted in cooperation and collaboration with the nurse manager to assess all oncology nurses' competence related to chemotherapy administration. The performance checklist used for instruction can be modified to collect data about each nurse over time as performance of each statement on the checklist is observed. This performance can be observed in a simulated or actual situation.

The next step in the process evaluates the data and makes judgments about the quality or conformance to requirements.

Evaluate the Data

The aggregated data is examined to determine if additional action is required. If the threshold for evaluation is not met, then no additional action is necessary. Quality, or conformance to requirements, is evident. However, if the data triggers an in-depth evaluation, discussions, analysis of patterns, or trends in service related to this study should take place to determine if the opportunity to improve service exists. In some cases, the power of the quantitative data provides an opportunity to shift the curve upward and further improve services. In a program of continuous improvement, one searches for opportunities to improve all processes.

Deming demonstrated that problems are more often within a system than due to an employee inability or lack of desire to do a good job. In fact, he illustrated this repeatedly and concluded that the employee has just a 20% chance of doing the job right and 80% of coming up against a system problem that will inhibit the completion of job done correctly. Using this information, the analysis of data should include the consideration of system problems. Perhaps a policy needs to be developed, modified, or enforced to improve the chances of doing the job in a way that conforms to requirements.

Problems may also be caused by insufficient knowledge and unclear expectations. If the data indicates that this is part of the problem, steps should be taken to resolve these problems.

Take Actions to Solve Identified Problems

When the data yields opportunities for improvement, staff development specialists should engage in a session that clarifies the problems and identifies potential actions that can be taken to resolve the issues. Commitment to these actions must be generated. This action plan identifies who or what is expected to change, who is responsible for implementing the action, and when change is expected to occur. These actions should be recorded.

An example of an action plan to solve identified problems relates to data collected that indicated lack of conformance to the requirement of current CPR certification. After analysis, it was discovered that it was unclear if all nursing personnel were required to conform, or just those in certain roles.

The *system* or policy needed clarification to monitor it accurately. Once the policy was clarified and the data was analyzed again, conformance to the requirement was still inadequate according to the threshold set of 85%. The action plan then was modified to identify who was expected to change (identified nursing personnel) and who was responsible for implementing the change (the nurse manager), and a deadline was set. A follow-up monitor yielded data that supported conformance to requirements by those nursing personnel identified clearly in the policy. This approach may also help staff development specialists target programs to appropriate personnel and use the scarce resources of specialist and staff time more efficiently.

Assess Actions and Document Improvement

Any actions taken should be assessed, usually through a repeated monitor. The monitor may be modified or not, depending on the data of interest. Improvements, or lack thereof, are documented, and as necessary, additional actions taken. Possible actions that improve services may include

- Revising systems
- Changing communication channels
- Changing organizational structure
- Establishing, revising, or clarifying policies
- Revising performance expectations
- Purchasing or repairing equipment
- Providing focused learning activities
- Counseling
- Disciplinary action
- Reallocating resources

Communicate

The final step in this ten-step process is communication. Relevant information should be communicated to the organization-wide quality management program. Organizations may vary in the formality of the communication structure and network, but an informal structure does not preclude the necessity of community quality improvement efforts. In some organizations, a summary report is expected on a scheduled basis. A sample report is provided in Chart 11-5.

Appropriate dissemination of information helps the overall quality improvement program. The problems and solutions of one department may affect another department, or they may be used as models to assist another department with their improvement efforts.

Expectations of Specialists

Quality management workshops were conducted throughout the country during 1988 through 1991 by the author, and much of this information

▐C hart 11-5
▮ Sample Guideline and Summary Report

**Nursing Staff Development Quality Monitoring
and Evaluation Guideline and Summary**

Date: ....

1. What is the aspect of practice or service that you will monitor?

2. What do you hope to accomplish with this monitor (or what is your objective or rationale for using resources on this monitor)?

3. What are the indicators of this aspect of practice that will tell you if you are doing a quality job?

4. What methodology will you use to collect data (include time frame, data sources, sample size, who will do the data collection and how will you collect the data)?

5. Dates of this review:

    .... First report   .... Follow-up report

6. Sample size:
   (No. learners, no. records, no. observations, no. other)

7. Findings:

8. Established threshold: ....
   Performance this review: ....
   Performance last review: ....

9. Conclusions:

10. Actions:

   Signatures:
   (Preparer of report) ....
   (Department Head) ....
   (Associate Director) ....
   (QA Coordinator) ....

*Source: Modified for staff development from form developed by Paula Swain of Paula Swain
Seminars, St. Petersburg, FL. Reproduce with permission.*

was shared. Staff development specialists were asked the following question during the early part of the activity: "What *expectations* do you have that would *indicate* that this was a *quality experience?*" Answers were shared readily and included

- Learn something new
- How to get it going
- Find out how to measure quality
- See or bring about positive change
- What I need to do now
- Getting unmuddled
- Making sense out of all the activities
- Find out how to make it routine, and fit into daily routines
- Validate current practices
- How to improve services
- How to monitor meaningful aspects of practice
- Learn how to define competencies
- Practical tactics

On reflection, it was interesting to note that these "indicators" could be used to measure the quality of many staff development activities. Further development of these "expectations of quality" may prove helpful to specialists who are attempting to define quality indicators for staff development programs. Measurements taken during the workshop included frequent checks by the author that information presented was clear and that application exercises seem to yield relevant and appropriate data. At the close of the seminar, the reactionnaire indicated a general shift to the positive side on the Likert scales provided to measure objectives. The opportunity to collect actual data was missed. This data collection may have yielded information useful in the continuing development of these ideas, themes, and principles. The measurement of the change in behavior as a result of this learning experience will be evident in future use of this and other information related to the management of quality in nursing staff development.

Summary

The concept of continuous improvement has been integrated throughout this chapter. It is the underlying theme to any quality improvement effort. Continuous improvement yields many benefits for the staff development department. Included in these benefits are justification of the department or program and evidence of the contribution to quality patient care that is supported by data. The use of quantitative data to improve the service delivery process is new to nursing staff development. Through practice and experience, consensus will be reached regarding standards of practice and the measurements used to determine conformance to those standards. This chapter has addressed a variety of models and approaches for quality management.

Staff development specialists share a common desire to use quality management principles in their work. To demonstrate this, specialist must engage in new behaviors and collect and organize data to monitor and evaluate their efforts. Then staff development specialists can use the words of Deming and say with authority and evidence that "I have done my best."

References

1. Kirkpatrick, D. (1960). *Program evaluation.* Alexandria, VA: American Society for Training and Development.
2. Joint Commission on Accreditation of Healthcare Organizations (1991). *Accreditation manual for hospitals.* Chicago: Author.
3. Swain, P. (1991). *Quality counts!* Seminar workbook. Paula Swain Seminars, St. Petersburg, FL.
4. Thompson, R. E. (Jan 1981). Relating continuing education and quality assurance activities. *Quality Review Bulletin,* 3–6.
5. Crosby, P. B. (1989). *Let's talk quality.* New York: McGraw-Hill.
6. McLagan, P. (1989). Models for HRD practice. *Training and Development Journal, 43*(9), 49–59.
7. American Nurses' Association (1991). *Standards for Nursing Staff Development.* Kansas City: Author.
8. Berwick, D. (1989). Sounding board: Continuous improvement as the ideal in health care. *New England Journal of Medicine, 320*(1), 53–36.
9. Wolgin, F. (1990). Improving patient care outcomes through education. In: Perspectives on Research. *Journal of Nursing Staff Development, 6*(6), 307–309.
10. American Nurses' Association (1976). *Guidelines for the review of nursing care at the local level.* Kansas City: The Association.
11. Schroeder, P., & Maibusch, R. M. (1984). *Nursing quality assurance: A unit based approach.* Rockville, MD: Aspen.
12. Joint Commission on Accreditation of Healthcare Organizations (1988). *Step by step through the montoring and evaluation process.* Chicago: Author.
13. Katz, J. M. (1991). Quality monitoring and evaluation in staff development. *Journal of Nursing Staff Development, 7*(1), 15–20.
14. Lewis, D. J., & White, L. A. (1991). Quality assurance: A staff development concern. *Journal of Nursing Staff Development, 7*(3), 120–125.

Bibliography

Ackerman, C. (1989, Feb/Mar). QA for educational programs and services: A customer-oriented approach. *Journal of Quality Assurance,* 16–18.

Berwick, D. (1988). Measuring health care quality. *Pediatrics in Review, 10*(1), 11–16.

Beyers, M. (1988). Quality: The banner of the 1980s. *Nursing Clinics of North America. 23,* 52–53.

Cocheu, T. (1989). Training for quality improvement. *Training and Development Journal, 43*(1), 56–62.

Coyne, C., & Killien, M. (1987). A system for unit-based monitors of quality nursing care. *Journal of Nursing Administration, 17*(1), 26–32.

Crosby, P. (1979). *Quality is free.* New York: McGraw-Hill.

Donabedian, A. (March 1986). Criteria and standards for quality assessement monitoring. *Quality Review Bulletin,* 99–108.

Foglesong, D. (1987). Standards promote effective production. *Nursing Management, 18*(1), 24–27.

Foster, M., Whittle, S., & Smith, S. (1989). A total-quality approach to customer service. *Training and Development Journal, 43*(12), 55–59.

Gillem, T. (1988). Deming's 14 points and hospital quality: Responding to the consumer's demand for the best value health care. *Journal of Nursing Quality Assurance, 2*(3), 70–78.

Hefferin, E. (1987). Trends in the evaluation of nursing staff development programs. *Journal of Nursing Staff Development, 3*(1), 28–40.

Holpp, L. (1989). Ten reasons why total quality is less than total. *Training, 26*(10), 93–103.

Kane, E., Evanczuk, K., Skorupka, P., & Cari, A. (1985). Staff development: A functional program. *Journal of Nursing Staff Development, 1*(3), 110–118.

Kunkle, V. (1987). Accountability standards balance quality and efficiency. *Nursing Management, 18*(1), 34–38.

Marchm, A. (1986). *A note on quality: The views of Deming, Juran and Crosby.* Boston: Harvard Business School Press.

Melum, M. M. (1990, December). *Total quality management: Steps to success. Hospitals,* 42–43.

Morton, P. (1985). A hospital's nursing education manual. *Journal of Nursing Staff Development, 1*(1), 61–67.

Morton, P. (1985). Standards-based evaluation of hospital nursing education services. *Journal of Nursing Staff Development, 1*(3), 97–104.

O'Leary, D. (1986, Nov/Dec). Joint Commission sets agenda for change. *JCAH Perspectives,* 6–8.

Oberle, J. (1990). Quality gurus: The men and their message. *Training, 27*(1), 47–52.

Patterson, C. (1988). Standards of patient care: The Joint Commission focus on nursing quality assurance. *Nursing Clinics of North America, 23*(3), 625–638.

Reichheld, F. F., & Sasser W. E. (1990, Sept/Oct). Zero defections: Quality comes to services. *Harvard Businesss Review,* 105–109.

Sagalla, E. (1989). All for quality and quality for all. *Training and Development Journal, 43*(9), 36–45.

Swierzaek, F. W., & Carmichael, L. (1985). The quantity and quality of evaluating training. *Training and Development Journal, 39*(1), 95–99.

Taguchi, G., & Clausing, D. (1990, Jan/Feb). Robust quality. *Harvard Business Review,* 65–75.

Tarcinale, M. (1987). The role of evaluation in instruction. *Journal of Nursing Staff Development, 4*(3), 97–103.

Tiessen, J. B. (1987). Comprehensive staff development evaluation: The need to combine models. *Journal of Nursing Staff Development, 3*(1), 9–14.

Watson, C., Bulesheck, G., et al (1987). QAMUR: A quality assurance model using research. *Journal of Nursing Quality Assurance, 2*(1), 21–27.

Zettinig, P., & Lang, N. (1981, July/August). Utilization of quality assurance concepts in education evaluation. *Nurse Educator,* 24–28.

Chapter 12

Forecasting the Future: Nursing Staff Development in the Next Century

Karen J. Kelly

To plan well today, the future must be considered. The future of the evolving field of nursing staff development lies solely in the hands of its specialists. Specialists who think and articulate carefully about nursing staff development will shape the next generation of practice. As more knowledge is unveiled through experience, research, and practice, the field will be refined. Nurses beginning nursing staff development practice will find an exciting field filled with enthusiastic, informed specialists who care about their work. These specialists will continue to inquire about this specialized field of practice and expand staff development knowledge using patterns of knowing described by Carper[1] such as personal experience, empirics, ethics, and esthetics to discover new learnings. Using methods described by Benner,[2] staff development specialists will reveal practice patterns and strategies used in practice that contribute to the development of nursing competence.

To continue to develop the practice of staff development, a plan is needed. To help staff development specialists look to the future and to the contribution they can make, a strategic planning approach is proposed. This method raises many questions to help the specialist consider the myriad factors that will influence practice throughout the nation and in the individual health care setting. Answers to these questions will help the beginning process requisite to shaping a vision of the future. This chapter focuses on the questions that will require answers to visualize future staff development practice.

Creating a Vision

It is difficult to imagine a future within the pandemonium of everyday staff development practice. It takes quiet time and thoughtful effort to visualize what work can be like in the future. Yet without a concerted effort to envision a future, the promise of quality staff development services will appear bleak.

The process of planning for a future begins with an affirmation that something that exists now will exist in the future. The steps involved in planning for that future are described in a strategic planning process that begins with a vision. To imagine future staff development practice, it is helpful to engage in an visioning exercise suggested by Simpson.[3] The following guidelines are suggested to gain the most benefit from the experience:

- **Eliminate distractions:** Suspend *internal* distractions that tell you to do something else, e.g., to stop daydreaming, to finish other projects, or to try to do other things at the same timed. Eliminate *external* distractions, such as noise, telephones, pagers, and interruptions from other people. This exercise is generally begun alone, in a quiet place, away from the usual commotion of an office.
- **Develop sensory awareness:** Focus attention on the body and its processes, such as breathing, temperature, and muscle tension. Awareness of these senses will help create a feeling of relaxation and comfort, and will help eliminate additional internal and external distractions.
- **Guiding images:** This step includes the use of imagination to move to other places in time or to see staff development from a different perspective. Music may be helpful during this phase, but the key to success is time. Creative imagining takes time, and it is important to allow time to let the mind wander and imagine a future.
- **Write it down:** This phase includes jotting down thoughts, fragments, symbols, and ideas that occurred during the imagery phase. These notes will serve as reminders to return to and continue the thought process and will aide in its evolution over time.

Shaping a personal vision of nursing staff development may involve subsequent exercises, but the beginning of any vision is quiet, thoughtful reflection about "what can be" in the future. Time taken to engage in visioning exercises will help build an innovative staff development future.

Focusing the Vision

While formulating a vision of staff development practice, it may be helpful to focus on three key factors:

- People
- Time
- Money

These factors relate to the reality of health care organizations and the economic environment. They also are the most significant variables that affect the ability of staff development specialists to effect change in the organization. An understanding of how each of the three key factors affects staff development practice within a specific agency is essential to shaping a vision that is also grounded in reality.

People

Consideration of what staff development specialists do now and what contributions they can make in the future are part of future forecasting. Questions to contemplate include:

- What unique skills do specialists have now, and how can those skills be enhanced to contribute to future needs?
- What expectations does the organization have for nurses and nursing practice in the future?
- What specifically do the specialists do to help the organization achieve goals and what else can be done?
- What outcome measures are currently available to demonstrate the effectiveness of staff development, and how can these outcome measures be improved?
- How many specialists are needed to conduct a quality staff development program?
- What services are provided and how can these services be improved?
- Are there other services that should be provided which would contribute to organizational goal achievement?
- Are there efficiencies that can be instituted to save scarce resources?

These questions and others will help the staff development specialist view the present from a variety of perspectives, an important element in any prediction of the future.

Time

Time is a constant, and yet we rarely are able to use the objectivity of time to help us accumulate data for future predictions. Questions that will help build data and plan a future include

- How much time does the average staff development specialist take to prepare for one hour of instruction?
- How much time is needed to assess the competency of a dozen clinical nurses?
- What productivity measures are used to illustrate the efficient use of resources?
- Are there other efficiencies in time that can be put in place?
- What qualitative measures support the use of time spent with certain programs or activities?
- How much time should be allocated by a specialist for a selected project?

Many time-related issues emerge with some reflection. The most common concern—that there is never enough time—should be set aside to consider the most constructive and productive use of this scant resource.

Money

Salary budgets represent the greatest proportion of money allocated to staff development. Often 90% of the departmental budget is dedicated to salaries. The need to carefully manage the integration of people, time, and money becomes evident with this observation. Questions that will help guide future considerations include

- What are reasonable salary expectations for specialists?
- What value is placed on the contribution of the specialist and how does it compare with the value of other members of the organization?
- Should salaries be an issue for the future?
- What are other money-related issues that need investigation and support?
- How is budgeted money accounted for? Are there other accounting methods that may provide better information?
- Are there costs that need to be monitored for comparison with other costs?
- Should salary dollars be shifted to contracted work to expand the service possibilities?
- Should additional money be allocated for other services that will strengthen the staff development program?

These questions will begin the process of consideration of the money factor. Money seems to be at the root of many of the perceived ills within the health care system. The use of money by organizations and staff development departments demonstrate the commitment to values and ideas that support the organization's mission and goals.

Nevertheless, rising costs, shifting service priorities and erratic funding assure that crises and change are inevitable forces shaping health services management in the foreseeable future.[4] Goals, services, and programs must be reassessed and new visions of the future must be created. What will staff development programs look like in the future? Limited resources and the management of these values will be an integral part of any future program.

Health care costs have risen to almost 13% of the gross national product and continue to rise. Health care reform is a banner waved by business and professional associations. How organizations respond to reforms and new directives is often determined by the response of individual units and departments within the organization. As a department or unit within the organization responsible for a variety of services, the staff development department or program administrator should consider how it will respond to new priorities and imperatives.

Each of the key factors of people, time, and money should be considered for future planning. Each element cannot be considered alone, as each one affects the other.

Staff development departments can operate in various ways within the organization. Kotler[5] described several types of organizations which can be adapted to types of staff development departments within organizations. They include

- **Responsive:** "Those that make every effort to sense, serve and satisfy the needs and wants of its clients and publics within the constraints of its budget." Kotler also categorized responsive organizations, or staff development departments in this case, into four levels including unresponsive, casually responsive, highly responsive and fully responsive.
- **Adaptive:** "One that operates systems for monitoring and interpreting important environmental changes and shows a readiness to revise its mission, objectives strategies, organization, and systems to be maximally aligned with its opportunities." Factors that affect the capacity of an organization (or staff development department) to change include size, funds, leadership, and constraints.
- **Entrepreneurial:** "One with a high motivation and the capability to identify new opportunities and convert them into successful businesses."

What kind of staff development department is present now and what kind might be envisioned for the future? Perhaps a blend of several types might work best in some organizations, while in others a more pure approach may be appropriate.

Consideration of the current and potential future of the staff development department and program within Kottler's descriptions is one part of a plan for the future.

Planning for the Future

To assist the futuring process, a strategic decision making and planning process is suggested. Many descriptions of this process have been advanced. For example, Drucker[6] describes the strategic planning process as a continuous, systematic process of making risk-taking decisions today with the greatest possible knowledge of their effects on the future. He goes on to say that strategic planning also includes organizing efforts to carry out these decisions. Finally, Drucker says this process also concerns itself with evaluating results of these decisions against expected outcomes through reliable feedback mechanisms.

Staff development specialists who recognize the continuous and simultaneous nature of the strategic planning process will avoid the frustrations of developing plans that cannot be altered as new data become available. Organizations and departments within organization must modify priorities in response to new data. Kottler[7] explains strategic planning as the managerial process of developing and maintaining a strategic fit between the organization's goals and resources and its changing marketplace opportunities. This definition emphasizes the changing situation, evident in the health care organizations, and the essential need to create a fit between opportunities and future plans. Specialists who ascribe to Kotler's description of strategic planning will use a marketing and positioning approach to advance the staff development program.

Goplerud[4] also provides additional insight into the strategic planning process and illustrates it as one that examines organizational goals, objectives, policies and strategies. He continues his explanation by including the process of developing means to guide the organization through its changing environment to achieve prescribed aims. Goplerud also advances the idea that there is no single, uniform procedure adaptable to any and all organizations.

The application of strategic planning principles to nursing staff development is the process by which members of the staff development department and others envision its future and develop the procedures and operations necessary to achieve that future. This process involves more than *anticipating* the future and planning accordingly, but rather helps staff development specialists *create* the future.

Strategic Planning for Staff Development

Many models to guide the strategic planning process exist. One approach useful to staff development specialists is the process described by Wheelen and Hunger[8] and modified here for application to nursing staff development. Thirteen steps are proposed and listed below. Each step will be discussed separately in the following section. The steps are

1. Evaluate current performance results.
2. Examine the current mission, objectives, strategies, and policies.
3. Review strategic managers.
4. Scan the external environment.
5. Scan the internal environment.
6. Select strategic factors related to strengths and weaknesses.
7. Select strategic factors related to opportunities and threats.
8. Analyze strategic factors in light of the current situation.
9. Review/revise the mission and objectives as necessary.
10. Generate, evaluate, and select the best alternatives and formulate the plan.
11. Implement strategies.
12. Evaluate and control.
13. Report results, reward yourself and continue.

It is helpful to get a gestalt view of the processes within this model. Figure 12-1 provides this view. Notice the first ten steps of this model could be considered strategy formulation. This is the thinking part of strategic planning. Steps 11 are considered strategy implementation and step 12 and 13 can be described as strategy evaluation and control.

These apparently neat, logical steps are helpful to organize and neatly

Strategic Decision-Making Process

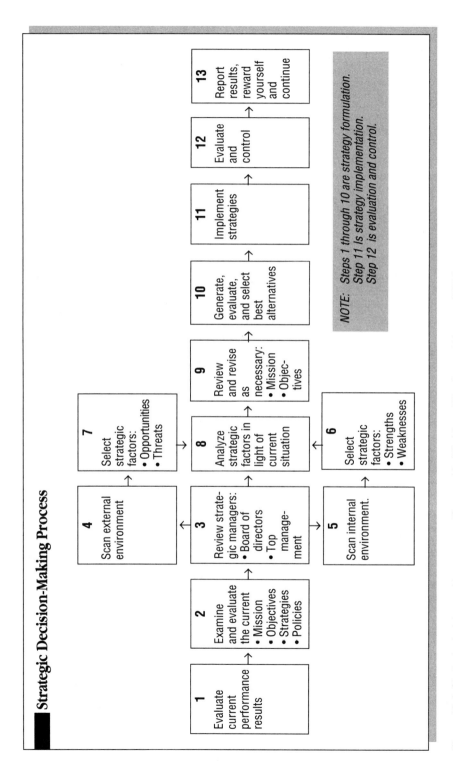

Figure 12-1 *Strategic decision making process. (Source: Modified from Wheelen and Hunger, 1986.)*

307

define this process. In the real world, however, strategic planning cannot be so neatly defined. Keller[9] makes the following observations about strategic planning:

- It is not the production of a blueprint, but rather a process of getting key people thinking innovatively with the future in mind.
- It is not a set of platitudes, but rather the formulation of succinctly stated operational gains.
- It is not a collection of individual program plans, compiled and edited, rather it is a plan for the whole department in relation to its long-term stature and excellence.
- It is not a substitution of numbers for important tangibles, but rather the introduction of these to sharpen judgments, analyses, and decisions.
- It is not an attempt to outwit the future, but rather an effort to make this year's decisions more intelligent by looking toward the probable future and coupling decisions to overall institutional strategy.

Finally, Keller remarks that strategic decisions are based on the best evidence available about the unpredictable future.

Strategic planning in nursing staff development involves formulation, implementation, and evaluation processes occurring and interacting simultaneously. While there will never be enough people, time, and money, strategic planning processes can nevertheless help staff development specialists and program administrators plan for a future that is managed by the profession. Engagement with this process takes time and effort, especially with resources already in scarce supply. Allocating time for strategic planning will give purpose and direction to the staff development program and provide confidence and resolve to program administrators and specialists as they implement the plan. The next several sections describe, through a series of questions, the steps in the Wheelen and Hunger strategic planning process. These queries are designed to guide the process and provide a broad perspective during strategy formulation.

Step 1: Evaluate Current Performance Results

Consider the following questions when evaluating the current performance of the staff development program or department.

What is the business of the staff development department or program? Competency development and maintenance should be part of this definition. The scope of service used as part of the quality management process also describes the "business" of the nursing staff development program or department.

What quantitative indicators are available to show that the "business" or services have been provided? Consider how many nurses were oriented last year and how many hours of instruction were provided. Add up the number of new graduate nurses that were socialized and how many preceptors were trained. Think about how many learning activities were provided in the usual categories, such as competency assessment, inservice education, continuing education, skills training, and leadership development. How many self-learning packages or modules were completed and how many hours of patient care were returned to the organization through these and other selected learning activities? How many hours of instruction were provided through these programs? Add up the number and hours provided related to quality management. Reflect on other programs, services, and activities that were provided and which can be quantified.

What qualitative indicators are available regarding the performance of the staff development department? Review the quality monitors and other indicators of value that provide data for analysis for the staff development program characteristics and features. Consider data gathered through consumer satisfaction surveys, particularly those collected by other departments such as the human resource department.

These data can be used for other purposes as well. For example, they may form the basis for the annual report. This compilation of data can then be reviewed and analyzed as a whole to gain a current performance perspective of the nursing staff development program or department.

Step 2: Examine Current Mission

The next step in the strategic planning process is the review of the mission, objectives, strategies, and policies of the organizations. The documents of the staff development department or program are also examined. The following questions should be considered:

Does the written philosophy match the practiced philosophy? Think about actions that support or refute the written philosophy and consider behaviors that may not support it. Consider how this philosophy is communicated, and if the typical consumers would agree that the philosophy can be observed through actions.

What message is projected through this philosophy? What is the *central idea* of the staff development philosophy?

Are there objectives that guide the program or department for a period of time? Think about the evidence available to show that work is being done toward accomplishing these objectives. Estimate progress made toward achieving each goal.

What strategies are used to help consumers understand how and when to use staff development services? Consider how new nurses and managers are apprised of staff development strategies and services and the effectiveness of these strategies.

What are the policies of the staff development department or program? Review the written policies and think about the need to add or delete. Reflect about the actual implementation of the polices and if practice matches policy. Revise as needed.

This step is often accomplished during preparation for accrediting and licensing agency visits. A periodic review of these polices is usually required. Some agencies, such as the Joint Commission on Accreditation of Healthcare Organizations (JCAHO) expect reviews of selected documents to occur at least once every three years. In some cases, more frequent review of these documents is warranted.

Step 3: Review Strategic Managers

During this step, the staff development specialist or program administrator should deliberate about the people significant to the program.

Who are the consumers important to the staff development operation? Think about head nurses and other nurse managers that provide the focus of the program. List all individuals who are vital for success.

Are there others in the division or the organization that are needed to assist the program? Consider all other individuals in the organization and determine who may be helpful as allies and collaborators. Think about specific administrators that may provide support and sustenance to the program and about others who may not.

The findings resulting from this step will give a broad perspective about the organizational players that may need to be influenced and those who can influence others for the continuing advancement of the staff development program.

Step 4: Scan the External Environment

Most strategic planning processes describe the external environment as those elements and communities outside the walls of the health care organization. For our purposes, consider the external environment to be everything outside the staff development department or program, including the organization, other departments within the organization, and the service area outside the building, as well as the global health care environment. Think about the following questions:

What are the new service and product lines offered by the organization? Consider new initiatives under scrutiny by the organization and if new competencies will be needed by nursing personnel. Think about potential changes in patterns of staff development services. Think about the typical services offered through the staff development department or program and how they fit with new initiatives.

What are the economic trends affecting the organization? Think about how health care is financed and how the organization is reimbursed for services delivered. Figure out how staff development is financed and what effect selected economic trends may have on the organization and the staff development program. Consider the potential effect of economic indicators, such as anticipated changes in reimbursement.

What are the organization's most dominant and important capabilities, skills, and relationships? Focus on how these skills and capabilities help or hinder the organization's movement toward goal achievement. Consider relationships with other organizations and how these affiliations can be enhanced.

What are the strengths and limitations of the staff of the organization as it relates to skills, productivity, turnover, morale, and flexibility? Appraise the strengths and limitations of the managers in such areas as leadership, planning, coordination, and staff development. Think about areas of improvement needed for various staff within the organization, particularly those associated with priority projects. Consider opportunities and threats to the organization and the staff. Concentrate on the actual and potential role of other organizations in areas such as competition, coalitions, cooperatives, and alignments.

What information is available regarding the service area and people in the community surrounding the organization? Focus on the role of the organization as a health care provider in its community and the essential services needed by the community to attain and maintain health. Consider programs that may be extended to the community of patients and nurses that may enhance the mission and goals of the organization.

Some of this information may be available through organizational planning and marketing departments. Other data may have to be collected through interviews with key individuals. During these exchanges, it may become evident that the implementation of new cooperatives and coalitions will advance the staff development program. The data collection and analysis that have occurred during the first four steps may or may not be linear as cited here. Often, an interview may yield data that fit into findings organized in all four steps discussed. This is common and illustrates again the sequential and simultaneous nature of strategic planning.

Step 5: Scan the Internal Environment

The internal environment, for staff development planning purposes, is the one within the staff development department and program. Queries that will enhance the program administrator's and specialist's knowledge base in this area include the following:

How do staff development personnel feel about who they are as a unit within the organization? Judge the general morale of the department and the future prospects. Think about how personnel view their purpose and contribution to patient care. Consider disagreements among staff about the purpose of the development program. Draw conclusions about differences in perceived mission and objectives and apparent disagreements with the mission and objectives.

What are the means and strategies used to carry out the staff development program? Assess the skills of staff development personnel and consider the need for additional or fewer personnel. Contemplate the need for new or different skills of personnel and the cost of developing these skills. Think about alternatives such as contracting for selected skills and projects.

This assessment will yield valuable information about the internal atmosphere and circumstances of the staff development department or program. Specialists and administrators will need to consider the collection and analysis of this data carefully, due to the personal nature of this material.

Step 6: Select Strategic Factors from Strengths and Limitations

Step six in this process requires an inquiry into the delineation of strategic factors related to the strengths and limitations identified in earlier steps. For example:

How can commitment to the staff development program be achieved? Consider ways to maintain a satisfactory productivity level for all parties involved. Think about systems and processes arranged to continually survey consumers. Analyze quality monitor results for system improvements. Consider technology as an asset and how it can be used to enhance staff development services.

What marketing strategies are needed? Decide what natural resources need to be developed and marketed. Think about the resources that are already available, but may need to be mined and refined. Assess what goals are reasonable regarding the size and growth of the staff development department or program. Estimate those features that are no longer necessary and those that need to be enhanced.

What can be done to improve the return on investment in staff development for the organization? Gauge the organizations desire for data about the investment in people through the staff development program and what information should be provided to demonstrate a return on that investment. Consider using monthly or quarterly reporting mechanisms, cost-benefit and cost-effectiveness analyses, and productivity formulas to support this inquiry.

This step requires shrewdness and astute perception by the program administrator and specialist to identify those strategic factors that are key to the continuing progress of the nursing staff development program.

Step 7: Select Strategic Factors from Threats and Opportunities

The seventh step requires a continuing selection of strategic factors related to threats and opportunities. The program administrator should consider the following:

What opportunities exist in the environment to help accomplish the staff development program mission and goals? Contemplate potential chances that are available that may contribute to goal achievement. Imagine potential funding sources for staff development over the next few years.

What are the potential threats? Consider worst-case scenarios and the organizational problems that may cause the staff development program to drift off course.

What new services or needs can be identified? Recollect earlier data about new initiatives within the organization and consider new staff development services that might enhance those services. Think about how to connect with individuals within the organization that are responsible for new projects and service line development. Consider new markets for staff development services. Reflect on current consumers and the opportunities provided through continuing service to these customers.

The wealth of data now available to the staff development program administrator and specialists is prodigious at this point and must be analyzed in order to make some sense of it.

Step 8: Analyze Strategic Factors

The factors identified and selected in earlier steps must now be analyzed in light of the current organizational situation. The following questions will assist this analysis:

What share of the market of consumers is desired? Think about what is reasonable given the economic situation and growth plans of the organization. Consider the organizational members and their commitment to staff development as a process to maintain competency. Assess opportunities that may be available in the years ahead that should be exploited or avoided.

How should the staff development program be cultivated so it is synchronized with organizational mission and goals? Examine the need to court selected members of the organization for information and support. Think about the need to establish links with designated parties to assist with this data analysis and collection. Consider validation and confirmation strategies that may reinforce the position of the staff development program. Think about any other data that may be necessary to this process to make it complete.

Thoughtful consideration of this step in the formulation phase of the strategic planning process is important. The program administrator who deliberates on all of these issues and the supporting information will find the process enlightening and productive. The next two steps conclude the formulation phase of the strategic planning process.

Step 9: Revise Mission and Objectives

Given the wealth of data available to the program administrator as a result of this ongoing inquiry, it becomes evident that selected documents may need revision and clarification. While these revisions may have occurred as a part of other processes, the administrator or specialist considers this need again. Consider the current documents that describe the staff development program. Does the mission statement include information about the basic business of the program or department? Do the documents identify the distinctive service that make the nursing staff development program different from other education departments in the organization? If other activities associated with the day-to-day operation of the staff development program have not caused a review of documents that support the service, the astute administrator will perform that task at this point in the strategic planning process.

Step 10: Formulate a Plan

The last step of the formulation phase of the strategic planning process is to generate, evaluate, and select the best alternatives and formulate a plan. The following questions will guide the development of that plan:

Of all the things that can be done, and given the data available, what are all the alternatives that should guide the staff development program in the future? Think about the strategic business units (SBUs) that should define the program. These are logical groupings of services such as orientation, competency assessment, leadership development, or other rational clusters of learning activities and services.

Is the plan based on realistic assumptions and accurate information? Validation by key members of the organization should answer this question adequately, but consider those sources and their reliability. Think about current resources and what resources will be needed to achieve the plan. Figure out if current skills, resources, and commitment are adequate or if new ones will need to be acquired; consider the timelines necessary for acquisition before the opportunity passes.

Is the plan internally consistent with other initiatives and goals of the organization? Judge the acceptability of the plan to managers who may be involved in the implementation. Assess the need to gain commitment or negotiate acceptability. Judge the flexibility of the plan

Will the strategy create economic or political value within acceptable risk limits? Judge the risks associated with the plan and the economic incentives that may be required. Assess the readiness of the organization to accept the plan and the ability to support it. Think about how the plan will need to be marketed to gain financial support if necessary. Given the above caveats, the program administrator selects the best alternatives listed in the first questions of this section. These alternatives are often ranked in order of priority and may be implemented as financial support becomes available.

At this point, the strategic plan is ready to be committed to paper and shared with others who become part of the common vision. The plan defines the future of the staff development program and should address several variables. Several pages are generally all that is necessary to effectively communicate this plan. A suggested outline is shown in Figure 12-1.

The final steps of the complete strategic planning process are concerned with implementation and evaluation, and are defined below in steps 11–13.

Step 11: Implement Strategies

Implementation of a strategic plan assumes that careful groundwork has been completed. This foundation may have been laid during the strategy formulation phase when key members of the organization were interviewed and cultivated for commitment to the staff development program. The astute program administrator will avoid the ten most common pitfalls associated with strategic planning as identified by Goplerud:[4]

C hart 12-1
Strategic Plan Document Outline

Your Strategic Plan

Some documentation is necessary to legitimize your strategic plan, though there is a wide variance regarding just how much you should write down. In my opinion, you should write down the least amount you need to communicate your vision. Following are some headings that can be used to guide a strategic plan that is probably more comprehensive than it needs to be in reality. The key to remember is the dynamic nature of this process, it may become outdated as you write it. However, it is a good idea to have a document of at least two or three pages that reflects all the thinking that is part of the strategic decision making process. Good luck with revisioning!

   I. Situation audit
      A. Current performance
      B. Internal environment
         1. Strengths
         2. Limitations
      C. External environment
         1. Opportunities
         2. Threats
  II. Strategic factors used to formulate plan
 III. Best alternatives/plan
 IV. Implementation schedule
  V. Evaluation plan
      A. Indicators for success
      B. Data collection
      C. Reports

Source: Kelly Thomas Associates, Alexandria, VA. Reproduced with permission.

1. Ignoring the power structure of the organizational setting while instituting the planning process
2. Assuming that planning can be delegated to a planner
3. Forgetting that planning is a political, social, organizational, as well as a rational process
4. Too much centralization of the planning so consumers feel little responsibility for the plan
5. Failure to develop overall staff development goals suitable as a basis for formulating long-range plans

6. Assuming that comprehensive planning is something separate from the entire management process
7. Becoming so engrossed in current problems that insufficient time is spent on strategic planning and the process becomes discredited
8. Failure to assume the necessary involvement of major line personnel in the process
9. Failure to review with departmental and division heads the strategic plan that has been developed
10. Assuming that a formal system can be introduced into a staff development department without a careful and perhaps agonizing reappraisal of current staff development practices and decision-making processes

Goplerud also lists some additional points for managers who are implementing strategic plans. He suggests that planning must have strong consistent involvement of top management in nursing to be worth undertaking at all. He further indicates that planning must be viewed as an integral part of management and that planning in health care organizations must take into account the complex organizational, political, and professional forces that affect their strategic actions. Finally, Goplerud advises the involvement of top nursing management in holding operational managers accountable for implementing plans as a critical element to the success of strategic planning. In nursing staff development, this element requires close and frequent communication between the staff development program administrator and top nursing management.

Pfeiffer and others[10] add additional insight to assist the staff development program administrator with understanding the strategic planning process. They counsel that strategic planning must be congruent with the identified values and mission of the organization and the nursing division. They further suggest that success is most likely realized when there is maximum creative output *within realistic boundaries.* Finally, Pfeiffer says it is probably a good rule to attempt to change only one significant item at a time!

Step 12: Evaluate and Control

To set up an evaluation system for the strategic plan, key indicators must be identified and monitored. Key indicators are those that would provide evidence that the plan is working, even as it is in progress. For example, if the strategic plan includes a marketing feature that will increase participation in a particular program, a key indicator of success could be number of attendees for the program. Following are some questions to consider when setting up an evaluation system include:

What critical success factors are essential to the attainment of the plan? Think about a few key areas of activity in which favorable results are essential to the success of the plan. These key areas may be program topics, outcome measures, or a particular strategy like self-learning.

What is strategically important data necessary for the evaluation of the plan? Figure out what data are necessary to evaluate the critical success factors and how to collect these data. Examine systems already operational for data collection and the need to improve or develop new data collection mechanisms.

What are three or four nursing division issues that need to be monitored as often as weekly? Think about what facts would give you information about the progress of your strategic plan. Consider those significant issues in process that may have an effect on the success of the plan. Appraise these data and the measures that may control the effect on the plan.

What are three or four areas in which failure to perform well may cause the greatest problems? Consider these areas and make efforts to assure that these will be monitored closely for good progress toward achieving the strategic plan. Set up monitoring systems that provide you with data to make judgments about progress.

The evaluation and control system designed as an integral part of the strategic plan also serves as a quality management tool, and data collected can be used to meet the quality assurance activities essential to any well run staff development program.

Step 13: Report Results

As part of the routine reporting process or a separate one, the staff development program administrator should document progress and results realized through the strategic plan. The following questions will help guide the development of the report:

Who needs to know about the results? Think about the members of the organization who have an investment in the staff development program. Estimate their needs for information and report accordingly. Assess what they may need and/or want to know—don't overburden these individuals with lengthy reports filled with data for their analysis, rather analyze the data and write brief and bright reports that communicate progress or modifications in the plan.

How will the report be delivered? Evaluate the usual means of communicating in the organization and use these methods and consider others. Consider reporting progress at meetings and other group gatherings. Keep reports brief and to the point.

When will results be reported? Judge the scope of the plan and develop a blueprint of reporting points. Set up a system of reminders to do the report.

These reports may be verbal, written, delivered with media, or a combination of these forms. The important issues with this final step of the strategic planning process are providing information about the progress of the plan to the appropriate people, and the form of communication chosen for transmitting this information. Different organizations have a variety of patterns of communication, and the staff development administrator must evaluate these patterns and choose the best one for communication.

Although this may seem to bring strategic planning to its final step, the dynamic nature of this process for nursing staff development causes this step to be a continuation of a process that is cyclic. The last step signals the need to begin again at the first step and continue to use this process to make decisions about the advancement of the nursing staff development program.

Efficiencies and Effectiveness

Strategic planning is characterized by six features.[11] First, strategic planning and decision making means that nursing staff development program administrators are proactive, rather than reactive, in determining the program's place in history. Second, strategic planning looks outward and is focused on keeping the staff development program in step with changing environments. Third, strategy making recognizes competition and the fact that staff development programs are subject to economic market conditions and increasingly strong competition. It also recognizes the time for coalitions and alliances to accomplish goals. Fourth, strategic planning is action-oriented, concentrating on decisions, not on documented plans, analyses, forecasts, and goals. Fifth, strategy making is a blend of rational and economic analysis, political maneuvering, and psychological interplay. It is participative and highly tolerant of controversy. Dissent is permitted, sabotage is not. The ultimate shaper of strategy is the staff development program administrator. Finally, strategic planning concentrates on the fate of the staff development program above all else. Therefore, it should be the first priority.

Staff development administrators can cite reasons for not getting around to strategic planning. Waltz et al.[12] identified some of these reasons:

- Crises-oriented management that focuses on putting out fires rather than developing a fire-proof environment
- Overemphasis on individuality that creates vested interests that override the common good
- Fear of change and the perhaps undesirable side effects of an otherwise desirable plan
- Fear of making mistakes because of the uncertainty of dealing with a rapidly changing environment
- Fear of the personal threat implied by the power and politics of the process
- Lack of leadership, preparation, vision, or interest

These reasons center primarily on fear of the unknown. The perceptive staff development program administrator will recognize this fear and overcome it with knowledge and insight about the process. All new concepts and methods require practice for refinement. Expectations for the perfect nursing staff development program strategic plan are unreasonable and probably fictional. During initial trials with the strategic planning process, select a portion of the total program for planning and change. With experience and success, the process can be extended to other areas. Achievements enjoyed can be directly associated to the use of a process that helps the staff development program administrator create a future that makes a contribution to quality patient care.

Summary: Peaks, Valleys, and Vista Views

Making strategic planning work requires endurance, practice, problem weathering, mistake corrections, and the development of mental muscle. Much wisdom can be gained through the strategic planning process. Everyday experiences in nursing staff development practice generate many highs and lows. When a particular activity in the program accomplishes what it sets out to do, great satisfaction for specialists is the result. When planned activities meet with delays, lack of support, or other logistical problems, frustrations result.

To develop a panoramic view of nursing staff development, reflection about the peaks and valleys of nursing staff development practice must occur. This contemplation of experiences can provide a rich tapestry for future practice. As experience is acquired and considered as part of the developing practice, it can be used to recognize patterns. These patterns can be woven into new practice patterns.

The use of exemplars to describe nursing knowledge embedded in practice is well demonstrated by Benner.[13] The use of similar approaches to discover our current practices and understand "how the best ones do it" will contribute to nursing staff development knowledge.

This text is a beginning attempt to define the practice of nursing staff development. The use of the various processes described within this text will help the novice staff development specialist and program administrator assess, maintain and develop the competence of nurses. The contributing authors have described their current practice. Future practice will be defined by the experience and knowledge development of specialists and program administrators in the field of nursing staff development in health care organizations.

References

1. Carper, B. A. (1978). Fundamental patterns of knowing in nursing. *Advances in Nursing Science, 1*(1), 13–23.
2. Benner, P. (1983). Uncovering the knowledge embedded in clinical practice. *Image: The Journal of Nursing Scholarship, 15*(2), 36–41.
3. Simpson, J. (1990). Visioning: More than meets the eye. *Training and Development Journal, 44*(9), 70–72.
4. Goplerud, E. (1990). Strategic planning in health care organizations. In Dienemann, J. (Ed.), *Nursing administration: Strategic perspectives and application.* Norwalk, CT: Appleton Lange.
5. Kotler, P. (1982). *Marketing for healthcare organizations.* Englewood Cliffs, NJ: Prentice-Hall.
6. Drucker, P. (1974). *Management: Tasks, responsibilities and policies.* New York: Harper & Row.
7. Kotler, P. (1982). *Marketing for non-profit organizations.* Englewood Cliffs, NJ: Prentice-Hall.
8. Wheelen, T., & Hunger, J. D. (1986). *Strategic management and business policy* (2nd ed.). Reading, MA: Addison Wesley.
9. Keller, G. (1983). *Academic strategy.* Baltimore, MD: Johns Hopkins University Press.

10. Pfeiffer, J. W., Goodstein, L. D., & Nolan, T. M. (1985). *Applied strategic planning*. San Diego, CA: University Associates.
11. Keller, G. (1983). *Academic strategy*. Baltimore: Johns Hopkins University Press.
12. Waltz, C. F., Chambers, S. B., & Hechenberger, N. B. (1989). *Strategic planning, marketing, and evaluation in nursing education and service*. New York: National League for Nursing.
13. Benner, P. (1984). *Novice to expert: Excellence and power in clinical nursing practice*. Menlo Park: Addison-Wesley.

ndex